# Dr. Patrick Walsh's
## GUIDE TO
## SURVIVING
## PROSTATE CANCER

### Second Edition

## Patrick C. Walsh, MD
*and* Janet Farrar Worthington

WARNER
WELLNESS

NEW YORK   BOSTON

This book is not intended as a substitute for medical advice of physicians. The reader should regularly consult a physician in all matters relating to his or her health, and particularly in respect of any symptoms that may require diagnosis or medical attention.

Warner Wellness
Hachette Book Group USA
237 Park Avenue
New York, NY 10169

Visit our Web site at www.HachetteBookGroupUSA.com.

Warner Wellness is an imprint of Warner Books, Inc.

Printed in the United States of America

First Revised Edition: June 2007
10  9  8  7  6  5  4  3  2  1

Warner Wellness is a trademark of Time Warner Inc. or an affiliated company. Used under license by Hachette Book Group USA, which is not affiliated with Time Warner Inc.

Library of Congress Cataloging-in-Publication Data
Walsh, Patrick C.
    Dr. patrick walsh's guide to surviving prostate cancer / Patrick C. Walsh and Janet  Farrar Worthington.—2nd ed.
        p.   cm.
    Includes index.
    ISBN-13: 978-0-446-69689-0
    ISBN-10: 0-446-69689-7
    1. Prostate—Cancer—Popular works.   I. Worthington, Janet Farrar.
    II. Title.

RC280.P7W365   2007
616.99'463—dc22
        2006025077

*To all the patients, past and present,*
*who inspired us to write this book, with deep*
*gratitude for the lessons they have taught us—*
*which we now share with others*

# Acknowledgments

This book would not have been possible without the work and experience of many people, too many to name here. We tried, but the result looked like a telephone book—and had about as much personal meaning. So instead of listing all, and inevitably missing one or two, of the sources upon which we've drawn to produce this guide, we would simply like to thank those colleagues, patients, friends, and family members who have helped us the very most, including:

Jonathan Epstein, Danny Song, Theodore DeWeese, Michael Carducci, Mario Eisenberger, H. Ballentine Carter, Misop Han, Alan Partin, David Rini, Robert Getzenberg, Donald Coffey, John Isaacs, William Isaacs, William Nelson, Angelo DeMarzo, Elizabeth Platz, Robert Veltri, Christian Palovich, Li Ming Su, Bruce Trock, Arthur Burnett, Ronald Rodriguez, Jonathan Jarow, David Chan, Mohamed Allaf, Craig Rogers, Anthony Schaeffer, Edward Schaeffer, Dan Stoianovici, Daniel Chan, Matthew Nielsen, David Hernandez, Daniel Makarov, Mark Gonzolgo, Karen Boyle, Philip Beachy, David Berman, Michael Zelefsky, Anthony Zietman, Stephen Freedland, Matthew Gretzer, William Roberts, Charles Pound, Joel Nelson, Janet Walczak, Vicki Sinibaldi, Gabor Fichtinger, and Lars Ellison.

We also acknowledge with deep gratitude the valuable contributions of these people: Peg Walsh; Barbara Downs; Mark, Blair, Andy and Josh Worthington; Bradley and Carole Farrar; Sally and Scott Worthington. A special thanks to Gayla Farrar, a cancer survivor whose gallant endurance has helped more people than she knows; and to Ronald Farrar, a rock in sickness and in health.

We would like to thank the late Leon Schlossberg, for his original illustrations; David Rini, for his superb ability to tell a story with pictures; Channa Taub, our literary agent; Diana Baroni, our editor; and Bob Castillo, our fine and careful copyeditor.

And finally, we would like to honor Tom Worthington, who died of prostate cancer when he was just beginning to live. Every man this book helps is a victory for you, Tom.

# Contents

# Introduction

Welcome. Maybe you're reading this book because, along with more than 200,000 American men this year, you've been diagnosed with prostate cancer—and found yourself a member of what many call the reluctant brotherhood, a club you never wanted to join. Or maybe you're in the reluctant sisterhood, and you're reading this so you can help your husband, father, brother, son, or a close friend. Or maybe you're not yet an official member of the club, but you've received the unwelcome invitation—a change in your prostate-specific antigen (PSA), maybe, or a prostate biopsy that turned out to be negative. In any case, we're glad that you have found your way here, because we want you to know that the world of prostate cancer is full of hope. More men are being diagnosed earlier than ever before, and more men are being cured of this disease.

This is a big change from the early 1990s, when Pat Walsh and I first started writing about prostate cancer. Back then, the PSA test—instead of being a mainstream screening tool for most physicians—was largely unheard of and was used mainly to monitor prostate cancer that doctors had already diagnosed. Many men who found out they had prostate cancer died of it, and the treatments were so variable that for many men, the side effects were at least as frightening as the disease itself. The picture for men with advanced prostate cancer was bleak, and if cancer had spread outside the prostate or had returned after treatment, the philosophy seemed to be to wait until everything else failed before even attempting chemotherapy. That fatalistic worldview has changed, largely thanks to oncologists such as Mario Eisenberger and Michael Carducci, of Johns Hopkins, who have helped develop and test many new drugs, some of which work in entirely novel ways. Now, oncologists have means of predicting who's at risk of a cancer recurrence—and instead of waiting for cancer to show up, they go after it as soon as possible, when it is most susceptible.

So much has changed. Thank God. Deaths from prostate cancer in the United States and other countries where there is an active approach toward screening and effective treatments for localized disease (curable disease, still confined to the prostate) are fewer every year. In fact, very soon now, it looks as if we may even be able to cheer that prostate cancer is moving down the ranks of fatal diseases. As this book is heading for the printer, the American Cancer Society estimates that prostate cancer may even fall behind colon cancer as the number-two cancer killer of men. Also, with this book, we celebrate something that doctors believed for many years. A landmark study from Scandinavia, discussed in chapter 7, proved that radical prostatectomy—for years the "gold standard" treatment for prostate cancer in America—saves lives. Are we out of the woods yet? Far from it; unfortunately, the burden of prostate cancer will not let up soon. As the huge baby boomer generation enters "the prostate years," the number of new cases is predicted to double, and the number of men dying from the disease may triple (see chapter 3). This is why we are also working harder than ever to learn how to prevent this disease.

One thing you'll learn from this book is that every single case of prostate cancer is different—as individual as snowflakes. The seriousness of a man's cancer depends on so many things. Some of it's the genetic deck of cards he was dealt—for instance, whether prostate cancer runs in his family, particularly if his father or brother developed it at an early age—and about half of it has to do with his environment. Environment here doesn't really mean the air he breathes (unless he happened to spray Agent Orange in Vietnam, in which case it does; see chapter 3). It may have something to do with where in the world he lives—how much sunlight he's exposed to, or the mineral content of the soil where his vegetables are grown, for example. But it has an awful lot to do with what he eats—whether, over the course of his lifetime, he's eaten a lot of vegetables, or red meat, or fish, or olive oil, or tomato sauce, or drunk red wine or green tea, and probably even whether today, for lunch, he picked tuna salad or a meatball sub. We are learning that every minute choice a man makes can affect his susceptibility to prostate cancer, and conversely, his ability to fight it off.

It makes sense, then, that the treatment for every man is different, too. My coauthor, Patrick C. Walsh, is one of the most respected prostate disease specialists in the world. In fact, he developed the revolutionary, now-standard operation called the anatomic radical retropubic prostatectomy, in which the prostate is removed, but potency and continence are preserved. (This operation is also known as the Walsh nerve-sparing procedure.) Does he, then, recommend surgery for every man? Far from it. He has operated on thousands of men with prostate cancer. He has also *not* operated on thousands of men with prostate cancer. That's why we say on the cover of this book "Give Yourself a Second Opinion"—not just from a surgeon, but from pathologists, radiation oncologists, and medical oncologists. Just as every man's disease is different, so is every man's ideal treatment. But first things first—do you indeed have cancer? And if you do, is it growing quickly or slowly? The right treatment starts with diagnosis, and there's nobody better at looking at prostate cancer cells, and understanding them (see chapter 6), than Jonathan Epstein of Johns Hopkins, one of the world's most gifted pathologists. Your second opinion from radiation oncology comes from two of the best in the business, Danny Y. Song and Theodore L. DeWeese—both in the Department of Radiation Oncology and Molecular Radiation Science at Johns Hopkins, and both people dedicating their careers to making external-beam radiation and brachytherapy better than ever (see chapters 9 and 10). The revolution in medical therapies for advanced cancer, with opinions from the renowned oncologists Mario Eisenberger and Michael Carducci, is discussed at length in chapter 12.

I've been writing about prostate cancer for nearly fifteen years, and I came to the subject in the worst way you can imagine. In 1991, I watched my fifty-three-year-old father-in-law, Tom Worthington, die of it. His death was horrible. Within a year of his initial diagnosis, after fleeting success with hormonal therapy, his tumor spread like wildfire. He died in a nursing home, castrated, hooked up to a catheter, in agonizing pain, pitifully thin, his bones so riddled with cancer that his arm snapped in two when a nurse tried to move him. I thought of him a lot as we wrote chapter 12. Now, new drugs are actually targeting prostate cancer in the bones even before it gets there, snatching up the welcome mat from this site that advancing prostate cancer seems to love so much. I try not to play the "what if" game, wondering if one of these amazing new treatments could have made the difference for Tom, but sometimes I can't help it.

Back to 1991 for a minute. It was in hopes of finding out how this could happen—how this "old man's disease" that men were supposed to die *with*, not *of*, could kill a man in the prime of life—that I found Pat Walsh. So unattuned was I to the world of prostate cancer that I didn't even know who he was, other than that he was the head of urology at Johns Hopkins Medical Institutions, where I happened to work as editor of the medical alumni magazine. (I must confess that, until all of this, I had never given much thought to the prostate at all and didn't even know what it did or where it was located. I knew that men had one and women didn't, but that was about it.) I had no idea that there was a cure for prostate cancer, that Walsh had invented it, and that his operation had been for years a gold standard for cancer control that maintained continence and potency. I didn't know, then, three very important things: One, that he developed the operation after years of intense, meticulous study of the anatomy of the prostate and male urinary and reproductive systems—a bedrock knowledge of the fundamentals, as athletes say. Two, that he is a consummate perfectionist, always working to improve his technique and the operation itself. About six years ago, for example, he spent his free time one summer watching hundreds of hours of videotape—of his hands performing the radical prostatectomy in dozens of patients. Why? He wanted to see whether some slight modifications in his technique could improve his patients' recovery of sexual function (it could; see chapter 8). Other surgeons have now started doing this; he was the first. And three, curing prostate cancer isn't just a job for him, the basis of a successful career that has won him every possible honor and award in the field. It's his life's mission. At Hopkins, Pat Walsh put together a world-class team of oncologists, radiation oncologists, molecular biologists, pathologists, urologists, and geneticists, who have been tackling this disease from every angle for the last two decades. The fruits of their labor appear throughout this book. Walsh, along with his longtime research director, a brilliant man named Don Coffey, is the driving force that made much of it happen.

I also had no idea that he would, within a few years, be the reason that prostate cancer was diagnosed early in my own father. What are the odds that this gifted surgeon with whom I would start to write books, would one day take out my dad's prostate and cure his cancer? That was seven years ago; Dad's PSA remains undetectable. In writing this book, our fourth, I have found myself feeling a bit like Charles Dickens must have felt as he wrote *A Christmas Carol*—introspective and personally haunted by three visions of my subject— the past, present, and future.

*Prostate Cancer Past:* The past is still too recent for me. It started with Tom, of course, but he's not the only man I've known whose life has been cut short by this disease. There was Sam, a successful banker, who was diagnosed ten years ago with prostate cancer at age fifty and opted for radiation because, newly divorced, he didn't want to face the recovery from surgery by himself (at that time, it was a bit longer and more difficult than it is today). What nobody knew then (again, things are different now; see chapter 10) was that he had a very aggressive cancer. When I met him, it had already come back locally. He fought the disease valiantly with hormonal therapy and then chemotherapy, but he died about three years later. I always think of him when I see a red convertible, because he bought one right after his wife left him as a symbol of his new life. Another man was Lester, a U.S. Marine drill sergeant, tough as a boot and also a wonderful cartoonist, who drew many pictures for me and my children. Les, a black man in his early fifties, had family history and race going against him. He had undergone a radical prostatectomy before I met him, but, as with Sam and Tom, the cancer had spread silently before he ever sought treatment, and he died less than five years later. He and his wife had an unshakeable faith in God that helped them tremendously throughout their ordeal. Because of his race (black men are more susceptible to prostate cancer—see chapter 3) and family history, Les should have begun screening for prostate cancer when he was forty. Nobody realized this then; we know it now.

And finally, close to home once again, my husband's maternal grandfather died of complications from radiation therapy for—you guessed it—prostate cancer, at age eighty-five. He had a number of health problems, including heart disease, had no symptoms of prostate cancer, and probably didn't even need to be treated. (We discuss this strategy, called expectant management, in chapter 7.) Another man who probably didn't need to be treated was my own grandfather, who died at age eighty-four of a heart attack, which I believe was caused by the heavy-handed regimen of hormonal therapy (five times the dose Walsh recommends in chapter 12) his uninformed family physician prescribed for prostate cancer. He had no symptoms of the disease and probably could have enjoyed his remaining years without even needing treatment; instead, the personality and physical changes caused by these hormones made his last months miserable.

*Prostate Cancer Present:* As in *A Christmas Carol*, this is the most joyful mode. I rejoice that for my father, prostate cancer was truly just a blip on the radar screen of his life and that he is around to love, and be loved by, his wife, two kids, and six grandchildren. It was the best example I know of an ideal scenario—prostate cancer detected early, treated, and cured. I am so happy for the many men I've met and kept up with over the years who have been treated for prostate cancer and who are doing fine now. I am as proud of Pat Walsh's ever-improving surgical procedure and stellar results as I would be if they were the result of my own painstaking study, years of experience, self-discipline, rigorous standards, and mission. He once told me something that got him through medical school, something one of his toughest professors used to tell all of his students: "You are not here to make friends. You are here to find the truth." And that's who he is. He doesn't mince words, doesn't gloss over anything, and doesn't pretend that all treatments are equal. But if he tells you something, you can trust him.

*Prostate Cancer Future:* And then there's tomorrow, which has a shadow lurking overhead. Despite the overwhelming amount of good news in this book, this edition of the book has been troubling for me personally because of a bombshell in PSA screening, which we talk about in chapter 5. Scientists have learned that having a low PSA level is no guarantee that a man doesn't have prostate cancer and that it isn't serious. In fact, 15 percent of men with PSA levels lower than 4 ng/ml have prostate cancer, and 15 percent of these men have aggressive disease. If some of these men were to wait until their PSA level reached the now-outdated magic number of 4, it might be difficult to cure their cancer. Scientists such as H. Ballentine Carter, a pioneer in making sense of PSA, now realize how crucial a factor a man's age plays in his PSA level. A man in his forties, for instance, who has a PSA level of higher than 0.6 that's consistently rising faster than 0.2 to 0.4 ng/ml per year may well have cancer and should have a biopsy.

Well, guess what? My husband, Mark, whose family history (on both sides) of prostate cancer first catapulted me into this reluctant sisterhood, had a PSA level of 0.7 ng/ml (that's certainly higher than 0.6) two years ago. We felt great about that low number at the time. We're not that complacent anymore. His PSA today is *still* 0.7. But we're watching it like a hawk now. (We were appalled that five years had gone by since his last physical. How did that happen?) He's forty-five years old. He doesn't smoke, takes selenium when he remembers, and enjoys a glass of red wine several nights a week. But he's a doctor, and like many of his colleagues, is excellent at caring for others and not very good at taking care of himself. He's a father of three active kids ranging in age from thirteen to three. We barely have time to cook dinner many nights, much less to figure out how to incorporate prostate-healthy foods into our diet. Have we blown it? Is it too late for us to lower his risk or perhaps delay or even prevent prostate cancer from forming in his body? We're praying that it's not. My husband and I each have a younger brother. What about them? We have two sons. What about them?

I'm telling you all of this to show that when I welcome you into this reluctant brotherhood and sisterhood, I mean it. I'm in it, too— which means that we're in it together. It's not an easy place to be, but again—believe me on this—it's infinitely better than it has ever been.

—Janet Farrar Worthington

# 1

# WHAT THE PROSTATE DOES: A CRASH COURSE IN MALE ANATOMY

## ▶▶▶ READ THIS FIRST

There's a "Read This First" in every chapter of this book. This is because prostate cancer—the last thing most men would ever choose to think about—is not just a scary subject to deal with, it's tough to understand. The disease itself is complicated, and the decisions about what to do next can be agonizing. Before you can chart your next course, you've got to sort through and attempt to make sense of many things.

If this were a potboiler novel, the kind of page-turner you start on page one and don't put down until you've savored the last word on the last page, you wouldn't need any guidance on how to read it; you'd just get going. If, on the other hand, this were an academic textbook, you might approach it with a highlighter in hand, emphasizing key points and take-home messages in bright yellow marker. This book falls somewhere in between, and people read it in different ways. They kick the tires, in effect—flip through the pages; maybe they head directly to a specific section, such as impotence, or biopsy, then backtrack and read about how prostate cancer gets started or jump ahead to chapters on treatment.

With this in mind, in every chapter we've done our best to give you the highlights—what you really need to know—up front. Consider this your briefing, or your "headline news." All of these overviews will familiarize you with the main ideas you'll be covering on the next pages.

That said, this is what you need to know about the anatomy of the prostate.

## WHAT IS THE PROSTATE?

The prostate is a small and probably expendable organ. Men can live quite comfortably without it. The prostate's biggest job, as far as we know, is to provide part of the fluid that makes up semen. But even this contribution does not appear to be crucial for reproduction—which is why some scientists think the prostate's main role may be to safeguard the reproductive tract from infection in the urinary tract. (In fact, its name in Greek means "protector.") It is not a vital organ. Thus, the major importance of the prostate is not what it does but what goes wrong with it—the problems it causes for nearly all men who live long enough. These are

- cancer of the prostate, the most common cancer in men;
- BPH (benign prostatic hyperplasia, also called enlargement of the prostate), one of the most common benign tumors in men and a major source of misery as men get older; and
- prostatitis, the most common cause of urinary tract infections in men.

## IF IT'S NOT A VITAL ORGAN, WHY IS IT IMPORTANT?

Although it's only as big as a walnut, the prostate is a miniature Grand Central Station, a busy hub at the crossroads of a man's urinary and reproductive tracts. It's at a highly strategic location, right at the outlet to the bladder. Urine and semen cannot leave the body without passing through the prostate. It is also tucked away, deep within the pelvis, surrounded by vulnerable structures—the bladder, the rectum, the sphincters responsible for urinary control, major arteries and veins, and a host of delicate nerves, some of them so tiny that we've only recently discovered them. This is why any form of treatment for prostate cancer can produce side effects including incontinence, impotence, and rectal bleeding.

## WHAT ELSE ABOUT PROSTATE ANATOMY DO I NEED TO KNOW?

The prostate is like a complicated sponge, with five distinct parts called zones. The two most important here are the peripheral zone, which is located next to the rectum, contains most of the glands in the prostate, and is the main site where cancer develops; and the transition zone, which surrounds the urethra and is the principal site where BPH begins. The prostate's growth and function are stimulated by hormones: testosterone, produced in the testicles, is converted to another hormone, called dihydrotestosterone (DHT)—the most active male hormone—in the prostate.

The bottom line: The prostate is a gland that does much more harm than good and is located in a terrible area that complicates any attempt to treat it. Despite this, as you will learn in this book, there has never been more hope in the treatment of all prostate disorders—especially cancer.

## The Prostate's Strategic Location

Welcome to the prostate—the bustling, walnut-sized hub at the crossroads of a man's urinary and reproductive tracts. What makes such a small, relatively obscure gland so important to men? The answer is not immediately obvious: the prostate is not, for example, a vital organ like the heart. Its biggest job, as far as we know, is to provide about one-third of the fluid that makes up semen. But even this contribution does not appear to be crucial for reproduction, leading some scientists to theorize that the prostate's main purpose actually may be to safeguard the reproductive tract from infection in the urinary tract. (In fact, its name in Greek means "stands before" or "protector.") The prostate has few other redeeming features, isn't necessary for life or even for sexual function, and is known primarily for the clinical problems it causes to nearly all men who live long enough.

What the prostate *does* have, however, is a highly strategic location, right at the outlet to the bladder. Urine cannot leave the body without passing through the prostate, via a tube called the urethra. (Think of the urethra as an expressway, and the prostate as the Lincoln Tunnel.)

## Nothing About the Prostate Is Easy

From a urologist's standpoint, even a routine checkup—to feel for lumps or hardness in a digital rectal examination—is more complicated and takes more skill than many of our patients realize. (For a detailed discussion of diagnosing prostate problems, see chapter 6.) The prostate is as tucked away—and as surrounded by booby traps—as any of the prizes sought by Indiana Jones in *Raiders of the Lost Ark*. It lies in the midst of vulnerable structures—the bladder, the rectum, the sphincters responsible for urinary control, major arteries and veins, and a host of delicate nerves, some of them so tiny that we've only recently discovered them—that can foil any physician who ventures into the area without exquisitely precise knowledge of the terrain. This is why *any* procedure to treat prostate cancer—surgery, external-beam radiation therapy, implantation of radiation "seeds," or attempts to kill cancer cells by cooling or heating the prostate—can produce side effects including incontinence, impotence, and rectal bleeding.

The prostate fits snugly within the pelvis; there isn't much "breathing room" there. Unfortunately, not only is the prostate packed tightly amid other structures, like pieces of a jigsaw puzzle, it is poorly insulated. The flimsy wall of tissue separating the prostate and the seminal vesicles is thinner than a piece of tissue paper—not much of a buffer zone for cancer. Consequently, once cancer reaches a critical size, it can easily penetrate the wall (also called the capsule) of the prostate and escape into this overcrowded region of the body, spreading to the nearby seminal vesicles or lymph nodes, or even further, into the bloodstream.

This is why—even though treatment for prostate cancer is improving dramatically—a man's best protection against this disease is to have it detected as quickly as possible. Ideally, for the American man at average risk of prostate cancer, screening should start at age forty with a physical and digital rectal examination (see chapter 5) and a blood test for prostate-specific antigen (PSA) (also see chapter 5). This first prostate checkup should establish a baseline, an essential comparison point for your doctor to refer to in future visits—in other words, it should be no big deal right now, but very important for later.

What happens next depends on your initial PSA level, but your doctor will probably want you to come back for another rectal exam and PSA test every two to five years. Like a suspicious character—but one on whom the police can pin no actual crime—the prostate is best put under observation at age forty and beyond. We used to recommend this only for men at higher risk—African Americans and men with a family history of prostate cancer (see chapter 3). Other men, we believed, didn't need to start worrying about their prostate until age fifty. But because of new research at Johns Hopkins led by scientists including H. Ballentine Carter and Alan Partin, we now believe that this is the best advice for all men.

## To Sum Up the Prostate

It's a gland that does much more harm than good and is located in a terrible area that complicates any attempt to treat it. Despite this, there has never been more hope in our field. At last, we are finding answers to the toughest questions of prostate cancer: Where exactly does it begin, and why? How does it spread? If we can't cure it, can we contain it—can we make advanced prostate cancer a chronic illness, like diabetes, instead of a fatal one? Can we change our thinking and try drugs that were once considered last-ditch measures sooner? Can we try adjuvant therapy, as doctors use successfully in breast cancer? Can we actually prevent cancer or somehow slow its progress with diet? If PSA comes back after surgery or radiation, what does it mean—and how much time do we have to find a more effective treatment? As for radical prostatectomy and radiation therapy, can we make these treatments even better, with fewer side effects and quicker recovery of potency and continence? How can we help men and their families get their lives back? How can we improve quality of life? All of these areas will be covered in detail in later chapters.

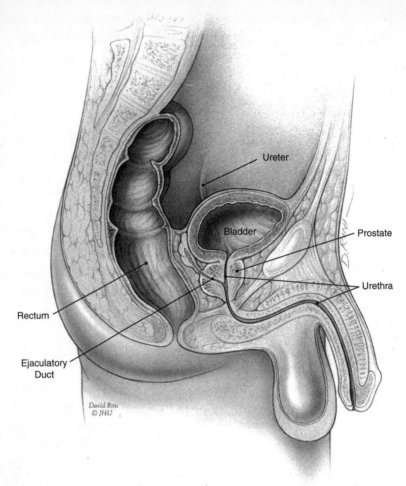

Ureter

Bladder

Prostate

Urethra

Rectum

Ejaculatory
Duct

David Rini
© JHU

**FIGURE 1.1   Crowded Territory**

There's the prostate, nestled deep within the male pelvis—at a highly strategic location, right at the outlet to the bladder. The prostate is surrounded by vulnerable structures—the bladder, the rectum, the sphincters responsible for urinary control, major arteries and veins, and a host of delicate nerves.

## A Brief Anatomy Lesson

Although we've tried to keep it brief, this crash course in anatomy may still be more than you ever wanted to know about the prostate and anything even remotely linked to it. But we believe it's essential that you understand where the prostate is and what it does, the two main systems it influences—the reproductive and urinary tracts—and how they can be affected when something goes wrong.

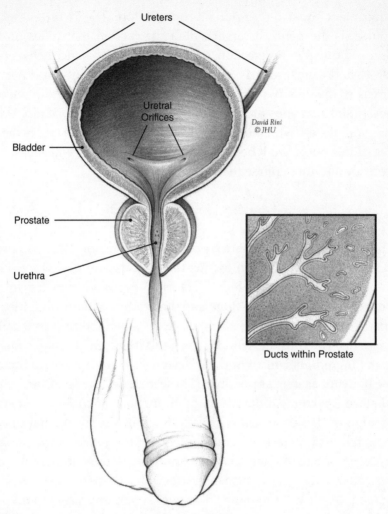

Ureters

Uretral Orifices

David Rini
© JHU

Bladder

Prostate

Urethra

Ducts within Prostate

**FIGURE 1.2   The Bladder, Prostate, and Urethra**

Urine flows from the bladder via a tube called the urethra, but it can't leave the body without passing through the prostate. Think of the urethra as an expressway and the prostate as the Lincoln Tunnel. *Inset:* Like a sponge, the prostate is made up of tiny glands. These drain into ducts that, in turn, transport secretions to the urethra.

## Reproductive Tract

For the reproductive organs, the basic act of sexual intercourse is as highly choreographed and synchronized as a NASA shuttle launch. First, the climate must be just right—in this case, the weather is a chain of coded chemical messages and hormonal signals. The equipment must be working properly, too. The main vessel, of course, is the penis, a remarkable construction that relies on hydraulic principles for erection, requires a delicate balance between arteries and veins, and is orchestrated by many intricate nerves. Orgasm, the climax of sexual intercourse, involves instantaneous, nearly simultaneous firings of fluid from the prostate, seminal vesicles, and testes (which make sperm). Because the prostate is the focus of this book, we'll begin there, although as you will see, sexual potency and intercourse really begin in the brain.

## Prostate

The prostate is a complicated, powerful little factory. Its main products, manufactured in numerous tiny glands and ducts, are secretions—components of semen. During orgasm, muscles in the prostate drive these secretions into the urethra (where it is joined by sperm and fluid from the seminal vesicles), which pumps it out of the penis. The prostate's fluid is clear and mildly acidic, and contains many ingredients, most of them designed to sustain sperm outside the body for as long as possible. (These include citric acid, acid phosphatase, spermine, potassium, calcium, and zinc.) Some prostatic secretions also protect the urinary tract and reproductive system from harmful bacteria that may enter the urethra. Here, the prostate truly lives up to its Greek name of "protector." Infections in this area can cause scar tissue to form in the ducts that drain the testicles, leading to infertility. If these infections were common, they would pose a serious threat to procreation—and this may be the major reason that all mammals have a prostate.

After ejaculation, the seminal fluid immediately coagulates—a key part of nature's "safety net" to maximize the odds of reproduction. If semen remained watery, it could not linger in the vagina. (In rats and other rodents, semen actually forms a pelletlike plug that effectively blocks other rats from depositing their semen in the same female.) The semen is gradually broken down again by an important enzyme made by the prostate—prostate-specific antigen (PSA). PSA's other great value is that it can be detected in a simple blood test. In recent years, this PSA test has become a crucial addition to medicine's arsenal for detecting prostate cancer and monitoring the success of treatment. (For more on what PSA can do and on other tests for prostate cancer, see chapter 5.)

Like New York City, the prostate is divided into five zones: Anterior, which takes up one-third of the space and consists mainly of smooth muscle; peripheral, the largest segment, which contains three-fourths of the glands in the prostate; central, which holds most of the remaining glands; preprostatic tissue, which plays a key role during ejaculation—muscles here prevent semen from flowing backward, into the bladder; and transition, which surrounds the urethra and is the epicenter of trouble in benign prostatic hyperplasia (BPH). For reasons not entirely understood, when a man reaches his mid-forties, the prostate tissue in the transition zone tends to enlarge, begins to push nearby tissue for room, and eventually starts to cramp the urethra. With this slow strangulation—think of a man's necktie slowly tightening around his collar—the prostate can make it exceedingly difficult for urine to get from the bladder through the prostate and out of the body. (For more on BPH, see chapter 2.) Most prostate cancer occurs in the peripheral zone. Fortunately, this is the region most likely to be felt during a rectal examination and tapped during a needle biopsy of the prostate (see chapter 6).

On a microscopic level, prostatic tissue is like a squishy sponge, riddled with tiny glands. These are the microfactories that produce the secretions, and they're connected by hundreds of ducts, which transport the fluid into the urethra. When these ducts become obstructed—as they do in BPH—PSA levels begin to rise in the bloodstream. Because prostate cancers don't make any ducts, glands in cancerous tissue become isolated. But these ducts still churn out fluid, which has nowhere to go—except into the bloodstream. That's why, gram for gram, prostate cancer contributes *ten times more* to blood PSA levels than does BPH.

Prostate cells come in two basic models—epithelial cells, glandular cells that make the secretions, and stromal cells, muscular cells that hold the epithelial cells in place. The stromal cells aren't just passive scaffolding; they also help the prostate grow. From the stromal cells, in fact, spring many growth factors. And growth factors, we have learned, play a pivotal role in the development and function of the prostate when it is healthy, and when it is cancerous.

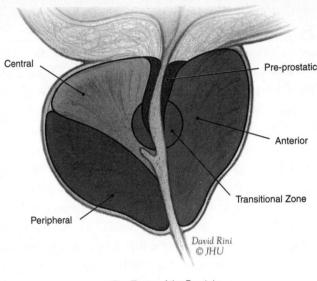

Central — Pre-prostatic

Anterior

Transitional Zone

Peripheral

David Rini
© JHU

The Zones of the Prostate
(viewed from the side)

**FIGURE 1.3   The Prostate's Five Zones**

The prostate is divided into five zones: *Anterior*, which is mainly smooth muscle tissue; *peripheral*, which contains three-fourths of the glands in the prostate; *central*, which holds most of the remaining glands; *preprostatic* tissue, which plays a key role during ejaculation—muscles here prevent semen from flowing backward, into the bladder; and *transition*, which surrounds the urethra and is the epicenter of trouble in BPH. *Most prostate cancer occurs in the peripheral zone.* Fortunately, this is the region most likely to be felt during a rectal examination and tapped in a needle biopsy of the prostate.

## How Do Hormones Affect the Prostate?

The prostate is very sensitive to hormones. In cancer treatment, this is a good thing: cutting off the supply of these sex hormones, or androgens, can shrink prostate cancer and delay its progression. The hormones that control the prostate originate in the brain: the hypothalamus makes a substance called luteinizing hormone-releasing hormone (LHRH), which it transmits using "chemical Morse code," or signal pulses, to the nearby pituitary gland. In response, the pituitary makes its own chemical signal, called luteinizing hormone (LH). LH, in turn, controls the testes, which make testosterone. Testosterone is the chief "male" hormone, the cause of—among other things—secondary sex characteristics such as body hair and a

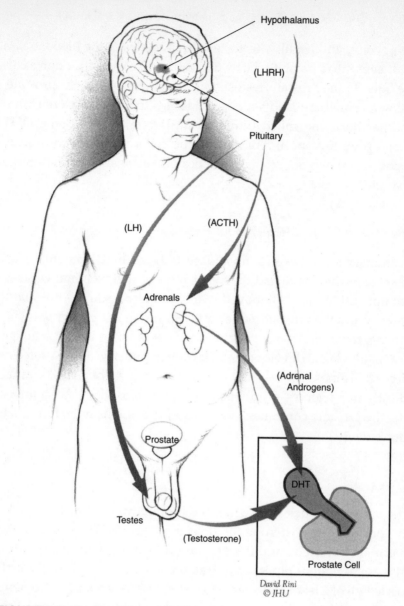

Hypothalamus

(LHRH)

Pituitary

(LH)

(ACTH)

Adrenals

(Adrenal Androgens)

Prostate

DHT

Testes

(Testosterone)

Prostate Cell

David Rini
© JHU

## FIGURE 1.4 The Prostate and Hormones

The hormones that control the prostate originate in the brain: The hypothalamus makes a substance called luteinizing hormone-releasing hormone (LHRH), which it transmits to the nearby pituitary gland. The pituitary then makes its own chemical signal, called luteinizing hormone (LH). LH, in turn, controls the testes, which make testosterone—the chief "male" hormone. Testosterone circulates in the bloodstream and seeps into a prostate cell by diffusion, like water through a coffee filter. The prostate, using an enzyme called 5-alpha reductase, refines testosterone into another hormone called dihydrotestosterone (DHT). Soon, DHT joins up with a specific protein in the cell's nucleus that acts like a key, switching on various genes within the prostate.

deep voice, and fertility. Testosterone circulates in the bloodstream and seeps into a prostate cell by diffusion—like water through a coffee filter. To the prostate, testosterone is a raw material: the prostate, using an enzyme called 5-alpha reductase, refines testosterone into another hormone called dihydrotestosterone (DHT). Soon, DHT joins up with a specific protein in the cell's nucleus and quickly becomes a powerhouse that switches on various genes within the prostate.

### The Prostate Is Not Required for Potency

In animals, it's not even a must for fertility; animals can remain fertile even if they have had their prostate—or their seminal vesicles, but not both organs—removed. We didn't always know this about potency and the prostate (see chapter 8), and the discovery was surprising, considering that the growth of the prostate clearly *is* linked to a man's sexual development. Starting at puberty, the prostate enlarges five times in size—from a weight of about 4 grams to 20 grams, the size of a walnut—by about age twenty. (For the rest of a man's life, the prostate continues to grow and become heavier, but much more slowly.)

### Testes

The testes, or testicles, are a man's reproductive organs. They make the hormone testosterone, as discussed above. They also make sperm, in hundreds of tiny tubes and threadlike, winding tubules. (If these miniature pipes were straightened out, each would stretch to a length of 2 feet.) There are two testes, each less than 2 inches long and about 1 inch wide. The testes, attached to blood-supplying lifelines called spermatic cords, are covered by the scrotum. Have you ever wondered why the scrotum is suspended in such a vulnerable position, below the body? Wouldn't it make more sense—and provide better protection—if the testicles were inside the body? Yes and no. If the testes were tucked away inside the pelvis, they would indeed be better protected—but there wouldn't be much to protect. The testes are located in the scrotum for the simple but expedient reason that it's a more temperate climate down there, by a couple of degrees. Sperm are delicate; they fare poorly when the temperature is too warm. The scrotum, in effect, is nature's cooler. (In fact, men who have undescended testicles—which are located inside the abdomen—cannot develop sperm because the normal body temperature is just too hot.)

## Epididymis

The sperm-making tubules in each testis converge to form the epididymis. Compared to the tubules, this is a river as large and serpentine as the Amazon: each tubule (one on each side), though only 1 millimeter wide, could be uncoiled to reach a remarkable length of 15 to 20 feet. This is one continuous tube—thus, it's easy to see why an infection here could cause scar tissue and blockage that would result in infertility. These tubules are packed side by side, top to bottom, to form the epididymis, an elongated structure about the size of a woman's pinky finger. This is the greenhouse where sperm mature until orgasm, when they shoot from the tail of the epididymis during a series of powerful muscle contractions. The epididymis clings to one side of each testis before turning yet again and heading upward to meet still another tube, called the vas deferens.

## Vas Deferens

This impressive tube (again, one on each side; together they are called the vasa deferentia), now grown to 3 millimeters in diameter, is a hard, muscular cord about 18 inches long. Its job is to pump sperm to the part of the urethra that lies within the prostate (the prostatic urethra). Because it is so thick, it can easily be palpated through the scrotum. (It can also be cut easily in an outpatient procedure—a form of male birth control called a vasectomy. When the cord is cut, sperm cannot exit the penis through ejaculation and instead are reabsorbed by the body.) The vas deferens travels to a space between the bladder and rectum, then courses downward to the base of the prostate, where it meets with the duct of the seminal vesicle to form the ejaculatory duct.

## Seminal Vesicles

The lumpy seminal vesicles, each about 2 inches long, sit behind the bladder, next to the rectum, hanging over the prostate like twin bunches of grapes. Arching still higher over them, on either side, are the vasa deferentia, which meet the seminal vesicles at V-shaped angles; these form the ejaculatory ducts, slitlike openings that feed into the prostatic urethra. The seminal vesicles are made up of caves called alveoli, which make sticky secretions that help maintain semen's consistency. (The vesicles got their name because scientists used to believe they stored sperm; they don't.) Like the prostate, the seminal vesicles depend on hormones for their development and growth and for the secretions they produce. Although the seminal vesicles are strikingly similar to the prostate in many ways, they're almost always free of abnormal growth—benign (as in BPH) as well as malignant. (This is covered in more detail in chapter 3.)

Lately, scientists at Johns Hopkins have begun exploring the relationship between the prostate and the seminal vesicles. What we have learned from their work is that the saga of human evolution is also a story of two male glands—both of which produce fluid that makes up semen. One gland, the prostate, is prone to cancer. The other, the seminal vesicle, is remarkably free of it. In nature, animals that are carnivores—meat eaters like dogs and lions—don't have seminal vesicles. The only animals that have both prostates and seminal vesicles are herbivores—veggie-eating animals, like bulls, apes, and elephants. There is only one exception to this rule: humans. Men have seminal vesicles, too. In other words, man, a meat lover, has the makeup of an animal that should be a vegetarian. For more on this research and what it means, see chapter 3.

## Penis

The penis—an engineering marvel built of nerves, smooth muscle, and blood vessels—has two main functions: sexual intercourse and urination. (Note: There is no bone in the human penis, although this is not the case in dogs and some other animals.) The penis works like a water balloon. Its basic structure is that of a rounded triangle; all three corners have cylinders of tissue (called the corpora cavernosa

## SEMEN IS MOSTLY . . . NOT SPERM

Semen is the ejaculate, and it's made up of seminal fluid and sperm. (One-third of the fluid originates from the prostate, two-thirds from the seminal vesicles.) Sperm makes up just a tiny fraction of semen (which is why a vasectomy does not reduce the volume of the ejaculate). Semen is surprisingly rich. Its components, mainly secretions from the prostate and seminal vesicles, include prostaglandins, spermine, fructose, glucose, citric acid, zinc, proteins, and enzymes such as immunoglobulins, proteases, esterases, and phosphatase. These other ingredients probably serve as a buffer to help sperm survive the trip and remain active and, in the case of sugars such as fructose and glucose, as a "snack for the road," to provide energy for a sperm's metabolism on its journey. Still other components—the zinc, for example, and proteases and immunoglobulins—may be cleansing agents there to help fend off infections and other harmful substances in the urinary tract.

Semen undergoes extreme chemical transformations after ejaculation, metamorphosing from a viscous liquid to a semisolid and back again. A few minutes after ejaculation, semen coagulates into a gel-like substance; then, within about fifteen minutes, it becomes a sticky liquid. In most animals, a substance made by the seminal vesicles is the cause of the coagulation; then PSA, an enzyme made by the prostate (see above), makes semen runny again. The character of semen varies greatly among species. For example, in bulls and dogs (which don't have seminal vesicles), semen does not coagulate at all. But in rats and rabbits, semen quickly coagulates to form a pellet; for these animals, a PSA-like enzyme is crucial in helping the sperm reach their destination. Because semen is a bodily fluid, like blood, it is affected by drugs and can be a carrier of sexually transmitted diseases, such as AIDS.

and the corpus spongiosum) that fill and become engorged with blood. In erection, as arteries pump a steady supply of blood into the penis, the veins (which normally pump it back out again) clamp down so the blood can't recirculate, thus keeping the penis "inflated" during sexual activity. All of this is made possible by the delicate nerves that lead to and from the penis. For years, these tiny nerves were poorly understood. The sad result was that removal of the prostate almost always meant impotence (see chapter 8). That is no longer the case.

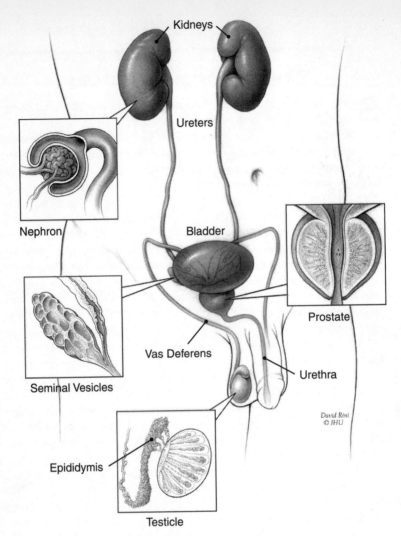

**FIGURE 1.5  How Urine Exits the Body**

From the top: The kidneys are the body's main filters. With more than a million tiny, wadded-up filters called nephrons, the kidneys sift through an incredible volume of fluid—about 45 gallons a day for a 150-pound man. Every day, the average man excretes about 2 quarts of urine. Urine exits the kidneys through ureters, pipelines that work like toothpaste tubes, squeezing urine downward toward the bladder. The bladder is a big bag. Stretched to its fullest, this muscular tank can hold about a pint of urine. Unlike the kidneys and ureters, the bladder—in normal circumstances—allows us some voluntary control; it generally obeys our decision to eliminate or hold urine. The next stop is the urethra, another muscular tube, which begins at the neck of the bladder, then tunnels through the prostate and continues into the penis.

Also seen here are the seminal vesicles, made up of caves called alveoli that make sticky secretions that help maintain semen's consistency, and the testes. The testes are a man's reproductive organs. They make the hormone testosterone; they also make sperm, in hundreds of tiny tubes.

## How the Urinary Tract Works

### Kidneys

The kidneys are the body's main filters. With each heartbeat, they cleanse the blood of toxic wastes, excess water, and salts and (among many other chores) help maintain the body's balance of fluids and minerals. With more than a million tiny, wadded-up filters called nephrons, the kidneys sift through an incredible volume of fluid—about 45 gallons a day for a 150-pound man (see fig. 1.5). Every sip of water we drink is refined, reabsorbed, and then processed again. (If the water and minerals weren't reabsorbed, our bodies would become seriously dehydrated within hours.) Not all of this material returns to the body, however; much of it passes out as urine. Every day, the average man excretes about 2 quarts of urine (a concentrated mixture of water, sodium, chloride, bicarbonate, potassium, and urea, the breakdown product of proteins).

### Ureter

Urine exits each kidney through a pipeline called the ureter. The ureters work like toothpaste tubes, squeezing or "milking" urine from the kidneys. Each ureter is about a foot long and narrow—less than a half-inch wide at its broadest point. Ureters are one-way streets: urine always flows the same way through them—straight toward the bladder.

### Bladder

The bladder is a big bag. Stretched to its fullest, this muscular tank can hold about a pint of urine (see fig. 1.2). Unlike the kidneys and ureters, the bladder, in normal circumstances, allows us some voluntary control; it generally obeys our decision to eliminate or hold urine. (The inability to control urination is called incontinence.) With intricately woven layers of muscle and connective tissue, the bladder can collapse or expand, depending on the amount of fluid it's asked to hold at a given time. A sophisticated backup system protects the bladder from extreme distention and the risk of rupture: when the bladder is very full, it signals the kidneys to slow down the production of urine. At the neck of the bladder is a gate called the trigone. The purpose of the trigone is to make sure urine flows only one way—downward, away from the ureters and kidneys. The trigone's valve makes a tight seal that prevents urine from backing up into the kidneys, even when the bladder is distended.

## Urethra

The next stop on urine's downward passage is the urethra, another muscular tube, about 8 inches long. This one begins at the neck of the bladder, then tunnels through the prostate at a 35-degree angle and continues into the penis. The urethra is divided into three segments—prostatic (the part that runs through the prostate), membranous (in between the prostate and penis—this is where the external sphincter is located), and penile. Like the prostate, it plays a role in both the urinary and reproductive systems; it serves as a conduit not only for urine but for sexual fluids. The prostatic urethra has its own gate to prevent fluid backup—a ring of smooth muscle located in the pre-prostatic zone. During ejaculation, this muscle ring contracts along with the bladder neck. This keeps semen from flowing the wrong way—up into the bladder—and directs its course downward, out the urethra.

That's it for the anatomy crash course. Throughout this book, as we describe diagnostic procedures, treatments, and complications, you may need to return to this chapter. That's what it's for—to give you a working familiarity with the territory we'll be covering in the next chapters. If it helps, think of these pages as your Michelin Guide to male anatomy. Now that we've discussed the context of the prostate—a significant gland in both the urinary and reproductive systems—it's time to explain why this tiny gland is so important and what can go wrong.

# 2

# LITTLE GLAND, BIG TROUBLE

## ▶▶▶ READ THIS FIRST

At some point in their lives, most men are going to have to come to terms with the prostate, because this little gland is the source of three of the major, common health problems that affect men:

- Prostate cancer, the most common cancer in men;
- Benign prostatic hyperplasia (BPH), also known as enlargement of the prostate, one of the most common benign tumors in men; and
- Prostatitis, a painful inflammation of the prostate and the most common cause of urinary tract infections in men.

   This news usually comes as an unpleasant shock, because most men don't even know that they have a prostate until something goes wrong. Worse, because there is no "statute of limitations" on prostate problems, some men are unlucky enough to endure more than one of these disorders. (In fact, some men find out they have prostate cancer during a routine procedure to treat BPH.) You may suddenly experience a bout of prostatitis or develop urinary problems because of prostate enlargement. Or your "wake-up call" to the prostate may be an abnormal prostate-specific antigen (PSA) blood test, or a suspicious lump felt during a rectal exam, raising the possibility that you have prostate cancer. Thus, it's important for you to understand all of the "Big Three" prostate disorders.

Here's what you need to know.

## PROSTATE CANCER

This is the most common cancer in men, and the third leading cause of cancer death in men. Because prostate cancer is the subject of this entire book, the only important point you need to know right now is that *when prostate cancer is small, it is curable.* However, because it is "silent" and produces no early-warning symptoms, routine testing is very important. How can we save lives from prostate cancer? The rest of this book is devoted to answering this question. The key is a four-pronged approach—prevention, early diagnosis, better treatment for localized disease (cancer confined to the prostate) with fewer side effects, and better control of advanced disease.

## BPH, OR ENLARGEMENT OF THE PROSTATE

BPH is so common that most men, if they live long enough, will develop it. By age seventy, 70 percent of men have it, and one-quarter of men with the disease require treatment. BPH is not prostate cancer, and having it does not mean that a man is more or less likely to get prostate cancer. BPH and prostate cancer are two different diseases that develop in different regions of the prostate—almost as if the prostate were two glands rolled into one. Prostate cancer begins in the outer, peripheral zone of the prostate and grows *outward*, invading surrounding tissues; that's why it rarely produces symptoms until it is far advanced. On the other hand, BPH begins in a tiny area of the inner prostate called the transition zone—a ring of tissue that makes a natural circle around the urethra, the tube through which urine and semen exit the body. In BPH, the growth is *inward*, toward the prostate's core, constantly tightening around the urethra and interfering with urination (which is why symptoms are almost impossible to ignore). BPH is a very common condition that affects most men. It is not cancerous, but it can mimic cancer. Today, there are many good ways to treat it, and most of them have few side effects.

## PROSTATITIS

Prostatitis is the most common cause of urinary tract infection in men, and an estimated 25 percent of all men who see a doctor for urological problems have symptoms of prostatitis. There are four conditions lumped under the umbrella name "prostatitis." The two least common and easiest to treat are caused by bacterial infection: acute and chronic bacterial prostatitis. These conditions are usually associated with fever, chills, severe burning on urination, increased frequency of urination, and, in some cases, a life-threatening infection in the bloodstream. Next, two forms of prostatitis fall into a category called chronic prostatitis/chronic pelvic pain syndrome. Nobody knows what causes these forms of prostatitis, and antibiotics do not help at all. The treatment here is largely aimed at relieving symptoms, with muscle relaxants such as alpha-blockers and other drugs, which ease muscle tension in the prostate and make urination easier. There's another, mysterious category known as asymptomatic inflammatory prostatitis, which produces no symptoms and is usually found by chance, when inflammatory cells are found in the prostatic fluid or inflammation is detected on a prostate biopsy. If it produces no symptoms, is it something we should even worry about? Maybe. We're still learning about this inflammation, and, although it is not cancer, it may be linked with the formation of cancer. In other words, whatever causes the inflammation may eventually cause cancer as well. (See chapter 3 for more on this.)

The best thing to know about prostatitis is that it is not cancer. The treatment for most prostatitis (except the bacterial kind, which responds to antibiotics) is often trial and error. Therefore, it helps if men and their doctors can work together, with much patience, to come up with the right plan. There is, however, some exciting new research that may help us find new ways to manage prostatitis. Many men have found that their symptoms improve when they change their diet and lifestyle.

## What Can Go Wrong With the Prostate:
## Cancer, BPH, and Prostatitis

For most young men, the prostate falls into the category "obscure body parts" that includes the spleen—that is, it's in there someplace, it probably does something useful, but it's best dealt with on a need-to-know basis.

Unfortunately, most men *are* going to need to know about the prostate sometime, because this little gland is the source of three of the major health problems that affect men: prostate cancer, the most common major cancer in men; benign enlargement of the prostate (BPH, or benign prostatic hyperplasia), one of the most common benign tumors in men and a source of symptoms for most men as they age; and prostatitis, painful inflammation of the prostate, the most common cause of urinary tract infections in men. Worse, because there's no "statute of limitations" on prostate problems, some men are unlucky enough to endure more than one of these disorders. For example, having BPH or prostatitis doesn't mean a man has "had his prostate trouble" and won't have further difficulty—either a return of symptoms or a new problem entirely, such as prostate cancer. Although this is a book about prostate cancer, when it comes to making the diagnosis and planning treatment, the other prostate disorders must be considered, too. Thus, it's important that men know about all of the "Big Three" prostate problems—what they are, how they are treated, and their telltale symptoms.

Fortunately, effective treatment and relief of symptoms is available for all of these prostate disorders. *Even prostate cancer, when caught early, is curable*—generally without causing loss of urinary control or sexual function. Better still, for the first time ever, we are very close to understanding how to keep advanced cancer in check, perhaps even for years.

### Prostate Cancer

Prostate cancer is the most common major cancer in men and the third leading cause of cancer death in men. Because prostate cancer is the subject of this entire book, we'll use this space only to make one point: when prostate cancer is small and curable, it is also silent—it produces no symptoms. That's why routine testing is so important—to detect cancer as early as possible. If it's caught too late, prostate cancer can be deadly, and if the disease is allowed to run its course, it can produce terrible symptoms and excruciating pain. But if caught in time, before the cancer spreads beyond the wall of the prostate, prostate cancer can be cured with surgery or radiation. For some men with small, slow-growing tumors, a process called expectant management—following the disease closely—may be a safe option (see chapter 7).

Treatment of prostate cancer is better than ever: we are now able to cure prostate cancer in more men, and with fewer side effects, than ever before. And, for the first time, groundbreaking research and novel methods aimed at stopping advanced prostate cancer in its tracks are starting to pay off, with promising new drugs now being tested in patients. Even though in some men we may not be able to cure prostate cancer, we may be able to stop it from growing further—which makes it very likely that, within a few years, men with advanced disease will die *with* prostate cancer but not *of* it. How can we save lives from prostate cancer? The key is a four-pronged approach:

- Prevention—to ward off prostate cancer entirely, or at least delay its onset for decades.
- Earlier diagnosis—with the help of highly sensitive tests and sophisticated models for analyzing the results, detecting prostate cancer at the earliest and most curable stages yet.
- Better treatment for localized disease—expanding and refining effective treatments, and working to minimize side effects even further.
- Better control of advanced disease.

Next, we cover the other two major prostate problems: BPH and prostatitis. Because none of the "Big Three" prostate diseases precludes the others, it is possible for a man to have more than one, even at the same time. However, if you don't have one of these problems, you may wish to go on to chapter 3 now and refer to the rest of this chapter—just like those young men we mentioned earlier—on a "need-to-know" basis.

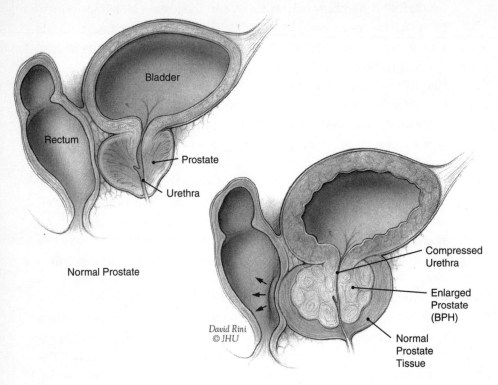

Normal Prostate

Prostate with BPH

**Figure 2.1** **How BPH Squashes the Urethra**

Here are two prostates—one with BPH, one without. What a difference! In the prostate with BPH, lumpy growths of glandular tissue plus tightening smooth muscle tissue act as a "double whammy" to choke the poor urethra and make urination increasingly difficult.

## Benign Prostatic Hyperplasia

Benjamin Franklin reportedly suffered from it; so did Thomas Jefferson. So will most men, if they live long enough. This almost inevitable condition is called benign prostatic hyperplasia (BPH), or enlargement of the prostate. The risk of BPH increases every year after age forty: BPH is present in 20 percent of men in their fifties, 60 percent of men in their sixties, and 70 percent of men by age seventy. One-quarter of men with BPH—more than 350,000 a year in the United States alone—eventually will require treatment, some of them more than once, to relieve the urinary obstruction BPH causes.

Before the 1990s, there was no effective medical (as opposed to surgical) treatment for this disorder. Men diagnosed with BPH were usually sent home and told to return when their symptoms were severe enough to warrant surgery. Just a decade ago, an American man had a 25 percent risk of undergoing prostate surgery for benign disease at some point in his life. In fact, BPH is still a common cause of surgery in American men over age fifty-five.

In recent years, as medical therapy has become available, more men have sought treatment to relieve their symptoms. Based on the figures mentioned above, it's likely that after age sixty, a majority of men will either be taking medication for BPH or considering it. However, not all of these men will be helped by the medicine: for men with severe symptoms or men who wait until the disease is far advanced before they seek treatment, surgery is still the best option.

Note: *Growth is not the same thing as cancer. BPH is not prostate cancer*, and having it doesn't mean a man is more or less likely to get prostate cancer. They're two different diseases—and in some ways, the prostate is almost like two different glands rolled into one. (However, because both BPH and prostate cancer are associated with aging, scientists are wondering if there are any other connections that we don't know about—see page 27.) Prostate cancer begins in the outer peripheral zone of the prostate (see fig. 1.3), and grows *outward*, invading surrounding tissue. BPH begins in a tiny area of the inner prostate called the transition zone, a ring of tissue that makes a natural circle around the urethra. In BPH, the growth is *inward* toward the prostate's core, constantly tightening around the urethra (the tube that carries urine from the bladder through the prostate to the penis) and interfering with urination (see fig. 2.1). This is why BPH produces such annoying, difficult-to-ignore symptoms—but why prostate cancer is often "silent," producing no symptoms for months or even years. The key word here is benign. (The word hyperplasia simply means an increase in the number of cells in the prostate, which causes it to become enlarged.) By itself, an enlarged prostate causes no symptoms and does no harm. If it weren't for the fact that the prostate encircles the urethra, BPH might never require treatment.

*What Causes It?*

The quick answer is, we don't know. Like wrinkles and gray hair, BPH just seems to come with the territory of aging. For reasons that are not clear, beginning at around age forty—in some men more than others—the inner zone of the prostate begins to grow. But even this is more complicated than it sounds. BPH involves two different kinds of tissue: glandular, made up of epithelial cells (the glandular factories that make the prostate's secretions) and smooth muscle cells (which contract to squeeze the secretions into the urethra). Somehow, BPH sets these two types of tissue at odds: it's the epithelial tissue that makes the lumpy lobes, but the smooth muscle tissue reacts to this buildup by tightening around the urethra.

Scientists suspect that the aging prostate somehow becomes more sensitive to testosterone, even though there's less of it floating around in the bloodstream. Why? As men age, testosterone production starts to fall—but the body's levels of estrogen (which normally are very low in men) remain about the same. We know that even a slight amount of estrogen can make testosterone more powerful; it may be that this imbalance in androgen and estrogen levels contributes to the disease. Also, the tissue changes in BPH may be triggered by substances called growth factors, possibly those made by muscle cells in the prostate.

Curiously, even though the tissue is growing—which normally would mean a big increase in the number of cells being made—the enlarging prostate makes about the same number of cells as always. How can this be? In any tissue, there is a finely tuned balance between the number of new cells and the number of cells that are dying. Apparently, the population boom in BPH isn't due to an increase in cell birth but to a decrease in cell death. For some reason, the cells in BPH are living much longer. Some process—perhaps an increase in growth factors—has altered their normal life span, creating a "fountain of youth" for prostate cells. Although the growth is not malignant, the process is similar to what's happening in prostate cancer—which suggests that, once we understand the factors that control cell death in BPH, we may have a better approach for controlling it in cancer as well.

## BPH: NEW MARKERS AND NEW QUESTIONS

**B**PH, Like Cancer, Can Be "Good" or "Bad." BPH doesn't just affect the prostate and, although it isn't cancer, it isn't always benign. It affects the bladder, and in severe form, its symptoms can be debilitating. "Until recently, all BPH was considered to be a single disease," notes Robert Getzenberg, Director of Research at the Brady Urological Institute at Johns Hopkins. But his research group has found a genetic marker called JM-27 that's associated with the most aggressive type of BPH. Further, Getzenberg and colleagues have developed a blood test that can determine whether a man has the most severe form of BPH or whether his case is mild. They hope that this test will even be able to predict how a man will respond to various treatments of BPH. "This is the first BPH-specific marker that has been identified, and we hope it will play a role in how men are treated for the disease," he says.

*BPH and Cancer—Any Connection?* BPH and prostate cancer affect different regions of the prostate, but they're both associated with aging. They may have other things in common as well, says Getzenberg. "We have identified a series of genes that appear to be altered in *both* BPH and prostate cancer. There may be much more connection between BPH and prostate cancer than we originally envisioned. Understanding more about the development of each of these diseases will help us develop better tools with which to attack them both."

### Does BPH Run in Some Families?

Several studies at Johns Hopkins suggest that it does. Hopkins scientists believe that for a small number of men—about 7 percent—age isn't the only major risk factor. These men probably have inherited one or more genes that somehow make them prone to BPH. In one investigation, scientists studied men aged sixty-four and younger with notable prostate enlargement. They also studied their relatives and family histories. They found that the male relatives of these men were four times as likely as other men to require a prostatectomy to treat BPH. And brothers of these men were six times as likely as other men to need surgery to treat BPH. Understanding how the disease works in these men—specifically, identifying the genes involved— may provide major insight into the far more common form of BPH (see box above) and one day may even help us prevent it. If you have a strong family history of BPH, scientists at Johns Hopkins would be very interested in hearing from you. (Send inquiries to the Hereditary Prostate Disease Study, James Buchanan Brady Urological Institute, Johns Hopkins Hospital, Baltimore, MD 21287–2101, Attention: Dr. Patrick Walsh.)

### What Does BPH Feel Like?

How does what's happening on the inside translate to the outside—into symptoms and their impact on a man's life? It varies: BPH is a different disease in every man, depending on a delicate interplay of factors, including the shape of the growth, the specific tissue involved, and how these variables affect the bladder. As the cell growth progresses, the tissue becomes lumpy. Bulbous nodules begin sprouting like mushrooms, forming characteristic clusters, or lobes.

These lobes tend to arrange themselves in one of three basic configurations. Lateral lobe enlargement features big knobs that sandwich the urethra. When a man urinates, these lobes can swing open and shut like double doors (think of a saloon in a cowboy movie), so despite their size, they may not produce much urinary obstruction. In middle lobe enlargement, the lobe bobs around the bladder neck, plugging it like a cork in a bottle and causing a man great difficulty with urination. (Because this form of BPH is much harder to ignore than lateral lobe enlargement, men who have it are far more likely to seek medical relief for their symptoms.) And in trilobar enlargement, the obstruction can happen in the bladder neck as well as in the urethra.

As the prostate squeezes the urethra, it impedes urine flow. This may manifest itself as frequent urination, needing to go to the bathroom several times an hour; hesitancy, or having to wait for the urinary stream to start; urgency, or the sudden sensation of needing to urinate, which may culminate in involuntary urine leakage before you reach the bathroom; repeatedly awakening in the night to urinate; starting and stopping during urination; and a constant feeling of fullness in the bladder. BPH can also lead to urinary tract infections and, rarely, can cause damage to the bladder or kidneys. It is often frustrating, annoying, and disruptive.

Think of a man's necktie slowly starting to tighten around his collar. This is what happens, over time, as the prostate's inward growth toward the urethra takes its toll. At first or in mild cases, this can mean an irritating but still tolerable change in quality of life. However, when it progresses beyond the nuisance point—when the bladder is never completely empty, or when the kidney or bladder become damaged—it needs to be treated.

At first, BPH is invisible. It causes few symptoms, because the powerful bladder muscle compensates for the narrowed urethra by making more vigorous contractions and forcing urine through the prostate. But over time, this extra effort takes its toll on the bladder, making it less efficient. This is when a man may notice a decreased flow rate and obstructive symptoms. The bladder, after months of heavy duty, also becomes a victim of its own powerful muscles: The muscle-bound bladder wall thickens and loses its elasticity. With all that extra muscle, the bladder can't hold as much as it used to; it becomes unstable and overly reactive. When this happens, a man feels the need to urinate more often—unfortunately, sometimes spontaneously. These are irritative symptoms: urge incontinence (when a man knows he has to urinate but can't make it to the bathroom in time) and nocturia (the need to urinate often during the night). Nocturia can also happen (or be made worse) if a man is unable to empty his bladder completely. If the bladder is always partly full with leftover urine, it doesn't take much—half a glass of water, even—to fill it all the way. Some of our patients joke that they've spent the first half of their lives making money, and they're spending the second half making water. Imagine how disruptive and frustrating it is for a man to have to go to the bathroom twice as often as he normally would.

## How Do You Know If You Have It?

Some men go right to a specialist, a urologist, for help with their urinary problems, but most men start out with a generalist—their family doctor or internist. Most likely, all of these doctors will approach your symptoms the same way: there should be a digital rectal examination and a PSA blood test. (These and other diagnostic tests are discussed in chapter 5.) You should be referred to a urologist if your doctor suspects BPH (or, for that matter, prostatitis or prostate cancer).

Because other conditions can mimic BPH, your doctor will probably begin by taking a detailed medical history and performing a physical exam. It is very important for your doctor to know your entire medical history, even if you have what appears to be a classic case of BPH. For example, an injury to the urethra (from having a catheter inserted into the bladder during a surgical procedure, perhaps) can create a urethral stricture—scar tissue that narrows the urethra—that has nothing to do with the prostate but does a great impersonation of BPH. Blood in the urine or pain in the bladder or penis could point to a bladder tumor or mean that a stone has developed in the bladder, prostate, or kidney. If you have a history of urologic trouble—recurrent urinary tract infections, for example, or prostatitis—it could be that an old problem has returned, but in disguise. BPH symptoms can also be produced by bladder cancer, prostate cancer, and neurogenic bladder (trouble with bladder function caused by a neurological problem, such as Parkinson's disease).

You will also be asked to score the severity of your symptoms and how much they bother you on a questionnaire called the International Prostate Symptom Score (IPSS), which appears below. This is a series of seven questions that can be answered on a scale from 1 to 5. (Briefly, symptoms are considered mild if the score total is 0 to 7, moderate if it's 8 to 19, and severe if it's 20 to 35.) The last question is the most important of all: How much do the symptoms bother you? This is critical, because BPH is not life-threatening. All of its treatments are directed at relieving symptoms—which means this symptom score will be the main basis for selecting therapy. (Thus, it is essential that you be brutally honest—rather than stoic and long-suffering or overly optimistic that this problem will go away by itself—in answering these questions.) The big question your doctor needs answered—and the one only you can decide—is whether you could live the rest of your life this way. Are you changing your life to accommodate BPH—giving up seats to a basketball game, for instance, so you won't have to tough it out in the long lines at the men's room? Are you planning your day around trips to the bathroom? If not—if you can put up with it for now—then you may choose to delay treatment. But if this problem is driving you crazy and disrupting your life, then it may be time to seek treatment.

The physical examination is discussed in detail in chapter 5. With

BPH—because the disease affects only the innermost core of the prostate—your doctor may not be able to feel anything out of the ordinary. It's important to keep in mind that the size of the prostate may have nothing to do with the degree of symptoms. Some men with major prostate enlargement have no urinary tract trouble, while other men with seemingly minor enlargement or even a small prostate can suffer terrible problems from obstruction. Again, it all depends on where the trouble is (see above for a discussion of the types of BPH).

You may also need other tests, including:

### Uroflowmetry
This test measures the speed of your urinary stream and the amount of urine you pass, and is done as you urinate (while you're alone in a testing room) into an electronic machine. (It's a urological version of the radar gun used to measure professional baseball pitchers' throws.) To ensure an accurate result, it's important that you urinate at least 5 or 6 ounces. This test can identify men whose maximum flow rate is not noticeably diminished and who may not benefit from treatment. (The normal peak urinary flow rate is 15 cubic centiliters or more per second.)

### Ultrasound
This is a painless imaging technique. It creates a picture by bouncing high-frequency sound waves off an object, like sonar on a submarine. It can be performed from the outside, through the abdomen, or transrectally, using a wand inserted in the rectum. Though not recommended for most men with BPH, ultrasound may be helpful in diagnosing such problems as obstruction of the kidney, stones, or a hidden tumor in the upper urinary tract; in estimating how well the bladder is emptying; and in determining the size of the prostate.

### Residual Urine Measurement
If you're not emptying your bladder completely, this important test will find out. Further, it will show how much urine you're leaving behind. This can be done indirectly by an ultrasound examination of the lower abdomen immediately after you urinate or directly by inserting a small catheter into the bladder (like a dipstick) and measuring

what's there. These measurements can be a helpful means of follow-ing the course of BPH and showing any change for the worse. If it turns out that you have large amounts of residual urine, your doctor will probably suggest that you seek treatment to avoid chronic uri-nary tract infection or damage to your kidneys.

### Urodynamic studies

Your urologist may want to do these studies if there is evidence that the primary problem is with the bladder, not the prostate. Cystome-try is a way to measure bladder pressure and function. It's performed by threading a tiny catheter into the penis, through the urethra, and into the bladder to monitor pressure changes as the bladder is filled with water. Pressure-flow studies, using a small catheter, check blad-der pressure as you urinate. (Note: Any time a catheter is inserted into the urethra, there is a slight risk of a urinary tract infection develop-ing a few days later. Be sure to tell your doctor if you experience any subsequent fever or discomfort.) In these tests, pressures within the bladder are compared with the rate at which urine is flowing. This can determine whether men with high peak urinary flow rates have ob-struction. Imagine squeezing water out of a balloon with a small opening. If you can squeeze hard enough, you can make the water flow, not just trickle. Similarly, some men with significant obstruction can produce reasonable urinary flow rates because they can generate high bladder pressure. These men will have relief of symptoms if their obstruction is treated. However, in some men, low urinary flow rates are caused by diseased bladders that can't produce much pressure. Relieving the obstruction in the prostate won't help these men, be-cause the true problem is the bladder.

### Cystoscopy

This test, usually performed in an outpatient setting, is uncomfortable but not painful; it is often used to assess the situation before an in-vasive procedure. A cystoscope is a slender, lighted tube (often flex-ible) that works like a periscope. It is inserted into the tip of the anesthetized penis and threaded through the urethra into the blad-der. This allows the urologist to see the bladder, prostate, and urethra and spot anything abnormal—such as a stone, stricture, or enlarge-ment. With cystoscopy, your doctor may also be able to see thickened muscle bands in the bladder. Like rings in a tree trunk, these tell a story—that a condition of bladder obstruction has probably evolved over months or even years. (Note: As with insertion of a catheter into the urethra, this test carries a small risk of urinary tract infection. Some men also experience blood in the urine or a temporary inability to urinate. Be sure to tell your doctor if you develop a fever or feel any discomfort.) Cystoscopy can also be used to rule out other conditions, such as the presence of a bladder stone or bladder tumor.

### How Is BPH Treated?

The first option is called watchful waiting, but it doesn't mean "do nothing." It means "wait and see." This is best chosen by men with mild symptoms—those who say they can live with it for the time being. The course of BPH is often hard to predict. Your symptoms could stay the same, improve, or get worse. Men who choose watchful waiting must make an extra effort to avoid any condition (such as constipation) or medication (including over-the-counter cold remedies) that could aggravate the problem. Beyond watchful waiting, there are two basic approaches—medical and surgical.

For men with moderate symptoms, the initial treatment should be medical. Here, again, there are several approaches: one class of drugs is called alpha-blockers. Remember the two kinds of tissue involved in BPH? One is glandular, made up of epithelial cells that secrete the prostate's fluids. The other is smooth muscle tissue— stromal cells that contract and squeeze this fluid into the urethra. As the glandular tissue enlarges and begins to narrow the urethra, the smooth muscle tissue tightens around it like a fist. In the normal prostate, there are two stromal cells for every epithelial cell. But in BPH, this ratio shifts. It's five to one, leading some scientists to describe BPH as a "stromal process." In other words, it's a smooth muscle problem. Alpha-blockers (the same drugs often used to treat high blood pressure) counteract this by causing this muscle tissue to relax. These drugs are helpful in men with small prostates and moderate symptoms.

For men who have a significantly enlarged prostate, it is reasonable to try another class of drugs called 5-alpha reductase inhibitors. These drugs block 5-alpha reductase, the chemical that changes testosterone into dihydrotestosterone (DHT), the active form of male hormone within the prostate. This is important because, scientists have learned, the trouble in BPH starts *after* testosterone is converted by 5-alpha reductase into DHT. There are two drugs—Avodart (dutasteride) and Proscar (finasteride)—that block the activity of this enzyme. Both appear to work equally well in shrinking the prostate and in decreasing obstructive symptoms. They may also halt the progression of BPH. These drugs neatly manage to block a hormonal process without affecting a man's levels of testosterone (the hormone responsible for libido and sexual function). However, the problem with these drugs is that the effect is gradual and very slow. To some men, the pace of change is agonizingly slow, with significant improvement coming only after several months to a year of taking these medications. Also, these 5-alpha reductase inhibitors work well only if the prostate is enlarged (men with smaller-sized prostates can have BPH symptoms, too). If the prostate is small, a prostate-shrinking drug isn't going to solve the problem. And the relief of symptoms lasts only as long as a man takes these drugs.

## Testing a Combined Approach

Could 5-alpha reductase inhibitors and alpha-blockers work better together? Is it possible that, for some men, two drugs are better than one? This idea was tested recently in a large, double-blind, placebo-controlled trial. Indeed, long-term use of both an alpha-blocker and a 5-alpha reductase inhibitor proved safe and reduced the risk of clinical progression—of symptoms getting worse—more than either treatment alone. Men taking both drugs had a lower risk of developing acute urinary retention (the inability to urinate) and were less likely to need invasive therapy. However, the combined therapy is not the miracle answer for every man with BPH. It's expensive, results are not immediate, and although the outcomes of this study were statistically significant, they amounted to only a few percentage points. Further, there is some concern that long-term use of 5-alpha reductase inhibitors may, by artificially lowering a man's PSA level, delay the diagnosis of prostate cancer until it has progressed into high-grade disease (this is discussed in chapter 4).

## *PROSTATE SYMPTOMS AND WHAT THEY MAY MEAN*

### *Symptoms of urinary obstruction . . .*

Weak flow
Hesitancy in starting urination; a need to push or strain to get
    urine to flow
Intermittent urinary stream (starts and stops several times)
Difficulty in stopping urination
Dribbling after urination
A sense of not being able to empty the bladder completely
Not being able to urinate at all

### *. . . could be caused by*

Benign prostatic hyperplasia (BPH)
Urethral stricture
Prostate cancer
Medication
Neurogenic bladder (bladder trouble caused by a neurological
    problem, such as Parkinson's disease)

### *Symptoms of irritation . . .*

Pain or burning during urination
Frequent urination, especially at night
A strong sense of urgency in urination; inability to postpone
    urination
Sleep disrupted by the need to urinate
Urgency incontinence

### *. . . could be caused by*

Thickened bladder, caused by obstruction from BPH
Infection in the bladder or prostate
Bladder tumor
Bladder stone
Neurogenic bladder

## *Surgical Options*

For men with severe symptoms or men who do not respond to medical therapy, there are many effective surgical options. The gold standard of these is a procedure called transurethral resection of the prostate (TUR or TURP), also described by patients (although it makes urologists cringe) as the "Roto-Rooter" procedure. It is a proven, effective way to improve BPH symptoms quickly and keep them at bay for years. The TUR is performed under anesthesia (usually spinal anesthesia). Although it is a surgical procedure, the abdomen is not opened up. (Only in rare cases—usually in men with very large prostates—is it necessary to perform an open surgical procedure to remove the prostate tissue surrounding the urethra.) In a TUR, surgeons reach the prostate via the urethra by placing an instrument similar to a cystoscope through the penis. This instrument, called a resectoscope, shines a powerful light that allows surgeons to view the prostate as they chip away at excess tissue. The prostate's core is removed in fragments by means of electrosurgical cautery or laser. These tissue chips collect in the bladder, and at the end of the procedure, they're flushed out, collected, and sent to a pathologist, who examines them and checks for prostate cancer. Because the resectoscope is threaded through the urethra, no skin incision is needed. In recent years, several promising new techniques have been developed. They all channel a form of energy—heat, radio waves, ultrasound, microwaves, and laser—to kill cells. Energy waves are generated, focused, aimed, and fired at the overgrowth of BPH tissue. Some waves work like a shotgun, blasting holes in the prostate. Others are as sensitive as a scalpel, delicately nibbling away at BPH tissue until the urethra is free of obstruction.

To sum up: BPH is a common condition that affects most men. It is not cancerous, but it can mimic cancer. Today, there are many effective ways to treat it, and most of them have few side effects.

### Prostatitis

Prostatitis hurts. This painful condition—an inflamed, swollen, and tender prostate—can be caused by a bacterial infection or by other factors. The major complaint in men with prostatitis is pain in the perineum (the area between the rectum and the testicles). They may also experience aches, pain in the joints or muscles and lower back, blood in the urine, pain or burning during urination, and painful ejaculation. In its own way, prostatitis is every bit as difficult and frustrating as BPH—not only because of the symptoms, but because there is not always an apparent cause. Prostatitis is a benign ailment—

it is not cancer, and it does not lead to cancer. It is not always curable, but it is almost always treatable.

The National Center for Health Statistics estimates that about 25 percent of all men who see a doctor for urological problems have symptoms of prostatitis. An estimated half of all men will experience some of these symptoms during their lifetime. Prostatitis is the most common cause of urinary tract infections in men; in fact, American men make about two million trips to the doctor each year seeking help for the symptoms of prostatitis or its siblings, "irritative prostatic conditions."

## What Causes It?

Sometimes we know, sometimes we don't. As one urologist commented in a review of this disorder, "Prostatitis is one of the most difficult clinical problems for men who suffer from it, as well as for the families of those men and their physicians. It is a particularly perplexing problem for urologists, who see many men with prostatitis and have difficulties with diagnosis and treatment." Fewer than 8 percent of men with prostatitis actually have a urinary tract infection (symptoms caused by bacteria, which can be helped by antibiotics). What about the rest of these men? There are actually four conditions lumped under the umbrella of prostatitis. Each one has distinct characteristics and responds differently to treatment. That's why getting the right diagnosis is so important.

The two least common forms of prostatitis are caused by bacterial infection. Note: Although these are sometimes referred to as "infectious" prostatitis, neither form is contagious and neither form can be transmitted to your sex partner. Acute bacterial prostatitis is a severe, debilitating condition that hits with all the subtlety of a Mack truck. No mystery here; men who have it know something is wrong, and they require immediate treatment. In addition to the symptoms described above, acute bacterial prostatitis is usually distinguished by chills and fever and extreme pain. It's difficult for a man to be stoic and try to "ride out" this condition. It's also a big mistake: if not treated, acute bacterial prostatitis can lead to more serious problems such as urinary retention (the inability to urinate), a life-threatening infection in the bloodstream (this is called sepsis), and development of an abscess (an accumulation of pus under pressure, like a pimple) within the prostate.

# INTERNATIONAL PROSTATE SYMPTOM SCORE (IPSS)

| | Not at all | Less than 1 time in 5 | Less than half the time | About half the time | More than half the time | Almost always | Your score |
|---|---|---|---|---|---|---|---|
| **1. Incomplete emptying** Over the past month, how often have you had a sensation of not emptying your bladder completely after you finished urinating? | 0 | 1 | 2 | 3 | 4 | 5 | |
| **2. Frequency** Over the past month, how often have you had to urinate again less than two hours after you finished urinating? | 0 | 1 | 2 | 3 | 4 | 5 | |
| **3. Intermittency** Over the past month, how often have you found you stopped and started again several times when you urinated? | 0 | 1 | 2 | 3 | 4 | 5 | |
| **4. Urgency** Over the past month, how often have you found it difficult to postpone urination? | 0 | 1 | 2 | 3 | 4 | 5 | |
| **5. Weak stream** Over the past month, how often have you had a weak urinary stream? | 0 | 1 | 2 | 3 | 4 | 5 | |
| **6. Straining** Over the past month, how often have you had to push or strain to begin urination? | 0 | 1 | 2 | 3 | 4 | 5 | |

|  | None | 1 time | 2 times | 3 times | 4 times | 5 times or more |
|---|---|---|---|---|---|---|
| **7. Nocturia** Over the past month, how many times did you most typically get up to urinate from the time you went to bed at night until the time you got up in the morning? | 0 | 1 | 2 | 3 | 4 | 5 |

**Total IPSS Score**

|  | Delighted | Pleased | Mostly satisfied | Mixed; about equally satisfied and dissatisfied | Mostly dissatisfied | Unhappy | Terrible |
|---|---|---|---|---|---|---|---|
| **Quality of Life Due to Urinary Symptoms** If you were to spend the rest of your life with your urinary condition just the way it is now, how would you feel about that? | 0 | 1 | 2 | 3 | 4 | 5 | 6 |

**If your total score is:**

0 to 7       your symptoms are considered mild
8 to 19      your symptoms are considered moderate
20 to 35     your symptoms are severe

Acute bacterial prostatitis is really an acute urinary tract infection (UTI). Fortunately, because the inflammation is so intense, this enables certain antibiotics—which normally wouldn't be able to penetrate the blood-prostate barrier, a shield designed to protect prostatic fluid—to reach the prostate. (Usually, in keeping out bad things like infection, this barrier also blocks helpful agents.) Acute bacterial prostatitis responds dramatically to antibiotics. However, many men are under-medicated—they either don't think they need (and therefore don't take) or aren't prescribed enough antibiotics to hit the infection hard and knock it out for good. A week to ten days of treatment may ease all signs of infection, and a man may even feel back to normal within a few days. But doctors have learned the hard way—from watching acute bacterial prostatitis return as a chronic infection—that it takes much longer, about six weeks of antibiotics, to get rid of the infection. In this sense, bacterial prostatitis is a lot like another stealthy infection, tuberculosis. The prostate is like a sponge, and if any trace of bacteria is not obliterated right away, acute bacterial prostatitis becomes much more difficult to cure. Eradicating acute bacterial prostatitis the first time around by relentless treatment with antibiotics is the best way to avoid developing chronic bacterial prostatitis.

Chronic bacterial prostatitis is also caused by bacteria and is also treated with antibiotics. It can be a recurring illness, coming back periodically for years after an initial episode of acute bacterial prostatitis. Its symptoms are usually milder versions of those seen in the acute form. Here, too, treatment with antibiotics should continue for six weeks. In many cases, the infection goes away every time with treatment; if, a few months later, it returns, it will vanish again after another round of antibiotics.

Both acute and chronic bacterial prostatitis are associated with UTIs, positive urine cultures that pinpoint the bacteria's location to the prostate, and the presence of inflammatory cells in prostatic secretions. (The hallmark of chronic bacterial prostatitis is that, when the infection returns, it's caused by the same type of bacteria that caused the previous infection.)

Chronic bacterial prostatitis, in fact, is so closely tied to UTIs that many doctors believe that if you don't have a UTI, and if you've never had one, you probably don't have chronic bacterial prostatitis. One explanation for persistent bacterial prostatitis may be lingering infection in tiny stones, called calculi, in the prostate. Prostatic calculi (the prostate's version of gallstones or kidney stones) are harmless and very common; about 75 percent of middle-aged men and 100 percent of elderly men have them.

The next category is called chronic prostatitis/chronic pelvic pain syndrome, and the cause here is a diagnostic puzzler: Nobody knows what causes the two forms of prostatitis in this group (which used to be named by what it was not, nonbacterial prostatitis), and antibiotics don't help at all. Men with chronic prostatitis/chronic pelvic pain syndrome may have many of the same symptoms as those with chronic bacterial prostatitis. However, in some men, the prostate may not even be the problem. The pain and other symptoms may be a result of spasms elsewhere in the pelvis, rectum, or lower back. This category has two subgroups: inflammatory and noninflammatory, based on whether any white blood cells (also called inflammatory cells) can be found in the prostatic fluid.

Treatment here is largely symptomatic. Your doctor may prescribe one or several medications, including antibiotics, alpha-blockers, 5-alpha reductase inhibitors, anti-inflammatory agents, and Elmiron (pentosan polysulfate sodium). All of these have been shown to help some men with these forms of prostatitis; the problem is determining which men will be helped by which drug or drugs. This may take a while—and plenty of patience—for you and your doctor to figure out. This is the "art" of medicine—your doctor thinking creatively, juggling and fine-tuning various treatments to find the best ones for you. Some doctors recommend anti-inflammatory drugs and sitz baths to ease muscle discomfort and make urination easier, and many men have been helped by changing their diet. Some foods—particularly spicy dishes, red wine, and caffeine—seem to make symptoms worse.

Then there's the mysterious "bonus" category known as asymptomatic inflammatory prostatitis. This condition produces no symptoms and is usually found by chance during a biopsy or when prostate tissue is removed for other reasons (for example, surgery for BPH or cancer). If it produces no symptoms, is this inflammation something we should even worry about? Maybe. We're still learning about this form of prostatitis, and, although it is not cancer, it may be linked with the formation of cancer. In other words, whatever causes the inflammation may eventually cause cancer as well. (This will be discussed at length in the next chapter.)

## How Do You Know If You Have It?

As described above, acute bacterial prostatitis leaves little room for guesswork. Other forms of prostatitis, however, cause milder symptoms (and asymptomatic inflammatory prostatitis doesn't cause any symptoms at all) that may not immediately suggest that the prostate is to blame. The constellation of symptoms of prostatitis includes pain in the perineum (the area between the rectum and testicles), testicles, the tip of the penis, the lower legs and back, and during or after ejaculation, as well as blood in the urine, the need to urinate frequently, and incomplete emptying of the bladder.

You are at higher risk of developing prostatitis if you recently have had a urinary catheter or other medical instrument inserted into your penis; engaged in rectal intercourse or oral sex; have had a recent bladder infection; or have other urinary problems, including BPH or an abnormal urinary tract. Stress also seems to play a role in prostatitis. (Note: If you have undergone recent surgery or any other surgical procedure, be sure to tell your doctor.)

## How Is Prostatitis Treated?

The easiest to treat is the most dramatic form, acute bacterial prostatitis. (The most likely cause of infection is *E. coli*, a form of bacteria that's common in the colon.) This can be cured with a course of antibiotics—usually one of a class called fluoroquinolones—that lasts for six weeks. Men with chronic bacterial prostatitis are helped by low maintenance doses of antibiotics. This is called chronic suppressive therapy and, as its name suggests, it is designed to *prevent* new UTIs from developing, instead of treating them after the fact. Men who do not have infections may be helped by drugs such as alpha-blockers (often used to treat high blood pressure; described above in the BPH section), antidepressants, and antispasmodics (drugs that help calm muscle spasms). The treatment for most prostatitis is often trial and error, and it helps if men and their doctors can work together—with much patience—to come up with the right plan. New evidence suggests that some nonbacterial prostatitis may actually be caused by an autoimmune condition that mimics the symptoms of prostatitis. This exciting new research may help us find new ways to manage the condition.

Finally, many men with prostatitis have found that their symptoms improve when they change their diet—eating a good balance of fruits and vegetables; avoiding spicy foods, alcohol, caffeine, and soft drinks that contain saccharin; and drinking enough water to keep urine running clear—and their lifestyle. A thirty-minute hot bath or sitz bath, twice a day, can relieve pain and make it easier to urinate. Getting daily exercise (but not riding a bike or an exercise bike, which can irritate symptoms) and resuming normal sexual activity may also be helpful.

# 3

# WHAT CAUSES PROSTATE CANCER?

## ▶▶▶ READ THIS FIRST

For American men—and men from all western countries—prostate cancer is something to worry about, because so many of us get it. This year, more than 200,000 American men will be diagnosed with prostate cancer, and 27,000 will die from it. An American boy born today has a 17 percent risk of developing prostate cancer and a nearly 3 percent risk of dying from it.

Although these numbers are high, the picture of prostate cancer today is far brighter than it's ever been—much more hopeful than it was even a generation ago. Consider these statistics: Of men diagnosed with prostate cancer in the late 1970s who did not die of other causes, only 70 percent survived five years, and more than half died of prostate cancer within fifteen years. How far we have come since then! Today, thanks to early diagnosis and screening, *more than 95 percent of men diagnosed with prostate cancer are alive ten years later.*

And yet, in terms of sheer numbers, there's a massive cloud on the horizon—the aging baby boomer generation, which makes up about 27 percent of the U.S. population. By some estimates, unless we can do something to prevent prostate cancer over the next twenty to forty years, the number of new cases will double. And unless we can find a better way to cure the disease, the number of men dying from it may triple. It's not that we're not doing a good job of treating prostate cancer, it's that we'll have so many more men to do a good job on!

That's why this book is more important now than ever. We hope to teach men and their families as much as we know about what causes prostate cancer, how to prevent it, and how we can treat it better.

### THE THREE MAJOR RISK FACTORS FOR PROSTATE CANCER: AGE, RACE, AND FAMILY HISTORY

- *Age:* Why is prostate cancer the bane of older men? Because, like many cancers, it takes years to develop. Mutations occur gradually, over decades, as oxidative damage—tiny changes within your cells—takes its toll. An American man in his mid- to late-seventies is seven times more likely to develop prostate cancer than is a man in his forties. What a difference a few decades makes: In men aged forty to fifty-nine, the risk of developing prostate cancer is one in fifty. In men aged sixty to seventy-nine, it's one in seven. And over the course of his lifetime, an American man's risk of developing prostate cancer is one in six.

- *Race:* African Americans have the highest risk of prostate cancer of any ethnic group in the world. Worse, black men seem to get more severe forms of prostate cancer, are more likely to have cancer recur after treatment, and are more likely to die from the disease than white men. Exactly why this is remains uncertain, although it may relate to genetic susceptibility, diet, and inadequate exposure to vitamin D (see below).

- *Family history:* If your father or brother has had prostate cancer, your risk of developing the disease is two-and-a-half times greater. If three family members (such as a father and two brothers) have developed prostate cancer, or if the disease occurs in three generations in your family (grandfather, father, son), or if two of your relatives have developed the disease at an early age (younger than fifty-five), then your family meets the criteria for hereditary prostate cancer, and your risk of developing prostate cancer may be as high as 50 percent. The genes responsible for this are under intense investigation, with the hope that when they are found, genetic testing will be available.

## A BALANCING ACT

Although you can't do anything about your age, race, or family history, there's another part of your life where you *can* make a difference: your environment. We know this from studies of identical twins. Genetically, they look the same, but their risk of prostate cancer varies, depending on the choices they make every day. Their risk of developing prostate cancer turns out to be 50 percent genetic and 50 percent environmental.

## WHAT ABOUT ENVIRONMENT?

Why is it that prostate cancer is common in western cultures and much less so Asia, but when Asian men migrate to western countries, their risk of prostate cancer increases over time? Scientists believe environment—mainly diet—must play a large role in determining who gets prostate cancer.

### Diet

Animal fat is bad for you, especially the fat found in red meat and dairy products. Men who eat a lot of these foods are more likely to develop advanced prostate cancer and die from it. Why? There is an enzyme in prostate cancer cells that craves the fatty acids in dairy products and red meat. Consequently, when a man with prostate cancer consumes a diet high in these foods, his cancer cells get nine times more energy than normal cells. Further, these cells produce hydrogen peroxide, which causes still more oxidative damage to DNA and more mutations, leading to further progression of the disease.

### Vitamin D, Sunlight, and Calcium

Vitamin D is a hormone that is known to protect us against cancer. We obtain vitamin D from two sources—10 percent from our diet and 90 percent from sunlight. When our skin is exposed to sunlight, vitamin D is synthesized from cholesterol. Ultimately, it's transformed in the kidney into its active form. This metabolized form of vitamin D has been shown to keep cells well differentiated; that is, to keep their shape intact and healthy and their growth slow and orderly. This is important because for cell growth, slow and orderly is good. When cells become cancerous, they become poorly differentiated; they lose their distinctive shapes and seem to melt together, and their growth becomes rampant.

## What About Hormones?

It makes sense that hormones must be a major cause of prostate cancer—after all, the male hormone testosterone is the major factor that causes the prostate to grow. But this correlation is still murky. It appears that it's not *how much* of a specific hormone a man has but *the way a man's genes respond to that hormone* that makes the difference. It may well be that in some men, a little hormone goes a lot further and has a much more powerful effect than in other men. Studies of hormone receptors in African American men have shown increased activity, and this may give us insight into why black men are so susceptible to prostate cancer.

## What Else?

There are a number of other factors that may or may not play a role in prostate cancer. The only occupation that has been found to be associated with a higher risk of prostate cancer is farming, and it is possible that this may be a result of farmers' increased lifetime exposure to agricultural chemicals, particularly herbicides. Although this link between herbicides and prostate cancer is not absolutely certain, it's strong enough that the U.S. government has agreed to provide service-connected disability for any veteran who was in Vietnam and who develops prostate cancer. What about vasectomy? The procedure itself doesn't increase a man's risk of getting prostate cancer, but it might give him a better shot at having it detected early, simply because he has a urologist and may be more likely to return to the urologist for checkups.

Does cigarette smoking increase a man's risk of getting prostate cancer? The quick answer is that it certainly doesn't help prevent it. But new research suggests that even if smoking cigarettes doesn't *cause* a man to develop prostate cancer, once that particular ball has been set in motion—once cancer starts to develop—it's more likely to be a rougher, more aggressive form of the disease that grows more quickly and is less likely to be caught in its early stages.

Drinking red wine in moderation seems to lower a man's prostate cancer risk. Frequent sexual activity may somewhat lower the risk as well. Having other prostate problems (bacterial prostatitis or BPH) doesn't appear to make prostate cancer more or less likely. And finally, there is conflicting evidence about whether a man's exercise or occupational exertion, or lack of it, has an influence on the development of the disease. So there you have it—a rundown of some of the factors that can increase a man's risk of developing prostate cancer. In chapter 4, we will take a look at things you can do to help prevent it.

## Who Gets Prostate Cancer?

If you are an Asian man who has lived all his life in, say, rural China, you will probably not need this book. That's because in your part of the world, few men ever get prostate cancer, and fewer still die of it.

This is not the case in America (or even in urban, increasingly "westernized" Asia), as we will discuss in a moment. One of the most remarkable things about prostate cancer is that throughout the world, there is a huge variability in the risk of getting it and of dying from it. The risk changes from place to place and, in many ways, from man to man. *The most common risk factor for prostate cancer is age; this is why men should begin screening tests for prostate cancer when they are forty.* But other factors are of major importance here, too, particularly race, geographic location—where in the world you live—and family history. There are others, but these are by far the most significant.

Thus, as far as prostate cancer goes, rural Asian men are lucky: the disease is not in the constellation of things they need to worry about. Men in western countries—Europe and North America—do not have that luxury. Prostate cancer is a very real menace on our horizon.

The statistics are sobering: This year, more than 200,000 American men will be diagnosed with prostate cancer, and nearly 30,000 will die because of it. In the United States, every three minutes or so, a new case of prostate cancer is diagnosed; about every nineteen minutes, a man dies from this disease. In men, it's the most common major cancer and the third most common cause of cancer death. As we've said, an American boy born today has a 17 percent risk of developing this disease and a 3.1 percent risk of dying from it.

Despite these numbers and despite all we've learned about this complicated disease over the years, many patients are still told by their doctors that "most men have prostate cancer, and few men die from it"—and thus, men shouldn't worry about prostate cancer. This is a gross and dangerous oversimplification. Some members of the medical community downplay the risk by fiddling with the numbers—dividing the number of new cases a year into the number of deaths. From this, they get the figure 14 percent: "Only 14 percent of men with prostate cancer die of it," they argue. "Therefore, most men don't die of it." Tell that to the wife whose husband died within six months of his diagnosis. Tell it to the families of the nearly thirty thousand American men who will die of prostate cancer this year. The truth is that some of these men—many of them in their eighties—found out they had prostate cancer and died not too long afterward of other causes.

On the other hand, we're getting better at spotting prostate cancer early; the average age of diagnosis has dropped from seventy-two to younger than seventy. Treatments are better than ever, and for the first time, we have hope of extending the lives of men with advanced disease. How far we have come in just a generation! In the late 1970s, of men diagnosed with prostate cancer who did not die of other causes, only 70 percent survived five years; more than half died of prostate cancer within fifteen years. Today, thanks to early diagnosis and screening, more than 95 percent of men diagnosed with prostate cancer are alive ten years later.

And yet, in sheer numbers alone, there's a massive cloud on the horizon. It's the aging baby boomer generation, which makes up about 27 percent of the U.S. population. Some 78 million men and women were born between 1946 and 1964; by the year 2030, they'll range in age from sixty-six to eighty-four. For prostate cancer, this is "prime time." Although we don't know all of the things that cause prostate cancer, we do know that it has the highest age-specific probability of diagnosis of any cancer. This means that a man's risk of getting it increases as he grows older (see box below). For a comparison, let's look at breast cancer in women: Before age sixty, breast cancer is more common in women than is prostate cancer in men. At age sixty, the risk of these two cancers is about the same. But after age sixty, prostate cancer seems to shift into high gear—and a man is three times more likely to develop it than a woman is to develop breast cancer. Can you see why the statistics of our aging population are worrying doctors who treat prostate cancer? By some estimates, unless we can do something to prevent prostate cancer over the next twenty to forty years, the number of new cases will double. And unless we can find a better way to cure the disease, the number of men dying from it will triple. It's not that we're not doing a good job of treating prostate cancer, it's that we'll have so many more men to do a good job on!

The point of these hard facts is to emphasize the need to cure this disease. Because if it is diagnosed late in the game or if men don't receive curative treatment, if they live long enough, prostate cancer does kill. Now, if you are an American man or someone who loves him, this doesn't mean you should panic. If you lived in a floodplain, a hurricane-prone coastal area, or an earthquake zone, what would you do? You would learn what you could, be vigilant, and remain prepared—because your knowledge and actions could save your life. The same is true for prostate cancer: what you learn from this book (and from your doctor, and—if you develop the disease—from other men and their families) may save your life, too.

TABLE 3.1

**WHAT ARE MY CHANCES OF DEVELOPING PROSTATE CANCER?**

| Age | Likelihood of Developing Cancer |
| --- | --- |
| 39 or younger | Nearly 1 in 10,000 |
| 40–59 | 1 in 45 |
| 60–79 | 1 in 7 |
| Lifetime risk | 1 in 6 |

## What Causes Cancer?

The answer to this question is just three letters—DNA. We hear about DNA all the time—at infamous criminal trials, for instance, and as a plot device on TV. But what is it? DNA is short for deoxyribonucleic acid. It is our genetic blueprint, and it's in every cell in our bodies—the "chemical Morse code" that directs each of our cells to make specific building blocks. These blocks are actually strings of chemicals, which scientists identify with letters. Changing just one letter can change everything.

A gene is a particular sequence of DNA that directs the production of a single protein. This genetic code is precious. It is the body's greatest treasure, the secret to life itself, and the body guards it jealously. Each cell has its own security systems designed to protect the integrity of this code. Every time a cell divides, this genetic code must be replicated perfectly. To guarantee that there are no errors in copying this vital information, every cell has a "spell-checker," which examines the code and repairs any defects it finds. The genes given this particular job are called mismatch repair genes—more on them in a moment.

### All Cancers Are Caused by Damage to DNA

In this sense, all cancers are genetic. (Note: "Genetic" doesn't always mean "inherited," although some doctors use the terms interchangeably. We'll talk about inherited, or hereditary, prostate cancer later in this chapter.) Their development—sometimes sparked by minor damage to a single gene—may be hidden deep within cells for years or even decades. Like a pothole that grows from one little crack in the pavement or a brushfire sparked by a lone bolt of lightning, cancer arises from one or a series of mutations in the DNA code. Incrementally, these changes create an environment that allows "bad" cells—cancerous or precancerous cells with hostile behavior and a disturbing tendency toward immortality—to flourish.

How does damage to DNA cause cancer? Actually, most of the time it doesn't; damage to DNA is incredibly common. It happens all the time, often at random, and it's almost always repaired instantaneously by the most efficient fix-it crews in the world. However, when mutations happen to transform a pivotal gene or several sensitive genes within a cell, the damage may overwhelm the body's normal defenses, and cancer may result. Think of an old movie in which a kid—like Mickey Rooney in *Boys Town*—"goes bad." Is there a genetic "Father Flanagan?" Can the errant gene be saved? Yes it can, sometimes, if the damage is reversible. In fact, scientists are learning that some foods may help block or even salvage injured genes that otherwise might become cancerous (see chapter 4).

Here are three major types of genes that are involved in cancer:

### Oncogenes

Some genes encode (provide the necessary information to make) growth factors, whose job is to make cells grow. They function as a chemical switch: click—turn on cell growth; click—turn it off and let the cells rest. However, when these genes are mutated, they become oncogenes, and normal cell replication can quickly turn into abnormal growth. Oncogenes speed up cell growth so much that this switch acts like a stuck accelerator in a car. If the switch can't be turned off, the cell's growth goes out of control.

### Tumor Suppressor Genes

These are checkpoint genes and they, too, are normally present in all cells. Their purpose seems to be to put on the brakes—to control cell division and prevent cancer from developing. Mutations here, too, can result in chaos. When these genes are disabled, the effect is like taking your foot off the brake of the car—giving oncogenes even more power and allowing growth to hurtle along even faster.

### Mismatch-Repair Genes

These are quality-control genes—the spell-checkers—that constantly monitor the genetic code as cells divide and fix any mistakes that crop up. If one or more of these inspector genes is mutated or the repair genes are defective, widespread mutations can occur, with disastrous results.

## What Causes DNA Damage?

Every day, our cells fend off countless threats from the outside—environmental factors as simple as sunlight (particularly ultraviolet light), which can lead to skin cancer, or as complicated as the chemical cocktail packed into each puff of a cigarette, which can cause lung cancer. The most common cancers of all—prostate, breast, and colon—most likely arise from oxidative damage, incremental damage accrued as carcinogens hammer away at our genes, like invaders with tiny battering rams. Familiar (for many of us) barrages from outside the body—for example, from each mouthful of chicken fried steak, bite of glazed doughnut, or slice of sausage-pepperoni pizza— result in minuscule changes within our cells. (For more on food and prostate cancer, see chapter 4.) Our bodies can withstand this gradual onslaught for decades, until the oxidative damage reaches a critical point. Even our everyday metabolism of nutrients and other chemicals produces a harmful by-product with a dangerous-sounding name: oxygen radicals, also called free radicals. These are highly reactive, unstable, electrically charged molecules that can surge with force enough to destroy tissue, melt membranes, and kill cells in an instant. Free radicals damage DNA. Like many key characters in causing disease, they start out with fine intentions and then go astray. Normally, they appear in small numbers as "hit men" for the immune system, wiping out bacteria and other foreign invaders. And normally, they are neutralized by riot-control police, called scavenger enzymes and antioxidant nutrients, within cells. However, if these scavenger enzymes are defective or if they're overloaded by too many free radicals, then the free radicals can attack the DNA in cells, causing mutations that lead to cancer.

## Molecular Causes of Prostate Cancer: The Double Attack of Oxidative Damage and Inflammation

The diagram on page 54 shows the decline and fall of a prostate cell— think of Anakin Skywalker in the *Star Wars* saga as he gradually crosses over to the dark side. (You can also compare this with the illustration in chapter 6 showing the modified Gleason grading system, which shows the progression of cancer, from not too bad to highly malignant, as it appears to a pathologist.) Normal, healthy prostate tissue shows little round shapes, which are tiny glands. Under the microscope, they appear orderly, harmonious, at peace with the world. The first sign of danger is prostatic intraepithelial neoplasia (PIN)— in which the glands are more disorderly but are not yet cancerous. In early cancer, the tissue still retains some normal structures. But as the cancer becomes more aggressive, begins to spread, and ultimately becomes unresponsive to hormones, all order deteriorates, and normal glands are overshadowed by dark, sprawling blobs.

And this all starts with oxidative damage. But, as always with prostate cancer, even this simple fact is more complicated than it

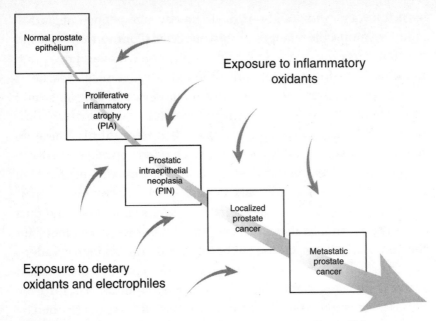

**FIGURE 3.1   How Oxidative Damage and Inflammation Cause Harm to the Prostate**

sounds. Oxidative damage can come from two sources. One, discussed above, is metabolic—our everyday metabolism of our food. The second arises from inflammation. (We mentioned this very briefly in chapter 2 in our discussion of prostatitis.) Look at those poor prostate cells. They're under attack from both sides. On one side, they're getting torpedoed by the body's processing of nutrients. On the other, they're being bombarded by inflammation. The overworked scavenger enzymes are supposed to be everywhere at once, protecting the cells from either kind of assault. (Electrophiles are electron acceptors, and oxidation is a process in which one or more electrons are removed.)

**Putting Out Fires**

One of these scavenger enzymes is called glutathione-S-transferase-π (pronounced "pie"), or GST-π for short. It serves as a genetic fire extinguisher, rendering free radicals into harmless, water-soluble products and providing toxin cleanup on a cellular level. GST-π, or the lack of it, is crucial in the development of prostate cancer. This noble protector is as essential—and as vulnerable—as the proverbial finger in the dike. Scientists at Johns Hopkins have discovered that although GST-$\pi$ is present in normal cells, it's been knocked out of prostate cancer cells right next to them. It's absent, in fact, in *all prostate cancer tissues*, and even in the telltale "funny-looking" PIN cells, which are not cancerous themselves but are strongly linked to prostate cancer and are considered by some to be precancerous. This suggests that the normal oxidative damage that occurs in cells has a much greater effect in prostate cancer cells because they lack this key enzyme. This is a great scientific finding, because it helps us understand how normal prostate cells are turned into cancerous ones. Now, Johns Hopkins scientists are searching for new ways to keep this enzyme from failing and seeking alternate ways to detoxify the free radicals generated by cell metabolism. The best "drug" for this—allowing the body's defenses to stand up to prostate cancer—may be nature's own: one or more cancer-fighting dietary agents, such as broccoli or tofu (both, coincidentally, present in the Asian diet), or an antioxidant (which neutralizes free radicals), such as selenium and vitamins C and E, and carotenoids such as vitamin A. (More on cancer-fighting foods in chapter 4.)

GST-$\pi$ protects against these free radicals and against oxidative damage that inflammatory cells can produce. So does selenium—a mineral found in the soil, present in some vegetables and in many over-the-counter vitamins, and available as a dietary supplement. So does soy. In fact, in one series of experiments, scientists found that rats given a soy-free diet were prone to prostate inflammation. Rats on a moderate soy diet developed very little inflammation, and rats on a high-soy diet developed none. *Diet can control this inflammation of the prostate.* Diet can also turn protective enzymes such as GST-$\pi$ on and off. (This is covered in more detail in chapter 4.)

## The Silence of the Genes

Within the last few years, the idea of methylation has become very important to scientists trying to unravel the intricate tapestry of the origins of prostate cancer. This genetic process was recently discussed by a trio of Johns Hopkins investigators—the oncologist

William G. Nelson, the molecular geneticist William B. Isaacs, and the pathologist Angelo M. De Marzo—in a landmark paper in the *New England Journal of Medicine.* My colleague Bill Nelson, whose pioneering work on the role of diet in prostate cancer revealed that oxidative damage is a major factor responsible for the development and progression of the disease, is the scientist who discovered that GST-π is knocked out of commission early in prostate cancer. He also discovered how the fatal blow to this gene is administered: GST-π is "hypermethylated." In chemical terms, it picks up an extra building block that changes its shape. Methylation is like adding an extra tooth to a zipper so it doesn't work properly, or changing the tumblers on a lock ever so slightly so the key doesn't fit it anymore. When this happens to any gene, it is silenced—rendered useless. When it happens to GST-π, this targeted hit, an assassination on the genetic level, allows prostate cancer to develop much more easily.

How does this fit in with what we already know about cancer and the genes? Above, we looked at some of the changes in how our genes work that can cause cancer—for example, how tumor suppressor genes can cripple a gene's ability to do its job, or how oncogenes cause a gene's function to be revved up, resulting in the out-of-control growth of cells. Interestingly, methylation falls into still another category of genetic troublemaking, causing what scientists call epigenetic change. Here, the genes aren't altered but turned into zombies. A gene is methylated and then boom—it's useless. In effect, it's put into a chemical straitjacket—think of Jack Nicholson in *One Flew Over the Cuckoo's Nest.* Nelson and colleagues have begun exploring the implications of this. "In addition to helping us understand what causes cancer," he says, "methylation is also being used to help detect it, as we identify new tumor markers." He is working to develop tests that can detect abnormal methylation of GST-π as a means of spotting cancer cells. Specifically, the tests look for altered clumps of DNA, called hypermethylated CpG islands, that aren't supposed to be there. One day, such tests might be used on biopsied prostate tissue or even urine specimens to help identify men who have cancer that has been missed by a prostate biopsy or to help predict how men will respond to radical prostatectomy or radiation therapy.

## Genetic Fire-Starters

If GST-$\pi$ is a genetic fire extinguisher, then inflammation is just the opposite—the gasoline that fans the flames. The Hopkins patholo-gist Angelo De Marzo believes that prostate cancer is driven by a bad combination of forces from within and without. From inside the prostate comes inflammation; from without come attacks by cancer-causing elements in the diet. Together, they cause damage that results in pockets of proliferative inflammatory atrophy, or PIA. With the help of the Hopkins pathologist Jonathan Epstein, De Marzo has made startling findings in studies of prostate tissue. He has seen cancer cells with the suspicious-looking PIN cells nearby. PIN cells aren't cancer, but they're not normal, either. The general feeling among pathologists is that PIN cells are cancer waiting to happen. Right in the thick of these cancerous and probably pre-cancerous cells, De Marzo has seen something else—hot spots of in-flammation. And sprinkled around this inflammation are areas of atrophy—cells that appear to be dying, but actually, under closer inspection, are seen to be proliferating rapidly. Basically, what De Marzo has witnessed is hodgepodge at a critical mass—a teeming goulash; chaos on a microscopic level. De Marzo has identified PIA as a specific precursor lesion of prostate cancer. He believes that these PIA spots represent evidence of a field effect change, "indi-cating that a very large region of the prostate has been exposed to something that causes cancer," and that these PIA lesions somehow pave the way—from there to PIN, and from PIN to cancer.

The concept that inflammation can cause cancer is not new. In-flammation is known to cause damage to cells and to DNA, and long-term inflammation is associated with many kinds of tumors. For example, chronic hepatitis causes cancer of the liver; chronic stomach inflammation, caused by a form of bacteria known as *H. py-lori*, causes stomach cancer; reflux esophagitis, over time, can cause cancer of the esophagus. Why is inflammation such a potent cause of cancer? It appears to act in two ways. The inflammatory cells pro-duce harmful forms of oxygen and nitrogen, which can mutate DNA directly. Inflammatory cells can also injure cells, prompting the body to crank out replacement cells as quickly as it can. This rapid turnover of cells is what we see in PIA, and it proves the adage "haste makes waste." Sometimes the replacement cells are churned out so quickly that the DNA isn't replicated exactly, and these mistakes can lead to further mutations. Either way, inflammation induces mutation of nearby cells, and this is the beginning of cancer.

### What Causes This Inflammation in the Prostate?

This is the $64,000 question, and for now, no one knows. The Johns Hopkins molecular geneticist Bill Isaacs and colleagues have been searching for the answer to this question in the genes of families with hereditary prostate cancer. How, they've wondered, do mutations in certain genes stack the deck toward cancer in some men? So far, they have found two genes that are responsible for the development of prostate cancer in small clusters of families. One, located on chromosome 1, is called RNASEL. The other, located on the short arm of chromosome 8, is called MSR1 (macrophage scavenger receptor 1). These genes have something very interesting in common: they're both involved in the body's defense against infection. When animals that lack the MSR1 gene are infected with bacteria or animals with a defective RNASEL gene catch the herpes simplex virus, 60 percent of them die. And this observation, says Isaacs, "raises the intriguing possibility that viral or bacterial infections might be the source of the chronic inflammation in some patients, and that this chronic inflammation might be responsible for the increased risk of prostate cancer." If it's true that some run-of-the-mill infection could trigger these events by producing the immune response of inflammation, "this will profoundly affect future studies of the causes of prostate cancer, and may ultimately lead to new approaches to prevent it."

One last word about this inflammation: if you have prostatitis, don't worry. Doctors have known for years that the prostate seems to attract inflammatory cells. De Marzo and Epstein tell us that pathologists were once taught to ignore them—to consider them an odd quirk of the prostate. What we've been talking about here is not the dramatic type of inflammation that comes with acute bacterial prostatitis or even with the chronic forms of prostatitis. Instead, it falls into the medical category of asymptomatic—it produces no symptoms—and the current consensus is that we know it's there, but we aren't sure what to do about it.

## PROSTATE AND BREAST CANCER:
## TWO SIDES OF THE SAME COIN?

Just as Asian men hardly ever die of prostate cancer, Asian women hardly ever die of breast cancer. Autopsy studies in the United States have found that between 20 and 40 percent of all women have microscopic amounts—just like the incidental prostate cancer—of breast cancer. (These microscopic clusters might be even more common but for the fact that women go through menopause. The decrease in female hormones probably makes these microscopic cancers shrink and become even more difficult to see. Men, however, keep making substantial amounts of male hormones until well into their eighties and nineties.) Both have benign forms of disease as well—in men, this is BPH (benign prostatic hyperplasia); in women, it's fibrocystic breast disease. Neither of these benign diseases will progress to cancer.

### TABLE 3.2

### PROSTATE AND BREAST CANCER: A COMPARISON

As these tables show, prostate and female breast cancer are remarkably alike. (Note: Men can get breast cancer, too, although very rarely. These statistics apply only to female breast cancer.) They share similar numbers of new cases and deaths per year, similar survival rates depending on when the cancer is diagnosed—whether it is localized or whether the cancer has spread—similar responses to hormonal therapy, and similar geographic patterns of distribution. (Note: You can see the latest American Cancer Society statistics online at http://www.cancer.org.)

|  | Prostate | Breast |
|---|---|---|
| Rank of all Cancers | No. 1 in Men | No. 1 in Women |
| Lifetime risk of developing it | 1 in 6 | 1 in 8 |
| Number of new cases in U.S. in 2006 | 234,500 | 213,000 |
| Deaths in the U.S. in 2006 | 27,400 | 41,430 |
| Lifetime risk of dying from the disease | 3.1 percent | 2.9 percent |
| 5-year survival (all stages) | 99 percent | 88 percent |
| 5-year survival if disease is diagnosed when it's localized (in men, this is T1 or T2 disease) | 100 percent | 98 percent |
| 5-year survival if disease is diagnosed when it has spread, or metastasized | 34 percent | 26 percent |
| Average age of diagnosis | 69 | 63 |
| Responds to hormone therapy | Yes | Yes |

TABLE 3.3

## WHO GETS PROSTATE AND BREAST CANCER?

|  | Prostate | Breast |
|---|---|---|
| Least likely to develop in: | Rural Chinese men | Rural Chinese women |
| Most likely to develop in: | African American men in Atlanta | Caucasian women in San Francisco |
| U.S. deaths per 100,000 African Americans | 69.2 | 34.6 |
| U.S. deaths per 100,000 Caucasians | 27.9 | 26.3 |
| U.S. deaths per 100,000 Hispanics | 22.5 | 17.7 |
| U.S. deaths per 100,000 Asians | 12.8 | 12.7 |
| More likely with migration from Asia to the West? | Yes | Yes |

## Risk Factors for Prostate Cancer

Of all the risk factors for prostate cancer, the three greatest are age, race, and family history (which is discussed later in this chapter).

### Age

Prostate cancer takes time to develop. Why? As we discussed earlier, the process of transforming a normal cell into a cancerous cell—one that can divide, grow, escape the prostate, and invade other tissues—requires a number of genetic mutations that alter DNA. Scientists have estimated that the number of mutations necessary to transform a normal cell into a cancerous one correlates with the number of decades it takes, on average, for cancer to develop. For example, there is a highly malignant form of cancer that occurs in the eye in infants and children called retinoblastoma. In those with the inherited form of this disease, only one mutation is necessary for this cancer to begin. In prostate cancer—where most men are not diagnosed until they are in their seventies—the number of genetic mutations necessary may be seven or eight. These occur gradually, over time, as oxidative damage takes its toll. Even if a boy is born with the deck stacked against him—if he has a family history of the disease, for example, or if he is African American—nothing will happen for many years.

Age is a risk factor for many illnesses because, no matter how physically or mentally fit, the body of a seventy-year-old man is just different from the body of a twenty-five-year-old. In men, the incidence of prostate cancer rises dramatically with age, more so than any other cancer. An American man in his mid- to late-seventies is seven times more likely to develop prostate cancer than is a man in his mid- to late forties. Look at the difference a few decades makes: In men aged forty to fifty-nine, the risk of developing prostate cancer is one in fifty. In men aged sixty to seventy-nine, it's one in seven. And over the course of his lifetime, an American man's risk of developing prostate cancer is one in six.

If you were just diagnosed with prostate cancer today, when did this cancer start? Scientists estimate that it takes roughly eleven or twelve years (about a year less in African American men) from the initiation of prostate cancer—when those first few cells go bad—to its clinical presentation—when it causes a significant change in PSA or when it's big enough for a doctor to feel during a digital rectal exam. There are, however, two groups in which prostate cancer strikes at an earlier age: African Americans and men with a family history of prostate cancer (this is discussed below).

### Race

African Americans and Africans in Jamaica have the highest risk of prostate cancer of any ethnic group in the world. If they get prostate cancer, they are more likely to die from it.

The number of black men per 100,000 who develop prostate cancer is about 60 percent higher than the number of white men, and of the men who get it, the number of black men who die is more than double. The statistics would be even worse, except African Americans also are at higher risk of developing other health problems, such as hypertension and coronary artery disease. Sadly, this means that most black men in this country don't live long enough to make it to what we call the peak incidence rates that occur with old age. That's why the lifetime risk of prostate cancer is about 17 percent for white men and 13 percent for black men. These statistics are misleading; the black man's risk is actually higher. The only reason that the lifetime risk of developing prostate cancer is lower in black men is the unfortunate likelihood that they will die too soon of some other illness.

African Americans, particularly young black men, seem to get more severe forms of prostate cancer and are more likely to have cancer recurrences and die from the disease than young white men. There are multiple reasons for this, and many of them relate to lower socioeconomic status. Many studies have shown that people of any race who don't have much money are less likely to undergo preventive health screening, are more likely to delay going to the doctor until the disease is advanced, and if they have prostate cancer, are less likely to be treated with radiation therapy or surgery because without insurance, these treatments are expensive. Hormone therapy is much cheaper. But, as we'll discuss later in the book, hormone therapy as a first-line attack on prostate cancer is not effective. Put all of these observations together and they suggest that prostate cancer kills many black men in this country because they didn't get the disease diagnosed in time to cure it. And although there may be an inherent biological aggressiveness in cancers in African Americans, information from "equal-opportunity" health care studies—places such as military clinics or HMOs, where the availability of medical care seems to be equal—suggests that black men seem to fare as well as white men when it comes to prostate cancer if the cancer is caught and treated early.

We now know that black men from any country are more prone to prostate cancer than any other men. We haven't always known this. Just a few years ago, scientists believed that black men living in Africa were at lower risk than black Americans—that somehow the African lifestyle was healthier or the diet was better, or vice versa. Evidence from recent studies shows that this is not true. In fact, prostate cancer is probably the most common cancer in African men. And a study from Johns Hopkins found that Kingston, Jamaica (which has a high concentration of men of African descent), may have the highest incidence of prostate cancer in the world—304 per 100,000 men, compared to 249 per 100,000 black men and 182 per 100,000 white men in the United States.

## Genetic Susceptibility

Why are black men hit so hard by prostate cancer? We don't know yet, but there are a number of leads: genetic susceptibility, inadequate levels of vitamin D (see below), and diet. The simple fact that the disease is so common in African and African American men strongly suggests that genes play a role. (Men of different races are known to have genetic differences in how they are affected by male hormones. This is discussed below.) Genetic susceptibility refers to a complex of genetic factors that creates a more hospitable atmosphere for cancer. The development of cancer is like a tumbling row of dominoes, in that a whole chain of genetic events must occur before a tumor can begin to grow. Inherited mutations in one or more genes probably speed up the process; presumably, in some men, a few of these dominoes are already knocked down at birth. (We'll talk about hereditary prostate cancer later in this chapter.) Environmental variables—what men eat and drink and how they live—may topple the rest. Genetic susceptibility is somewhere in the middle of all this: not exactly a mutation that causes cancer but a genetic makeup that creates a more hospitable atmosphere, which makes it easier for cancer to set foot in the door. In the domino analogy, maybe genetic susceptibility tilts the table slightly, making the dominoes more likely to fall without actually knocking them over.

## Hormones and Race

Prostate cancer is strongly affected by hormones. For years, it was believed that the levels of male hormones in African Americans were higher than those in Caucasian and Asian men. However, when scientists looked at the levels of male hormones in African American men, they found no consistent difference. Recently, genetic research has shed new light. Hormones exert their effect on specific tissues by communicating with particular proteins called receptors within cells. A portion of the receptor for male hormones known as the CAG repeat (because it appears over and over), on average, is larger in Asian men. It's intermediate in white men and shorter in black men. The result of this slight variation is that for any given level of hormone, the shorter the CAG repeat, the more active the receptor. This short repeat makes testosterone more efficient in prostate cells, so that the same amount of testosterone goes farther and has more of an effect in African Americans than in other men. Men with longer repeats have less of this stimulation. In related research, Caucasian men with prostate cancer who turn out to have micrometastases—minuscule offshoots of prostate cancer in the lymph nodes (and thus more aggressive and more advanced cancer)—also have this same overactive androgen receptor. This short CAG repeat may help explain why black men are more susceptible to developing prostate cancer and, particularly, to developing more aggressive disease. One study by Harvard researchers concluded, "Men with shorter repeats were at particularly high risk for distant metastatic and fatal prostate cancer."

Another contributing factor for black men may be inadequate levels of vitamin D. The major source of vitamin D is the effect of sunlight on the skin, which transforms cholesterol into vitamin D. As we'll discuss later in this chapter, vitamin D protects against prostate cancer. Because black skin is more efficient at blocking out sunlight, black men are known to have lower levels of a form of the vitamin called 1,25-dihydroxyvitamin D. This may make black men more susceptible to prostate cancer. Still other research suggests that black men get more animal fat in their diet. This is important, because substantial evidence links diets high in animal fat to a greater risk of prostate cancer, and in particular to aggressive disease. (For more on dietary fat, see below.) Undoubtedly, scientists will discover other factors—and it is almost certain that some of them will be genetic—that will shed new light on this major racial difference in susceptibility to prostate cancer.

### Environment: Prostate Cancer and What You Eat

We move from body fat to the other kind of fat—dietary fat. The idea that "you are what you eat" is, for prostate cancer and other diseases, where the rubber hits the road. Here, every day, you make hundreds of choices about what to put, or not put, into your body. Nobody's saying that diet alone can cause or prevent prostate cancer. (For one thing, prostate cancer is too complicated and cantankerous a disease to have one simple, easy-to-remedy cause.) But it can hurt by weak-

## CALORIES, EXERCISE, AND PROSTATE CANCER

What do caloric intake—the number of calories you eat per day—and exercise have to do with cancer? The answer may be quite a lot. Studies have found that restricting caloric intake greatly reduces the development of breast tumors in animals. The impact can be profound: a 30 percent reduction in caloric intake can reduce the development of breast tumors by as much as 90 percent. But calories are just part of the picture. Just as important is energy expenditure—what happens to those calories in your body. Do they get burned up or turned into muscle, or do they just accumulate as flab? For example, a marine in boot camp wolfs down about 3,000 calories a day and burns every one of them. But a sedentary man on the same diet would gain weight.

If you're overweight, you're in good company—more than one-third of American adults are in the same boat. But being obese doesn't just mean having excess body fat. Eating more calories than your body needs and the resulting accumulation of body fat changes your blood's concentration of many hormones, including androgens, estrogen, leptin, and insulin-like growth factor. It also increases the risk of developing several major cancers.

How closely linked are obesity and prostate cancer? We don't know; the evidence is mixed. Although some studies have suggested that obese men are more likely to develop prostate cancer, other studies have found just the reverse. There may be some good reasons why fewer overweight men are diagnosed with prostate cancer. As we'll discuss more in chapter 5, PSA levels are lower in men who are obese—a factor that may delay diagnosis. Another reason relates to simple mechanics: in some obese men, it is more difficult to feel the prostate.

However, when we look at statistics on advanced disease and death from prostate cancer, obesity's effects are easier to see. Several studies have shown that heavier men (with a body mass index, or BMI, greater than 30–35; see below) have a greater risk of developing an elevated PSA level after radical prostatectomy. Further, a number of epidemiological studies have found significant links between an increased BMI and the risk of dying from prostate cancer. One study by the American Cancer Society found that men with a BMI greater than 30 were 20 to 25 percent more likely to die of prostate cancer than thinner men. Another study of 135,000 construction workers in Sweden found that men with the highest BMIs were 40 percent more likely to die from prostate cancer. In studies involving more than one million men, obesity has been shown to increase the risk of prostate cancer death. Still another study of men with prostate cancer, reported in the *New England Journal of Medicine*, found that the heavier men are, the greater their risk of dying from the disease. For example, for a 6-foot-tall man weighing between

225 and 260 pounds, the risk of dying increased by 20 percent. For a heftier man of the same height, weighing between 270 and 300 pounds, the risk increased by 34 percent.

It may make a difference, too, *when* a man starts carrying around the extra weight. One interesting study found that men who were overweight in their teens and early twenties were less likely to develop prostate cancer later in life. This may be, the researchers reasoned, because these young men have lower testosterone levels and that the hormonal atmosphere somehow keeps cancer from gaining a foothold during this critical, formative time. Another study showed that men who gained the most weight in the twenty-five years before being diagnosed with prostate cancer were more likely to have a rising PSA level (which signals the return of cancer) after radical prostatectomy. These authors, too, link obesity to hormonal changes: men who gain a lot of weight in adulthood often have higher levels of growth factors such as IGF-1, and this may actually stimulate cancer, if it happens to be developing and progressing during this same time.

What does this mean for you? If you weigh more than you should, now's the perfect time to shed some pounds. Every little bit helps. Look at it this way: millions of men are investing in vitamins, health-food supplements, and other remedies that may or may not lower their risk of prostate cancer. Here's one proven way to lower your risk. What have you got to lose?

ening the body's defenses. In a disease that develops in countless incremental building blocks—think of a very tall house of cards—little things matter very much indeed.

*Dietary Fat*

Evidence from many animal studies suggests that dietary fat may not only help *cause* cancer, it may affect the way that cancer *progresses*—among other things, the rate at which cells proliferate, the ability and likelihood of cancer to invade other tissues, and the body's ability to defend against this invasion. For example, scientists have linked the increased intake of saturated fat to a higher risk of prostate cancer. Another undesirable class of fats, usually described on food packages as partially hydrogenated oil, can be found in fats that remain solid at room temperature. These and similar oils—often hidden in

TABLE 3.4

## WHAT'S YOUR BODY MASS?

Or, more accurately (perhaps too accurately), how fat are you? How much you weigh is only part of the equation; it's your weight in relation to your height that matters here.

Doctors use a measurement called body mass index (BMI) to help them figure this out. You can use it, too. This chart will tell you if you are overweight (a BMI between 25 and 29) or obese (a BMI of 30 or above). (Note: Men who are very muscular may have a high BMI as well.) To determine your body mass index,

- Multiply your weight in pounds by 704; then
- Multiply your height in inches by itself.
- Divide the result of step one with the result of step two.

For example: If you are 5 feet, 10 inches (that's 70 inches) tall and weigh 150 pounds, 150 × 704 is 105,600. 70 × 70 is 4,900. 105,600 divided by 4,900 is 21.55. Your BMI, then, is 21.5, and you are not overweight.

### BODY WEIGHT

| Height | BMI = 25 | BMI = 30 |
|---|---|---|
| 4'10" | 119 lbs. | 143 lbs. |
| 4'11" | 124 | 148 |
| 5'0" | 128 | 153 |
| 5'1" | 132 | 158 |
| 5'2" | 136 | 164 |
| 5'3" | 141 | 169 |
| 5'4" | 145 | 174 |
| 5'5" | 150 | 180 |
| 5'6" | 155 | 186 |
| 5'7" | 159 | 191 |
| 5'8" | 164 | 197 |
| 5'9" | 169 | 203 |
| 5'10" | 174 | 207 |
| 5'11" | 179 | 215 |
| 6'0" | 184 | 221 |
| 6'1" | 189 | 227 |
| 6'2" | 194 | 233 |
| 6'3" | 200 | 240 |
| 6'4" | 205 | 246 |

cakes, doughnuts, cookies, and many packaged snack foods—can also increase free radicals and thus damage DNA. In chapter 4, we will talk about carotenoids (the most famous of these is beta-carotene), which are metabolic precursors of vitamin A. Some studies have associated vitamin A with an increased risk of prostate cancer, but again, like so many issues regarding diet, it is more complicated than it sounds. In Asia, vitamin A in the diet comes almost entirely from green and yellow vegetables. But Americans get most of their vitamin A from animal fat. This correlation between vitamin A and prostate cancer, as one Canadian study concludes, "may be due solely to increased fat intake."

The first thing we should tell you about fats is that *not all fats are bad*, particularly the kinds found in vegetables, nuts, and fish. In fact, some of these are downright good for you. Because this issue is so difficult, and because there is such a variety of fats and fatty acids, some patients wonder if they should shun fat altogether. Confusingly, many diets simply advise reducing total fat without making the distinction between "good" and "bad" fats. That would be throwing out the baby with the bathwater, because some "good" fatty acids—particularly some present in vegetables and fish—may slow or even inhibit the growth of prostate cancer cells. Thus, simply emphasizing these "good" fats may make a big difference in your body's ability to fend off cancer. In one Finnish study, men aged forty to forty-nine reduced their total fat consumption from 40 to 25 percent of total calories and increased their ratio of dietary polyunsaturated to saturated fats. (What the heck are these? See page 69). Although the men did not change their total caloric intake or otherwise alter the diet (to add more fiber, for example), this simple change produced significant decreases in the total level of testosterone.

### Eat More Fish
The Health Professionals Follow-Up Study, involving 51,000 men, found that those who ate a lot of fish had a lower risk of prostate cancer and especially of metastatic prostatic cancer. Although marine fatty acids accounted for part of this effect, there may be other beneficial factors in fish as well. Another study, published in the British journal *Lancet*, followed the health of 6,000 Swedish men for thirty years. They found that men who ate no fish had a two- to threefold higher frequency of prostate cancer than those who ate moderate to high amounts of fish.

## DIETARY FAT: HOW DO YOU KNOW WHAT'S WHAT?

The words are long, and even worse, they all sound alike. Who can tell the difference between saturated, polyunsaturated, and monounsaturated fats? And yet, somehow you're supposed to make sense of these similar words, decipher labels on packaged foods, seek out the good fats, and avoid the bad. Does your fat consumption really have anything to do with prostate cancer?

Yes, it does, although scientists are still learning exactly how it all works. Fats are complicated, and although these terms can be frustrating, you can learn enough about them to get by in the grocery store. Here's a quick primer of the good, the bad, and the ugly, starting with the worst:

*Saturated Fats:* We should call these the "All-American" fats, because the average American diet is full of them. These are the ones found in red meats and dairy. The traditional Asian diet has hardly any saturated fat in it.

*Polyunsaturated Fats:* These are found in vegetable oils (corn oil, safflower oil, and other cooking oils), nuts and seeds, fish oils, and margarine. There are a lot of these polyunsaturated fats, and some are worse than others. Some, called omega-3 fats, are found in fish oils and may be helpful in preventing coronary artery disease. (The main source of these, obviously, is the fish themselves; however, you can also buy fish-oil supplements at health-food stores.) Others are called omega-6 fats. (These names simply refer to the chemical makeup of these fats.) One of these is arachidonic acid, which is found in red meat, whole milk and cheese, and egg yolks.

Food processors use a preservation method called hydrogenation. The most annoying thing about this, for our purposes, is that it introduces a whole new set of terms, all of which sound alike, for us to learn. Hydrogenation helps keep fat solid at room temperature. Unfortunately, the process seems to have a similar effect in your arteries, and people seeking "heart-healthy" foods are learning to avoid words like "partially hydrogenated," "hydrogenated," "transhydrogenated," and "trans fat" because these foods raise cholesterol levels. What do they do to the prostate? Well, they're known to damage DNA and may contribute to oxidative damage.

*Monounsaturated Fats:* Finally, some of the safe ones. Olive oil is a monounsaturated fat; so is canola oil. Neither is linked to prostate cancer. In fact, the Mediterranean diet is rich in olive oil, and Mediterranean men have a much lower risk of prostate cancer than American men. (This may be due to other things, too—more exposure to sunlight and vitamin D, fewer dairy products and calcium, and more tomatoes and lycopene.)

The bottom line? Basically, the message is the same: Avoid red meats and whole dairy foods, and limit your intake of processed, hydrogenated snack foods, cake mixes, and the like. Eat more vegetables and fruits. And become a label-checker. Read what's in there before you buy anything, even a candy bar. You may be surprised at the hidden fats you're putting into your body every day—and how easy it is to cut fat intake and calorie consumption simply by watching what you eat.

## DIET, EVOLUTION, AND PROSTATE CANCER

In the grand scheme of things—since humans first appeared on Earth—prostate cancer is an illness of fairly recent evolution. Like heart disease, it is an apparent by-product of the sedentary western lifestyle and its notoriously unhealthy diet—rich in animal fat, processed fare, and fast and other junk food, and poor in fresh vegetables and fruits.

In other words, it's the dark side of progress. As resilient as we are, as remarkably adaptable as the human body is, there are some forces—the cheesesteak, for instance—that nature never equipped us to handle. How ironic that we who have learned to defy gravity can be brought down, incrementally, by years of supersized bacon burgers and meat-lover's pizzas. Today's man is far more likely to spend hours hunting for Web sites or TV channels than foraging for food, his fingers more likely to be stained by Cheetos than by the juices of nuts and berries.

We did not evolve to eat this way, says the Johns Hopkins scientist Don Coffey, who took a four-million-year detour in his attempt to explain prostate cancer and learned that somewhere along the way, man took an evolutionary wrong turn. Consider, he says, two male glands: the prostate and the seminal vesicles. They are similar in function (both provide fluid that makes up semen) but have one crucial difference: cancer of the prostate is all too common. Cancer of the seminal vesicles is so rare that it almost doesn't exist.

Only mammals have prostates; by definition, only mammals have breasts as well. Breasts and prostates seem to have evolved on parallel tracks: the prostate appeared in the male at about the same time the female developed breasts and fed her children with breast milk. Today, countries with high rates of breast cancer tend to have similar rates of prostate cancer; countries with low rates of prostate cancer have relatively few cases of breast cancer. When people migrate from areas with little breast or prostate cancer to places with high rates, their own odds increase over time.

In nature, meat-eating animals such as dogs and tigers don't have seminal vesicles. The only animals that have both prostates and seminal vesicles are herbivores—vegetarians such as horses. But men have both of these glands. Shouldn't we be vegetarians, too? The fact that men eat meat seems to be a mistake that nature never accounted for. How can this be? In exploring this question, Coffey looked a few rungs further down the evolutionary ladder and found the pigmy chimp, also called the bonobo. Bonobos and humans have many things in common, except for diet. Bonobos are, as humans probably were, very long ago, vegetarians. They don't get prostate cancer.

About twelve thousand years ago, Coffey says, humans stopped being scavengers and started producing their own food. This brought about a major change in diet and lifestyle: Instead of chasing after animals, humans started herding them and then breeding them in captivity. As this happened, we became increasingly sedentary. We quit eating a great variety of fresh vegetables and greens—from three thousand types down to about twenty. "We started smoking our meat, salting it, putting nitrates on it," says Coffey. "Now we get everything from the store, nothing from a farm. We call it fresh, but it's not fresh, especially our meat," which most of us prefer well done, not raw.

For decades, the American Cancer Society and National Cancer Institute have urged Americans to lower their cancer risk by changing their diet: Eat fewer animal fats and dairy products. Eat more fiber, fresh fruits, and vegetables. Exercise more.

If breast and prostate cancer have indeed developed from our evolutionary wrong turn, how can we prove it? Coffey pored over zoo records from around the world and found that no animal kept in a zoo dies from prostate cancer or breast cancer. There are only three cases of cats dying of prostate cancer. Horses do not die of prostate cancer, bulls do not die of it, and only a very few primates have ever died of it. Yet one out of every six American men gets prostate cancer. And the only animal to develop clinical prostate cancer with any significant incidence is the dog— sedentary, like many humans, and the pet that eats most from our table.

## The Asian Diet: East vs. West

If you live in a western country—in North America, for example, or western Europe, New Zealand or Australia—your risk of developing cancer and dying from it is higher than it would be if you live in a less developed part of the world, such as Asia, India, or the Middle East. The four horsemen of our cancer apocalypse, the most common cancers we face, are prostate, breast, lung, and colorectal. In the United States, a man's lifetime risk of developing one of these "Big Four" cancers is 45 percent; the risk is 38 percent for an American woman. Now, if you live in a less industrialized part of the world, your risk of dying from cancer is much lower, and the four horsemen are different as well. The "Big Four" to worry about in developing nations have traditionally been cancers of the stomach, liver, esophagus, and cervix.

But this may not always be the case. Look at China as an example. Fewer people in rural China are dying of cancers of the stomach and esophagus, and more people in urban China are dying from cancers of the lung, colon, breast, and prostate. What's happening here? Scientists believe the keys to this change are in the diet. With better sanitation and more readily available fresh foods, cancers of the esophagus and stomach are declining. Lung cancer is now number one, unfortunately, because cigarette smoking in China has tripled over the last twenty years. And look what's available—for the first time ever—in grocery stores and restaurants: western goodies! Foods that are high in fat and sugar, and more meat. Another big change—a more sedentary population. It's no coincidence that there has also been an increase in obesity and diabetes in China. There's more: We have known for years that when Chinese men and women move to the United States or another western country and live there for at least twenty-five years, their likelihood of getting our "Big Four" cancers rises, approaching that of native westerners. Now, because of this huge environmental change in their own country, the Chinese don't even have to travel to raise their cancer risk; they can raise it right there at home. Currently, prostate cancer is the eleventh most common cancer in Chinese men and the sixteenth most common cause of death. But between 1985 and 1995, the age-adjusted death rate for prostate cancer more than doubled. In Korea, between 1993 and 2003, it quadrupled. This rise in prostate cancer is expected to increase over the next twenty years.

### Does Diet Trump Race?

This brings us to the interesting fact of "incidental" prostate cancer—a phenomenon that might also be called "The Two Faces of Prostate Cancer." It is the story of significant cancer—the kind that kills, the subject of this book—versus its good twin, "insignificant," or incidental, cancer—small clusters of the earliest stages of prostate cancer in an apparently latent, or harmless, form that reside in millions of men. These are minuscule spots of prostate cancer, most of them so small that they would never pose a danger, that are generally detected at autopsy. It is highly unlikely that these cancers would even be diagnosed; for example, they don't make enough PSA to warrant a biopsy. For all practical purposes, this cancer doesn't count. The very fact that it's found only at autopsy tells us that: it means these men lived to a ripe old age and died, and they were never troubled by the presence of cancerous cells in their prostates. There are millions of men out there who manage to dodge the proverbial bullet. This is why some doctors erroneously conclude, and report to their patients, "If you live long enough, you will get prostate cancer." What they fail to say or may not realize is that these are cancers so small and insignificant that they are never diagnosed.

Until very recently, scientists believed that Asian men who lived their entire lives in Asia developed these incidental cancers at the same rate as western men, and that because of their environment (specifically, their diet), these tumors did not progress to the point where they were detectable. The belief was that whatever causes prostate cancer in the first place—the initiating factors or events—happens everywhere, and that the crucial difference is what happens next—whatever promotes these small cancers to grow and become potentially lethal. In the United States, for example, those cells seem to progress into cancer that needs to be treated in 10 to 20 percent of men as they age. In Asia, scientists believed, the cancer just sits there like a freckle as opposed to a cancerous mole.

But we now realize that this is wrong. Autopsy studies have found incidental prostate cancer in about 30 to 40 percent of American men. But it's in far fewer Asian men—ten times fewer. Also, inflammation and atrophy (which we talked about above) are found in the prostates of many Caucasian men, but they occur five times less frequently in Asian men.

To sum up: In general, the rate of prostate cancer is high in western cultures and low in Asia. But that's about as straightforward as it gets. Asian men are also much less prone to incidental cancer and its precursors, inflammation and proliferative atrophy. When these same men move to the West and live here for at least twenty-five years, their risk for prostate cancer draws closer to that of western men. And yet, genetically speaking, Asian men still hold better cards than other men do. Even though their risk of developing prostate cancer goes up when they move to the West, Asian men are still somehow protected by genetic factors. Their cancer risk reaches only about half that of Caucasian men born in the United States and even less than half that of African American men, which tells us that environment is not the whole story. (One subtle but important racial difference may be in the CAG repeat, discussed above.)

When we break this down into specifics, determining the worldwide rates of prostate cancer get a lot more complicated. The incidence of prostate cancer varies from place to place and group to group more than probably any other cancer in the world. So, although China has the lowest reported rate of prostate cancer, for Chinese men living else-where in Asia, particularly Singapore and Hong Kong, the rate is nearly five times higher. And for Chinese men living in the West, particularly Los Angeles and Hawaii, it's twelve to sixteen times higher. The prostate itself, interestingly, seems to react to a change in location or diet: the size of the prostate of men in China is significantly smaller than that of Chinese men who migrate to Australia. (For that matter, men of every race in Australia have larger prostates than do men in China.) However, after a Chinese man has lived in Australia for ten or more years, his prostate increases to the same size as an Australian man's. The difference in prostate volume is almost completely due to changes in the transition zone, where BPH, benign enlargement, develops (see chapter 2). And these prostates became more beefy within a relatively short time—just a decade—after the Chinese men migrate to Australia. What's going on here? Again, it's got to be the environment.

The risk of developing prostate cancer increases tenfold when native Japanese men move to Hawaii. Although scientists have re-cently noted a rise in prostate cancer in Japan, there has also been an increase in screening for the disease, so it's not clear whether prostate cancer is actually on the upswing there or whether this is just an ar-tifact of more intensive attempts to diagnose it. Similarly, in Taiwan, the rate of prostate cancer has doubled over the last thirty years, but scientists attribute this mainly to the aging of the population.

It's also important to note that when Asians migrate to the United States, the increase in the development of prostate cancer doesn't happen overnight; it takes years. This suggests that whatever the environmental risk factors are that make a man more prone to cancer, they act late in life—and this, in turn, gives us great hope that once we understand just what these factors are, we may be able to prevent the disease.

## Sins of Omission and Commission

What is it about western countries that makes our men so suscepti-ble to prostate cancer and our women so prone to breast cancer?

Why, in fact, are there such striking parallels between those two cancers—with countries having roughly the same high or low levels of both (see tables 3.2 and 3.3). And why, in comparison, are those diseases so rare in Asian and some Middle Eastern countries? What are they doing right, and what are we doing wrong? The answer must lie, in large part, in what we eat. By unfortunate coincidence, the western diet probably provides the worst of both worlds. Notorious for its overabundance of animal fat, it also lacks many substances— soy products, citrus fruits, vegetables (particularly tomatoes), green tea, and a lot of fish—that may actually prevent cancer.

Are Americans and Europeans—whose rate of prostate cancer is ten times higher than that of men from many Asian countries—eating foods that cause these cancers? Or does the Asian diet somehow protect the prostate and breast from them? Are we dealing with sins of *commission*—eating too many french fries and hamburgers—or *omission*—not eating enough broccoli and carrots? Or is it an unlucky combination of both? As we will discuss later in this chapter and in the next, it is becoming increasingly obvious that a poor diet triggers a specific chain of events in the genes. Each subtle mutation brings us one step closer to cancer. In chapter 4, we will examine some possible acts of omission—foods that show great promise in protecting the body and preventing prostate cancer. Right now, let's talk about some sins of commission.

### Fat, Red Meat, and Dairy Products

The greatest danger in the western diet seems to come from animal fat. Indeed, as far as animal fat goes, the traditional Asian and western diets could not be more different. In the United States, 30 to 40 percent of our calories come from fat, and most of that fat comes from animals. But in China—where for centuries, people have eaten mainly rice, vegetables, and soy, washed down with many cups of unsweetened green tea—only 11 percent of the calories comes from fat, and of that, slightly less than half is from animal fat.

Many studies of large groups of men followed for years or even decades have shown a consistent link between consumption of fat-containing animal products—primarily red meat and dairy products— and advanced prostate cancer and death from prostate cancer.

Although there is confusing information on whether a high-fat diet increases the risk of being diagnosed with prostate cancer, there is a clear consensus that men who put away large amounts of calories from animal fat—especially red meat and dairy products—are more likely to be diagnosed with advanced disease and to die from it.

Scientists at Johns Hopkins who were looking at the genes expressed in prostate cancer found a gene expressed nine times more in cancerous tissue than in normal tissue that may explain what's happening here. This gene is called *alpha methylacyl CoA racemase* (AMACR or racemase for short), and it's not a particularly "new" gene; for years, scientists have known that it plays a key role in the body's metabolism of fatty acids. It makes an enzyme that breaks down complex fatty acids, especially phytanic acid, which is found in dairy products and red meat. Phytanic acid comes from phytol, which in turn is derived from chlorophyll. Which means, says the molecular geneticist Bill Isaacs, "that animals that eat a lot of grass end up incorporating a lot of phytanic acid into their milk and meat." Think cows, and think—as Isaacs, the pathologist Angelo De Marzo, and colleagues are thinking—of the known links between red meat and dairy products and prostate cancer. The presence of great amounts of racemase in prostate cancer actually helps feed the cancer; it's like having the chuck wagon on site to cook up some grub for cowboys on the go. When men with prostate cancer eat red meat or dairy products, the cancer cells have the potential to gain and use more energy from these foods than do normal cells. And something else happens, too. When the body (with or without prostate cancer) metabolizes phytanic acid, it makes a toxic by-product—hydrogen peroxide. Hydrogen peroxide is known to be one of those agents that increase oxidative stress in cells, attacking the DNA, causing mutations, and helping cancer to progress. The identification of racemase may be the best scientific evidence yet to prove that dietary factors influence the growth and progression of prostate cancer.

In one study of more than 51,000 health professionals, a positive association was seen between the intake of red meat, total fat, and animal fat and the risk of prostate cancer. A follow-up to the Health Professionals study showed that a high-fat diet (processed meat in particular) appeared to be associated *only* with advanced cancer, not with localized, slow-growing cancer. In that study, saturated and monounsaturated fats were associated with advanced prostate cancer. Another study of men in Hawaii found that the risk of prostate cancer went up in step with the consumption of beef and animal fat. In one study, men who ate five or more servings of red meat a week had a 79 percent higher risk of developing prostate cancer.

### The Arabian Paradox

Here's an interesting statistic: Saudi Arabian men eat a diet that's rich in saturated fat, but they have a very low incidence of prostate cancer. A nutritional study of 2,300 Saudi men found that their daily fat consumption was greater than four ounces each; of this, about 40 percent was from red meat (such as lamb) and dairy products. Saturated fat made up about half of the total fat intake, and there was no difference in the amount of fat in the diet of men who got prostate cancer and men who didn't. So why can these men get away with eating a lot of red meat and dairy products and remain largely unscathed by prostate cancer? Almost certainly, genetic or racial factors offer some protection. In addition, these men have abundant exposure to ultraviolet light (which means they're getting a lot of vitamin D—see below). But perhaps more important for those of us at higher risk is to see what else is eaten in large quantities at mealtimes: high-fiber cereals, cooked tomatoes, rice, fruits, vegetables, and dates—all washed down with copious amounts of tea.

It's hard to make sense of conflicting results. For scientists, food studies are something of a nightmare—tough to carry out and tougher still to analyze. For researchers, a finding that red meat is associated with an increased risk of prostate cancer easily raises as many questions as it attempts to answer. For example: Is it the meat itself that raises the risk of cancer? Or some specific fat within that meat? Or maybe it's the way the meat is cooked—are carcinogens, or cancer-causing agents, created when the meat is fried or charred? We know, for instance, that charred meat is bad. Every time we fry a pork chop, grill a steak, or cook a hamburger, we generate a few unwanted extra ingredients—carcinogens. One of them is PhIP. PhIP is what scientists call a procarcinogen. It's benign enough by itself—like a werewolf before the full moon comes out—but when it's metabolized, it becomes something far more dangerous. And it's not just fried meat, either; the by-products of PhIP in fried chicken can be just as bad. In the liver, PhIP is transformed into a chemical called N-hydroxy-PhIP. For some cells in the body, including prostate and breast cells, this new chemical is far more dangerous, because it attacks DNA. In laboratory animals, the PhIP carcinogen can even cause breast cancer and prostate cancer. Johns Hopkins scientists are working to use PhIP as a marker: PhIP causes telltale changes, or adducts, in the DNA—picture barnacles on a sailboat—that can be monitored. If scientists can figure out which foods protect against prostate cancer, these adducts should decrease. Among other things, a test counting these adducts could confirm that scientists are on the right track in preventing prostate cancer.

### Fat and Breast Cancer

One large Harvard study looking for connections between fat intake and specific fatty acids (including total fat, animal fat; saturated, polyunsaturated, and trans fats) and breast cancer in thousands of women couldn't find a specific link—even in women with a family history of breast cancer. "In this large prospective study, we found no evidence that higher total fat intake was associated with an increased risk of breast cancer, even though the relationship was assessed many different ways," the researchers said. "These findings suggest that reductions in total fat intake during midlife are unlikely to prevent breast cancer, and should receive less emphasis. Rather, women's decision about fat intake should be guided primarily by risk of heart disease, which is strongly influenced by the type but not total amount of fat."

In another study, these Harvard scientists made an important point: "The lack of association of total dietary fat with breast cancer, and probably other cancers as well, should not be confused with the relation of excess body fat to cancer risk. Higher body weight has been associated with increased risks of cancers of the endometrium, colon, and (among post-menopausal women) breast." Dietary fat intake, the researchers noted, doesn't necessarily determine a person's body fat, which "is largely determined by the balance between physical activity and total caloric intake, which in almost all diets derives mainly from carbohydrates."

---

### *ENVIRONMENT JUST MEANS DIET, RIGHT? WRONG!*

If only it were as simple as a direct cause-and-effect relationship. Then we could say, "Eat this and you'll never get cancer," and "Don't eat this, or else." But it doesn't always work that way. In fact, if it does, we should view any such evidence with a healthy dose of caution. For example, for years, scientists assumed that the high frequency of stomach cancer in China was caused by dietary factors—until we learned that it was instead caused by bacterial infection with *H. pylori* (which also causes stomach ulcers). Oops!

Is the Asian diet the key? We just don't know. Here's one line of thought that my Johns Hopkins colleague William Nelson is just starting to pursue: In many areas of the Far East, there is excessive crowding, often in areas with poor sanitation. Many children are exposed to a host of bacterial and viral illnesses when they are very young—and when their prostates are not yet developed. It may be that these same infections happen in adulthood to western men, at a time when injury to the prostate might induce chronic inflammation—which, in the long run, may be the breeding ground for the development of prostate cancer.

In other interesting work, scientists from the University of Maryland Department of Epidemiology and Preventive Medicine have examined the effect of diet on the intestinal microflora (gut bacteria). They have shown that by varying the diet, they can change the bacterial groups that thrive in the gut. Eating a diet high in fat, they found, results in higher numbers of the kind of bacteria that can live in the absence of oxygen; eating a diet high in protein results in just the opposite. These researchers have also shown that drinking black tea (for more on tea, see chapter 4) can also affect which bacteria do well.

What does this mean for us? It might be that the microflora themselves produce compounds, such as butyrate, which may shield us from cancer or other compounds, such as methane derivatives, which may be harmful. Eating protective foods might enlist a previously unknown battalion of soldiers—the gut bacteria—to fight off cancer.

---

### *Vitamin D, Sunlight, and Calcium*

Where in the world you live determines, in large part, how much vitamin D you get. Vitamin D is a hormone known to protect the body against cancer through a mechanism that could be called "taming the lion." We know from studies on cell cultures done in petri dishes that when vitamin D is added to cancer cells, it slows down their growth and causes them to climb a few rungs up the cancer ladder toward civilization—to revert to a less aggressive state. It seems like this is what happens in humans, as well.

Where does vitamin D come from? Ninety percent of it comes from the everyday exposure of our skin to the sun's rays. The rest of it can come from our diet. Milk, the main dietary source, is fortified with modest amounts of vitamin D, as are orange juices and a few breads and cereals. Unfortunately, the amount of vitamin D added to fortified foods is notoriously unreliable, and the only significant natural food sources are oily fish, such as salmon, mackerel, and sardines, and fish oil. The Japanese diet is rich in fish that contain vitamin D.

In the skin, dehydrocholesterol is converted into something called cholecalciferol vitamin D and then into a compound with an even longer name, 25-hydroxycholecalciferol. Vitamin D then changes into its active form (called 1,25-dihydroxyvitamin D) in the kidney. (More on how this works when we talk about calcium, below.) This form of vitamin D has been shown to keep cells well differentiated—to keep their shape intact and healthy and their growth slow and orderly.

### Sunlight

People who live in southern climates get a lot more sun than do people in the north. Several years ago, researchers looked at the geographic distribution of the sun's ultraviolet (UV) rays and the number of prostate cancer deaths throughout the United States. After adjusting the data to account for the South's higher concentration of older men, the scientists uncovered a striking North-South pattern, with the highest concentration of prostate cancer death in the North and the lowest in the South. But when they looked at sunlight exposure, they found just the opposite—the heaviest exposure in the South and the least in the North. Areas getting the least UV radiation had the most prostate cancer deaths, and vice versa. They concluded that UV radiation may protect men from getting clinical prostate cancer, and that vitamin D somehow slows or prevents incidental prostate cancer from becoming clinical. This might explain why prostate cancer death rates are highest in Scandinavian countries, Canada, and the United States and lowest in Asia. Also, it may explain a key racial difference. Vitamin D is mostly formed in the skin. People with dark skin absorb less sunlight and are known to have lower levels of vitamin D. In one study, African scientists compared blood levels of vitamin D in black men in Zaire (now Democratic Republic of the Congo) with Zairian black men living in Belgium and found significantly lower levels of vitamin D in those who had left sunny Zaire.

The best way to help your body produce vitamin D is to spend some time outside in the sunlight every day for at least fifteen to thirty minutes. Note: Be cautious about trying to duplicate the sun's rays with megadose supplements from the health-food store; too much of anything, including vitamin D, can be toxic. If you do take supplements, the recommended dose is 400 to 800 IU (international units) daily. The reason for this became quite clear in a study from Scandinavia in which scientists found that men with normal levels of vitamin D had the lowest risk of prostate cancer, while men with the highest levels had nearly twice the risk of developing the disease! This is an extremely important point. Many of us feel that "if a little bit is good, a lot is better." Wrong. The authors of this study speculated that the men with the highest levels may have been overenthusiastic in their embrace of vitamin D–rich foods or supplements, and this, they suggest, may have led to vitamin D resistance. Again, moderation in all things is a good way to live. More is not always better.

Yet another explanation—one that deserves further study—for the observation that prostate cancer risk correlates with sunlight may be quite simple. Where do fruits and vegetables grow best? In the sunlight. Fifty years ago (before greenhouses and hydroponic gardening, and before world markets and the widespread importation of foods), it was much easier for an Italian man to eat fruits and vegetables year-round than a Scandinavian man. Today, even with the great availability of food, this is still the case, and there is much less prostate cancer in Italy than there is in the Scandinavian countries. Conversely, men in Scandinavian countries tend to eat more dairy products, which brings us to our next risk factor.

## Calcium

Remember Elsie the cow? Picture a whole herd of happy-looking black-and-white cows just like her, grazing in the countryside in a field full of buttercups, little bells tinkling around their necks. In the list of things that are considered wholesome and good, dairy products rank right up there with apple pie. How is it, then, that milk, which according to the ads "does a body good," could possibly be linked to cancer? This makes the following all the more surprising: In a series of case-control and cohort studies, there was a direct association between dairy intake and the risk of dying from prostate cancer. Furthermore, it may be that calcium—stalwart preserver of strong teeth and bones—is in large part to blame. Scientific evidence has linked a higher daily intake of calcium (well beyond the recommended daily amount for older men) with advanced prostate cancer—and, more commonly, with metastatic disease. A meta-analysis of eleven case-control studies showed an increased risk of prostate cancer associated with drinking milk. In another study, conducted in Seattle, men who consumed the most calcium had a twofold higher risk of developing cancer that spreads beyond the prostate.

It seems that calcium interferes with the antitumor effect of 1,25-dihydroxyvitamin D (discussed above). Normally, your kidneys take vitamin D and convert it to its active form, 1,25-dihydroxyvitamin D. But the kidney's ability to transform vitamin D is regulated by the amount of calcium in the bloodstream. If you have low levels of calcium, your body makes more 1,25-dihydroxyvitamin D; if you have high levels of calcium, your body makes less of it—which means that vitamin D doesn't have the oomph that it should. Thus, calcium can effectively block vitamin D from becoming a helpful cancer fighter in your body and make it more likely for prostate cancer to develop.

But here's something interesting: fructose (the sugar found in fruit and in sodas that contain high-fructose corn syrup) may help counteract the calcium. Fruit is a major source of phosphorus. Phosphorus binds calcium, reducing its bioavailability—in other words, it makes it inactive in your body. A study conducted at Harvard found that a high fructose intake was associated with a decreased risk of prostate cancer. "We hypothesize," the Harvard researchers said, "that diets high in dairy products and meat and low in fruits are associated with increased risk of prostate cancer because these diets tend to be high in calcium . . . and low in fructose, and thus associated with lower circulating [1,25-dihydroxyvitamin D] levels."

How much is too much calcium? What's a body to do? We're

supposed to get a lot of calcium to protect our bones and even to take calcium supplements if we don't get enough. How can we do right by our bones without endangering our prostates? Unfortunately, the scientific evidence is mixed. One study found that consuming more than 1,000 mg (1) a day increased the risk of prostate cancer. However, a report from the Baltimore Longitudinal Study of Aging suggested that the cutoff was closer to 2,000 mg (2) a day. In another study, a randomized clinical trial of calcium supplementation, men consumed 1,200 mg of calcium a day for four years and later showed no increased risk of prostate cancer.

Also confusingly, it seems that calcium supplementation has different effects in various stages of prostate cancer. The Health Professionals Follow-Up Study showed that men who took high levels of calcium (2,000 mg or more daily) were three times more likely to develop high-grade, potentially fatal prostate cancer than low-grade tumors—the early, most curable kind of prostate cancer. Some scientists speculate that calcium may have a different effect on early cancer, perhaps preventing it from getting worse, than it does on later-stage cancer, perhaps even helping it to progress.

What if you prefer to get your calcium the old-fashioned way, from milk and dairy products? Scientists leading the first National Health and Nutrition Examination: Epidemiologic Follow-Up Study, a large American study, found that men who consumed an average of twenty-one servings of dairy products a week—this works out to dairy products at breakfast, lunch, and dinner—had twice the risk of prostate cancer as men who consumed a weekly average of five to eleven servings. So here we are again, back at moderation. And rather than overdoing vitamins and supplements, it makes better sense just to be certain that you are not deficient in calcium or any other vitamins or minerals. There is strong evidence for this explained in the next chapter.

## Family History

Does prostate cancer run in the family, or did a lot of men in your family just happen to have it? About 25 percent of men with prostate cancer have a family history of it. But only about 3 or 4 percent of men have hereditary prostate cancer—an inherited, genetic form of

---

### *WHAT IS HEREDITARY PROSTATE CANCER?*

Of all the men who will be diagnosed with prostate cancer this year, about 3 or 4 percent of them will be men born with a head start—one or more bad genes (discussed below) that greatly increase their odds of developing cancer and of developing it at an earlier age.

Although purely hereditary cases of cancer make up only a small percentage of all the men with prostate cancer, we believe that understanding hereditary prostate cancer may help us crack the genetic code of how this disease works. The defective gene or mechanisms involved in hereditary cancer are almost certainly the same ones that somehow go wrong in the far more common sporadic cancer, which develops over the course of a lifetime.

In most men, cancer probably happens because of an unfortunate chain of events—at least one genetic aberration, plus one or more environmental things, such as a poor diet. Say it takes three strikes in order for cancer to begin. Being born with a faulty gene might be worth one or two strikes. Add a lifetime of eating the wrong foods (or not eating the right ones), and bingo—strike three.

An estimated 250,000 American men may carry one of these defective genes, which can be inherited from either parent. Briefly, if your father or brother has prostate cancer, your risk is two and a half times greater than the average American man's, which is about 17 percent. It goes up from there: depending on the number of affected relatives you have and the age at which they developed the disease, your risk could be as high as 50 percent. If you are in a family that meets the criteria for hereditary prostate cancer—if you have at least three close relatives, such as a father and two brothers affected; or two relatives affected if both were younger than fifty-five years old when diagnosed; or if your family has disease in three generations—a grandfather, father, or brother, your risk could be 50 percent. Members of families with hereditary prostate cancer should have a digital rectal examination and PSA test every year, beginning at age forty.

To learn more or to enroll in our hereditary prostate cancer study, visit our Web site (http://urology.jhu.edu/) or write to us: Hereditary Prostate Cancer Study, The James Buchanan Brady Urological Institute, Johns Hopkins Hospital, 600 North Wolfe Street, Baltimore, Maryland 21287.

---

the disease (involving mutated genes that can be passed on by either parent) that develops at a younger age. Simply having a family history of prostate cancer raises your own risk of developing the disease, but it doesn't necessarily mean you have the hereditary form of prostate cancer.

## TABLE 3.5

### PROSTATE CANCER RUNS IN MY FAMILY: WHAT'S MY RISK OF DEVELOPING PROSTATE CANCER?

Having a family history of prostate cancer doesn't mean that you are definitely going to develop the disease. After all, prostate cancer affects millions of men worldwide, and it may just be coincidence that your father or brother developed the disease. However, the likelihood of this happening goes up if one of your family members develops it at a young age or if several members of your family have prostate cancer. Say your father developed prostate cancer at age seventy, and nobody else in your family has the disease. Although your risk is probably somewhat greater than that of someone without a family history of prostate cancer, in this example we'll set your relative risk at one. Note: These risks are relative. They are not absolute, but are designed to give you an approximation. Now, if your father developed prostate cancer at age sixty, your risk would be 50 percent higher; if he developed it at age fifty, your risk would now be twice as high.

What if your father developed prostate cancer at age seventy but your brother also developed it? Your risk would now be four times higher. And if your father developed it when he was fifty and your brother has it, your risk would be seven times higher. This is why it's so important to know not only who in your family has had prostate cancer but how old he was when he developed it. And remember, the increased risk of prostate cancer can be passed on by both sides of the family, so it's important to know the health history of your mother's father and brothers, too.

| Age at Diagnosis | Additional Relatives | Relative Risk |
| --- | --- | --- |
| 70 | None | 1.0 |
| 60 | None | 1.5 |
| 50 | None | 2.0 |
| 70 | 1 or more | 4.0 |
| 60 | 1 or more | 5.0 |
| 50 | 1 or more | 7.0 |

How can this be? How can prostate cancer run in families and not be inherited? We see this in other forms of cancer (breast cancer, for example), and the explanation is complicated—or, as scientists put it, multifactoral. In other words, there are several reasons. One is that there could be shared environmental factors, such as eating the same foods or living in the same geographic location. Another is that if a man's brother, uncle, or father develops the disease, he may be more likely to get his own PSA tested and begin regular screening.

However, there are some aspects of a family history that make it more likely that a family is dealing with the inherited form (see What Is Hereditary Prostate Cancer? above). We now understand that men with a hereditary tendency toward prostate cancer actually inherit a mutated gene (possibly one of the same genes that, in "regular" prostate cancer, mutate over the course of a lifetime). This has two important implications: First, because a man inherited one of these faulty genes, he is more likely to develop prostate cancer and—because he has a head start—to develop it at a younger age. Thus, men with a family history of prostate cancer need to start yearly screening early. Second, because prostate cancer can be inherited from either the mother or the father, it is crucial that men know as much as they can of the medical history of both sides of their family.

Note: Even though hereditary prostate cancer starts earlier, it is still every bit as curable as "regular," or sporadic, prostate cancer. In a Johns Hopkins investigation, patients with hereditary prostate cancer and patients who had no family history of prostate cancer were matched based on the pathology of their cancer (all of these terms, signposts for cancer that pathologists look for when they examine the surgically removed tumor, are discussed in chapter 6). The scientists compared the Gleason score, lymph node status (whether cancer had penetrated the lymph nodes), seminal vesicle status, extracapsular penetration (whether cancer had gone beyond the prostate wall), and surgical margins of the men in both groups. They then studied the men's follow-up data for ten years after surgery, looking for a detectable PSA level or any other evidence that cancer had returned. They found no significant difference in either group. Thus, if you have a family history of prostate cancer, you are more likely to develop the disease but are not more likely to die from it. The key is to get the jump on it; to realize it's a possibility, and to start looking for it.

### Confoundingly Common

Scientists didn't always know this much about hereditary prostate cancer. In fact, it took the medical community a long time to recognize that prostate cancer could be inherited at all. In this chapter, we've discussed the various risk factors—including simply getting older—that can make men more prone to prostate cancer. We've seen that prostate cancer is very common—confoundingly so, as a matter of fact. That's why for decades, researchers downplayed the idea that (just like more conspicuous illnesses, such as hemophilia) it could be inherited, even though it was known to run in families. Forty years ago, genealogists in Utah noted that prostate cancer seemed to cluster in families. They found that if a man's father died of prostate cancer, his own risk of dying of prostate cancer was two- or threefold greater. Even more striking, they found that, among familial cancers, this clustering of prostate cancer was actually more common than the clustering breast or colon cancer, yet both of these diseases were recognized much earlier to have a hereditary predisposition. In order of familiality (an index of how likely it is for a cancer to run in families), the common cancers are ranked in this order: melanoma, ovarian cancer, prostate cancer, colon cancer, and breast cancer. This observation was reinforced recently by a large Scandinavian study of identical twins; researchers found that hereditary factors were highest for prostate cancer, explaining 42 percent of the risk of developing the disease, and lower for colon and breast cancer (35 and 27 percent, respectively. For more on twins and prostate cancer, see below).

### Wrongly Stereotyped

Yet for some reason, prostate cancer got lumped in the category of ailments that happen to come with old age—part of the baggage of aging, in effect. With this perception muddying the water, these observations went relatively unexplored for a couple of decades. Scientists just couldn't get past the commonness of prostate cancer. In the 1980s, I began to see increasingly younger men with prostate cancer and was struck by how many of them had a family history of the disease. Then, in 1986, I met a forty-nine-year-old man with an unforgettable legacy: Every male in this man's family had died of prostate cancer—his father, his father's three brothers, and his grandfather. At that time, virtually every physician in the United States could reel off the statistics for breast cancer—that a woman's risk increased twofold if her mother or sister had it. It seemed odd to me that there was no similar information available on prostate cancer.

These questions launched the first of a series of studies at Johns Hopkins. The first question: Would the observations that had been pretty much limited to Utah Mormons hold true with a larger, more diverse group of men? A study of 691 patients who had come to Hopkins for radical prostatectomy confirmed that having a family history of prostate cancer did indeed increase a man's risk of developing the disease. When we ruled out environmental factors, our results strongly suggested that increased susceptibility to prostate cancer could be inherited from either parent (which we have since proven— see below). We then went on to define and characterize hereditary prostate cancer, showing the clear link between family history and a man's probability of developing prostate cancer (see box, page 91).

Over the last two decades, there have been many studies on family history and the risk of prostate cancer. This is what they've shown:

- If your first-degree relative (father or brother) has prostate cancer, your risk is increased two and a half times.
- Your risk is higher if that relative was younger than sixty when diagnosed.
- Your risk is also higher if it's your brother rather than your father (because you can inherit the defective genes involved in prostate cancer from your mother as well as your father).
- If you have two first-degree relatives with prostate cancer (brother and father), your risk is three and a half times higher.

**The Genetics of Prostate Cancer**

Where are these faulty family genes located? How do scientists find them, and what do we know about them? The standard way to look for genetic "sore thumbs"—bits of DNA that stick out as odd or unusual—is to look at the genes in families that meet the criteria, in this case, for hereditary prostate cancer. We do this using a technique called linkage analysis, looking for patterns of association between certain portions of chromosomes and the presence of cancer in multiple members of a family or families that couldn't possibly happen just by chance. In this way, we can link cancer to a small segment on a chromosome. (More on this below.)

Sadly, the best families to study are the ones hardest hit by prostate cancer—so there can be no mistaking hereditary cancer for terribly bad luck—in which several men in the same family just happened to develop the disease. The families fill out detailed questionnaires about their health, occupations, and family history and send blood samples from which scientists extract their DNA. We have been fortunate, working with investigators from the National Human Genome Research Institute, Wake Forest University, and the University of Umeå in Sweden, to put together a large group of more than two hundred such families.

And we were very lucky, in 1996, to show the first linkage between prostate cancer in families and a gene located somewhere on the long arm of chromosome 1. Since that time, linkage to more than eight chromosomal areas has been reported. These include four areas on chromosome 1, one on chromosome 8, one on chromosome 17, one on chromosome 20, and interestingly, one on the X chromosome—a milestone in cancer research. This is the first time the X chromosome (which sons inherit only from their mothers) has been definitively linked to a major cancer.

### Linkage

This exhaustive search for the gene or genes probably won't turn up some weird-looking mutant that instantly calls attention to itself as a cause of cancer. The genes involved here are genes that everybody has. For example, everybody has a BRCA-1 and BRCA-2 gene, both of which are involved in breast cancer. However, everybody doesn't have the *same sequence* of those genes. The sequences fluctuate, like ingredients in a recipe—just as both bread and salt dough have the same ingredients, depending on the recipe, one is edible and one is not. This is a daunting task, like trying to find one misspelled word in twenty sets of the *Encyclopædia Britannica*—and each set contains twenty volumes! The first job is to try to narrow down the search—to figure out which books are most likely to contain this mistake. That's linkage. The next step is to go through those books, page by page.

### The Genes in Question: What We've Learned So Far

So far, four "prostate-cancer genes" have been identified. Unfortunately, none of them will be useful for screening large groups, because the mutations have been found only in small clusters of families. However, they have given us helpful leads as to what might cause prostate cancer. The first gene, identified on chromosome 17, is called HPC2/ELAC2. We don't know exactly what this gene's normal job is, but it may be involved in cell cycle regulation—the orderly birth and death of cells. If it doesn't work, abnormal growth may result. The next two genes are involved in the body's response to infection.

These genes provide tantalizing support for the idea that some hidden infection may be responsible for the inflammation that ultimately leads to PIA and then to invasive prostate cancer. One of these, found on the long arm of chromosome 1, is called RNASEL (the acronym for ribonuclease-L). When this gene is inactivated in animals and the animals are infected with certain viruses, as many as half of them die. Another gene, found on chromosome 8, is called MSR1 (the acronym for macrophage scavenger receptor 1). This gene also plays an important role in the body's response to bacterial infections—and again, when animals don't have this gene and get infected with certain types of bacteria, about half of them die. The fourth gene is NKX3-1, which has a role in the normal development of the lining of the prostate before a boy is even born. In laboratory animals, scientists have shown that knocking out this gene allows prostate cancer to start.

Undoubtedly, these first four are just the tip of the genetic iceberg. Scientists believe that, because no single, common gene has been found after a decade of intense searching, there are many roads that lead to Rome—many mutations in pathways that, when interrupted, cause prostate cancer. It would be nice if these mutations, however many there are, turn out to occur on some of the same pathways. This would make it easier for scientists to develop strategies—such as changing the environment or supplementing the diet—to help spare the men who have these mutations from getting prostate cancer.

### Inherited Risk: Am I Just More Likely to Get Cancer, or Is It Already a "Done Deal"?

Although it's not always clear when scientists talk about genetics, there are two kinds of genetic influences. One of them is what we've been talking about here—true hereditary prostate cancer, which is relatively rare and accounts for only about 3 or 4 percent of all cases of prostate cancer. Hereditary prostate cancer and other inherited diseases are what geneticists call "highly penetrant": if you inherit a specific gene or genes, that's it—you get the disease. It's a done deal.

But there's a second type of hereditary influence that is much more common, much more subtle, and leaves the door open to *not* getting cancer. In this case, your genetic makeup may have one or two chinks in it that may have a bearing on whether you get a disease,

---

### GENETIC RESEARCH: WHAT DOES THE FUTURE HOLD? HOW TO IDENTIFY POLYMORPHISMS

The future is very bright. There are many advances right on the horizon, just months or a few years away. First, genetic sequencing is getting faster, easier, and less expensive—to the point where the National Cancer Institute is contemplating sequencing the entire human genome in a large number of men and women with different kinds of cancers, with the hope of finding common variations that involve common pathways. This would have been unheard of even a decade ago, when sequencing the entire genome of a single human was a monumental task. Imagine if we could have made the leap—which took half a century—from those early computers that used punch cards and took up an entire room, to the ones roughly the size of a Buick, to personal computers, to laptops in just a few years. Technology is moving faster.

Another dramatic breakthrough was made in 2005, with the publication of the HapMap. This refers to haplotypes—a set of closely linked markers on a single chromosome that appear to be inherited, undisturbed, in large chunks of DNA. It's like the difference between random notes of music and stretches of recognizable tunes. The same songs get passed down, unchanged, from generation to generation. This map is, if you will, the highly sophisticated, genetic version of *Name That Tune*. It recognizes those exact pieces of DNA. A recent editorial in the *New England Journal of Medicine* explained it this way: "In the mid-1960s, George Harrison, Paul McCartney, John Lennon and Ringo Starr were often found together. If you looked for Harrison, there was a high likelihood, but not complete certainty, that you would find the other members of the Beatles. That's exactly what the HapMap will do." Because these developments are happening so quickly, geneticists are confident that within the next decade, we will have a much clearer picture of the genetic defects responsible for most cancers. And because prostate cancer appears to have the greatest heritability of the common cancers, this should provide great insight into how this cancer gets started.

---

may increase your susceptibility to it somewhat—but cancer may not be a predestined conclusion. One example of this increased susceptibility—scientists call this a polymorphism—we discussed above: a specific "short repeat" of CAG, a protein sequence most likely to be found in African American men and in Caucasians with metastatic cancer. Another is a variation in the vitamin D receptor gene, which can affect the body's response to vitamin D, and still another is a variant for producing 5-alpha reductase type II, an enzyme in the prostate that converts testosterone to DHT, the active male hormone in the prostate. The 5-alpha reductase-II enzyme seems to be more active in white and black American men than in Japanese men. Some scientists have speculated that levels of male hormones correlate with a man's risk of prostate cancer. These studies by and large have been disappointing, providing no consistent conclusions. Instead, a more likely explanation is that it's not *how much* of a specific hormone a man has but *the way a man's genes respond* to that hormone. It may well be that in some men, a little hormone goes a lot further and has a much more powerful effect than it does in other men. This is how variations in the genes coding for androgen and vitamin D receptors and 5-alpha reductase enzyme may influence risk of prostate cancer.

There are other polymorphisms, and still more will be discovered. It may well be that it is gene-gene interaction—a complicated mix of genes, with each polymorphism increasing a man's susceptibility to prostate cancer just a little bit.

### What Can We Learn from Twins?

Two boys have exactly the same DNA. They're identical twins, and when they grow up, one eventually gets prostate cancer; the other doesn't. How can this be? The only answer is that although genetics are important, environment may help turn the tide. In other words, even if you've been born with the same bad deck of cards as someone who develops prostate cancer, if you play your cards right, you may still win the game.

This is why geneticists love to study identical twins. (Fraternal, or nonidentical, twins are no more alike than brothers.) If being born with the same DNA were the only factor that made a man susceptible to prostate cancer, then we would expect that every time one identical twin developed prostate cancer, his brother would, too. If genetics played no role, then identical twins would be as likely to develop prostate cancer as any other brothers who share the same environment but not the same DNA. By comparing how often a disease develops in identical twins with how often it occurs in nonidentical twins, we can estimate the influence of genetic and environmental factors. There have been two major studies of twins and prostate cancer, one from

Sweden, and the other a study of American World War II veterans. These studies found that in the vast majority of cases, both identical twins did not get cancer. The likelihood of both identical twins developing prostate cancer was 19 percent in one study and 27 percent in the other. In both studies, the likelihood of nonidentical twins both developing cancer was much lower—only 4 percent in one study and 7 percent in the other. These studies showed that DNA isn't everything: Although identical twins were four to five times more likely to develop the same disease, it was by no means inevitable. Other factors, presumably environmental, must play a stronger role. Indeed, these studies concluded that the relative role of genetic versus environmental factors is fifty-fifty.

If these men had the same DNA—basically, the same body—why didn't genetics count for more? Because what happens to that body is critical. This means that if you are an identical twin and your brother has cancer, you are not destined definitely to get the disease. If you and your brother have not made exactly the same lifestyle choices, then your risk of getting prostate cancer is not exactly the same. This message is extremely important: *environment changes your risk of developing prostate cancer.* If, in future studies, scientists could determine *how* the twins' lifestyles were different—what good or bad choices these men made along the way—we might be able to understand why the disease occurs in the first place. Studies like this and of men who inherit the susceptibility genes (in hereditary prostate cancer) but do not get the disease may tell us much about prostate cancer.

## Association with Other Tumors

Cancer researchers have known for years that some families don't just have a higher risk of a particular cancer but a "cancer syndrome," such as hereditary breast/ovarian cancer syndrome, in which cancer develops at more than one site. (Note: This is different from cancer that starts in one place and then metastasizes, or spreads, throughout the body.) There is no evidence to suggest that hereditary prostate cancer is strongly associated with cancers at other sites or that it is part of a significant hereditary cancer syndrome, with two exceptions.

Two genes that are mutated in breast cancer are repairmen. Their job is to find genetic errors and fix the DNA mutations that cause them.

They are called BRCA-1 and BRCA-2, and men who inherit defects in these genes can also develop prostate cancer. For example, for men in families that carry the BRCA-2 mutation, the risk of developing prostate cancer is increased two and a half times. (The risk is also higher for prostate cancer in these families if a female relative is diagnosed with breast cancer before the age of thirty-six.)

Also, investigators from Utah recently reported a higher risk of colorectal cancer, non-Hodgkin's lymphoma, multiple myeloma, cancer of the gallbladder, and melanoma in some families with hereditary prostate cancer. For most men with hereditary prostate cancer, these risks are not increased. But there can be isolated families with a certain genetic makeup (which we haven't yet figured out) that may raise the risk of their developing these other tumors.

## What About Hormones?

Scientists have known for a long time that prostate cancer is under the control of hormones—that men who are castrated before puberty rarely develop prostate cancer, and that men with advanced prostate cancer can be helped by hormone therapy (shutting off the supply of male hormones to the prostate). The complicated relationship between hormones and prostate cancer is discussed in much greater detail above.

Having said that, there is no good evidence to suggest that the level of testosterone in the blood can be used to estimate whether a man is more or less likely to develop cancer. (In fact, as we'll discuss below, some men with low testosterone levels have a higher risk of developing the disease.) Instead, the way the body *responds* to hormone levels may be more important.

### What About Hormone Replacement?

If there is no association between hormone levels and the development of prostate cancer, is it okay for a man to "pump up" his testosterone levels? The answer here is categorically no! Dehydroepiandrosterone (DHEA) is a dietary supplement; you can buy it at any health-food store. Many men do because DHEA levels drop as a man ages, and the hope is that boosting DHEA will be the proverbial fountain of youth.

It isn't. Worse, there's a risk involved with taking hormones. If a man has latent prostate cancer (the "incidental" kind discussed above), it is possible that taking DHEA could be like pouring kerosene on a fire. It should go without saying that any man who has had prostate cancer should never take any form of male hormone supplementation. As a recent review of DHEA concluded, "There is no convincing evidence that DHEA has any beneficial effect on aging or any disease. Patients would be well advised not to take it."

### Supplemental Testosterone: The Fountain of Youth?

With the development of new ways to replace testosterone using gels that can be rubbed on the skin, there has been a flurry of marketing encouraging men to pursue this fountain of youth. There is no question that as men age and their testosterone levels go down, they have many of the signs and symptoms associated with low levels of testosterone in younger men—low sex drive, loss of muscle strength, weakening of the bones, and osteoporosis. But we don't know which is the cart and which is the horse. In other words, are these conditions caused by the diminishing testosterone, or are these symptoms and the lowered testosterone both caused by aging? The Institute of Medicine, after an extensive review of all these studies, concluded that no one knows the answer to this question. And, before a large-scale study is undertaken to determine the safety of testosterone replacement in older men—and whether it increases their risk for prostate cancer—we should first find out whether it even works. The authors of this review proposed that older men with low testosterone levels take part in a clinical trial to see if testosterone replacement reverses these problems. This makes great sense. Obviously, if it turns out not to help—and it might increase the risk of prostate cancer, to boot—then testosterone replacement is not the great antidote for aging it's cracked up to be.

But what if your testosterone is borderline low, and your doctor wants to treat you with supplemental testosterone? Is this okay? Again, it's probably not a good idea unless you are tested first to be sure you don't have cancer. *Having low testosterone levels doesn't mean you won't get prostate cancer; one study, in fact, showed that a number of men with low testosterone levels did have prostate cancer.* Thus, if you are a man at risk of developing prostate cancer because of your age or family history, and if a doctor tells you that you need extra testosterone because your own levels of this male hormone are low, you should probably have a needle biopsy of the prostate first, just to rule out cancer. PSA levels are driven by testosterone, and if your testosterone level is low, your PSA level could be falsely low—low enough to "fake out" your doctor. Although there is not a wealth of scientific information on this subject, there are enough red flags to suggest *taking extreme caution when tampering with hormones.*

What if your testosterone is definitely low? Is supplemental testosterone okay now? Not without further testing. We've recently learned that prostate cancer—especially, extensive, high-grade cancer—produces a substance that suppresses the hypothalamic-pituitary axis (more on this chemical pathway in chapter 12) and lowers testosterone. We know that when the prostate is removed in these men, their testosterone returns to normal levels. Thus, if your testosterone is low, before you start testosterone replacement, you should have a PSA test, a rectal examination, and a biopsy, just to make certain that prostate cancer is not the cause. This is a good idea for another reason, too. Evidence from a study of eight hundred men in the Baltimore Longitudinal Study of Aging showed that men with the highest levels of free testosterone in their blood were more likely to develop prostate cancer. That study's authors, too, recommend that men who take extra testosterone be regularly monitored for the development of the disease.

Another class of hormones, called insulin-like growth factors (IGF), may also influence the development of prostate cancer. These growth factors—which can make prostate cancer cells grow and proliferate—are found in the prostate's epithelial and stromal cells, which have specific receptors for insulin-like growth factor type 1 (IGF-1). IGF-1 receptors are found in advanced prostate cancer cells that can function without help from hormones (called androgen-independent cells). IGF can be counteracted by particular proteins that bind to it and block its action in the cells. One study found that prostate cancer risk was higher in men with elevated levels of IGF-1. (For more on IGF as a possible predictor of prostate cancer, see chapter 5.)

## Other Risk Factors

This section is a compilation of loose ends that scientists haven't yet figured out what to do with. For example:

### Occupation—Farming and Exposure to Agent Orange

The only occupation that has been found to have a higher risk of prostate cancer is farming. This has been shown in a number of studies. For example, one University of Iowa study found Iowa farmers to be at a higher risk of dying from certain cancers, including prostate cancer. The question, however, is why. Is it due to lifestyle? It is very hard to know what to do with information from this type of study, because it is so difficult to separate what people are—their family history—from what they do—their eating habits. For example, in some studies, farmers have been shown to have more fat in their diet and to eat fewer fruits and vegetables. (The Iowa study found that farmers had a higher total energy intake, consumed higher levels of protein, fat, and saturated fat, and ate more red meat than other men; in addition, older farmers ate fewer fruits and vegetables than did other men their same age.)

Nonetheless, one plausible explanation for a link between farming and prostate cancer may be an increased lifetime exposure to agricultural chemicals, particularly herbicides. (Some of these concentrate in fat; also, some affect body chemistry by causing a drop in estrogen levels.) Researchers from the National Academy of Sciences looked at agricultural exposure to herbicides and concluded that there was some evidence that this made men more susceptible to prostate cancer. As a result of this study, the U.S. government agreed to provide service-connected disability to any veteran who was in Vietnam and who develops prostate cancer. More recently, the first study of cancer incidence in American Vietnam veterans was published. Doctors looked at the individuals who actually did the spraying of Agent Orange and found an increased risk of prostate cancer and melanoma that correlated with their degree of exposure to dioxin (the chemical believed to be the culprit here). According to the Department of Veterans Affairs, "Vietnam veterans who believe they have health problems that may be related to their exposure to Agent Orange while serving in Vietnam, or their survivors should contact the nearest VA medical center or regional office. VA's nationwide toll-free number (for benefits) is 1-800-827-1000." The VA Web site is www.va.gov. Vietnam veterans interested in finding out more may also want to contact the Vietnam Veterans of America, 8605 Cameron St., Suite 400, Silver Spring, MD 20910; or call 1-800-VVA-1316; http://www.vva.org (click on "Agent Orange"). The VVA is a nonprofit, congressionally chartered organization dedicated to helping veterans and their families receive benefits and services. Veterans Benefits and Services also offers many services, which can be found on this Web page dedicated to Agent Orange: http://www.vba.va.gov/bln/21/benefits/herbicide/.

### Cigarette Smoking

Although there is no good evidence that cigarette smoking increases a man's risk of developing prostate cancer, there is accumulating evidence that men who smoke cigarettes are more likely—if they do develop cancer—to have aggressive disease and to die from it. In a Johns Hopkins study of men under the age of fifty-five who developed prostate cancer, *only smoking* was connected with the development of aggressive disease. Why could this be? Remember the protector enzyme GST-π, which fends off oxidative damage and is inactivated early on in prostate cancer development? This enzyme also combats the major carcinogen in cigarettes, a chemical called benzopyrene. Thus, if a man has embarked on the path toward prostate cancer and loses the protection of GST-π, he'll not only suffer greater oxidative damage but also the additional effects of a bunch of toxic chemicals injected into every cell of his body with each puff.

### Things That Do Not Increase the Risk

### Vasectomy

Why is it that so many men who are diagnosed with prostate cancer are men who have had a vasectomy? One reason is that vasectomy is very common; a lot of men have had one. It is felt that these men, having established a professional relationship with a urologist, are more likely to go back to a urologist—and urologists are probably more likely than other physicians to look for prostate cancer.

## Sexual Activity

Some people worry that increased sexual activity can cause prostate cancer because of the mistaken belief that ejaculation causes an increase in testosterone levels. This is not true. There is no good reason to believe that having an active sex life will stimulate the prostate to grow or cause prostate cancer. In fact, at least one conclusive study has shown that priests have the same risk of prostate cancer as do married men. Some researchers speculate that men who have sex more often may be more likely to acquire a sexually transmitted disease, which may infect the prostate, cause inflammation and other damage, and increase the risk of prostate cancer.

But other scientists reckon that sexual activity may actually *decrease* the risk of prostate cancer—that regular ejaculation "cleans house," if you will, in the prostate, making it a less welcome harbor for cancer-causing agents, infection, and stagnant materials that could lead to inflammation. Recent results from the Health Professionals Follow-Up Study, led by researchers at Harvard, support this idea. The scientists found that men who reported more ejaculations—more than twenty-one a month, on average, across their adult lives—had two-thirds the lifetime risk of prostate cancer of men who reported fewer (four to seven) ejaculations a month. The authors suggested that frequent ejaculation may alter the composition of the prostatic fluid, lower the concentration of potentially harmful chemicals, or reduce the number of intraluminal prostatic crystalloids, tiny stones that have been linked to prostate cancer in some studies. The main message, says the Johns Hopkins epidemiologist Elizabeth Platz, one of the authors of this study, is that "men should not be worried that frequent ejaculation will cause prostate cancer." The next step, she adds, is to figure out why it seems to have this protective effect and the role inflammation plays here.

## Alcoholic Beverages

Unlike breast cancer in women, where a definite link has been shown, there is no evidence that drinking alcohol makes a man more likely to develop prostate cancer. Actually, one study done in King County, Washington, uncovered good news for red wine drinkers: although there was no overall connection between the development of prostate cancer and alcohol consumption, scientists found that men who drank red wine had a 24 percent reduction in their risk of being diagnosed with the disease—a 6 percent decrease for every 2 ounces of red wine consumed a week. And for men who drank four or more glasses a week, there was a 50 percent reduction. Furthermore, the researchers found a 60 percent reduction in the diagnosis of high-grade, aggressive disease. What's happening here?

Red wine's secret weapon may be a chemical called resveratrol, a polyphenol (see chapter 4) that is concentrated in grape skins. Interestingly, it's produced in response to a fungus that shows up on grapes; the level is higher in red wines made in rainier years. Resveratrol appears to be an antieverything—antioxidant, anti-inflammatory, and antiangiogenic (it discourages new blood vessels that could help cancer cells grow from forming). It also reduces cell proliferation. Note: This effect was not seen with white wine or with other alcoholic beverages. Is it possible, the authors wonder, that this is why France has half as much prostate cancer as the United States and why Italy has 20 percent less?

### Physical Inactivity

The jury is still out on this one. No strong proof has been found to link a man's exercise or occupational exertion—or lack of it—to prostate cancer. In fact, the evidence is simply contradictory; one recent study stated that cardiorespiratory fitness and physical activities may protect against the development of prostate cancer. In this study, men completed a questionnaire in 1986, detailing their physical activity. Men who were sixty-five years or older in 1986 and who exercised vigorously for more than three hours a week had a 70 percent decrease in their risk of developing high-grade, advanced, or fatal prostate cancer. But a recent study from the Health Professionals Follow-Up Study suggests the opposite. Younger men got no benefit from vigorous exercise. In fact, these authors reported in another article that young, lean men who were more physically active had a *higher* risk of developing metastatic and fatal prostate cancer.

How could it be that exercise helps if you're older but hurts if you're younger? I had an interesting conversation with Dr. Kenneth H. Cooper, the president and founder of the Cooper Aerobics Center in Dallas—a strong advocate of exercise and antioxidants. He described anecdotal evidence of marathon runners who died from prostate cancer and gave me his explanation for this. When the body works very hard, as it does during vigorous exercise, it also makes more free radicals. To counteract this, he believes, athletes need to take higher doses of antioxidants.

### Other Prostate Problems

There is no evidence that having BPH increases or decreases the risk of prostate cancer unless a man undergoes surgical treatment. In that case, because tissue samples may be examined by a pathologist, there could be a slightly higher chance that cancer will be found. Again, because BPH starts in the prostate's transition zone and cancer begins in the peripheral zone, the two conditions are probably not related.

What about prostatitis? Several studies have suggested a weak link between prostatitis and prostate cancer. However, this may be similar to the explanation for the increased risk in men who undergo vasectomy: men who go to a urologist and have prostate symptoms are more likely to have a biopsy. However, as we noted earlier, asymptomatic inflammatory prostatitis—the kind you know about only if your prostate is biopsied—does appear to be associated with the development of prostate cancer. But men who have this inflammation never know they have it. This means that if you do have symptoms of prostatitis, you shouldn't worry. You don't have the kind that could lead to cancer.

Now that we've talked about what causes—and doesn't cause—prostate cancer, the next step is to turn this around and see how we can prevent it. The main focus of prevention is diet: not only avoiding those "sins of commission"—keeping away from foods that probably encourage cancer—but reversing those "sins of omission" by identifying and eating foods that actually fight cancer. On to chapter 4.

# 4

# CAN PROSTATE CANCER BE PREVENTED?

## ▶▶▶ READ THIS FIRST

Ultimately, the way we'd prefer to treat all cancers is to prevent them from happening in the first place. One day in the not too distant future, we hope to look back on the era of cancer just as we now reflect on the eras of polio and smallpox—as a plague of the past. It sounds like wishful thinking—an ideal right up there with eliminating poverty and crime. And yet scientists firmly believe that one day this will happen. Until then, what do we do?

In the last chapter, we talked about what most likely causes prostate cancer—oxidative damage to DNA. It's a domino effect—a cascade of genetic changes through which a normal cell is transformed into a cancerous cell. These changes can happen before birth in men with hereditary prostate cancer, or—as is the case with most men who get prostate cancer—they can happen over the course of a lifetime.

When we talk about the environment causing cancer, mostly we mean diet—the high-fat, low-vegetable-and-fruit western diet that clogs our arteries and also, it seems, makes us more prone to cancer. Thus, if a man's diet—every bite of cheeseburger, or hot dog, or sausage and bacon biscuit—can contribute to these incremental changes that somehow push a cell over the edge and make it cancerous, is it possible that changing what he eats can also lower his risk of developing prostate cancer? Yes. The problem now is determining what do we eat instead. And for how long do we have to eat these other things or supplement our diet with chemopreventive agents? This is what scientists are trying to do now—figure out the specifics of a cancer-fighting diet.

Scientists worldwide are working to isolate specific cancer-fighting substances in the hopes of making nutraceuticals, drugs extracted from specific nutrients. This is very exciting work. And yet, to put it in perspective, much of this research is simply confirming something scientists have known for decades. The best way to prevent cancer is to eat more fruits and vegetables, eat less red meat, consume fewer calories in general, and burn off a few of those calories with regular exercise. This is why the American Cancer Society has made the following recommendations for years: Make sure most of what you eat comes from plants. Eat five or more servings of fruits and vegetables a day and other foods from plant sources, including breads, grains, rice, pasta, or beans, several times a day. Eat foods low in fat, and limit your consumption of meats, particularly meats high in fat. Stay within your healthy weight range (see the body mass index table in chapter 3), and get at least moderate exercise for thirty minutes or more on most days of the week.

Finally, eating all of the broccoli and good things in the world—though it may well make a difference in the long run—doesn't take away your risk of developing prostate cancer right now. If you are age forty or older, if you have a family history of prostate cancer, or if are African American, you need more preventive measures than a good diet can guarantee. You need a yearly rectal exam and PSA test.

## A Word on Preventing Prostate Cancer

In the last chapter, we talked about the demographic nightmare looming on the horizon of prostate cancer—aging baby boomers.

Millions of American men, all at once, entering prostate cancer's "prime time." The sheer numbers alone tell us that over the next forty years, the number of men being diagnosed with prostate cancer and dying from it will double or even triple unless we can do something to stop it. The simplest, most effective, and least costly solution is prevention. If we could prevent prostate cancer or significantly lower men's risk of developing it, we wouldn't have to worry so much about what's called secondary prevention—treating the disease as soon as possible after it's been detected. Prevention could spare us this worrisome game of catch-up; it could also lower the chances that we'll find prostate cancer when it's too advanced to be cured. Prevention could save men the cost of expensive procedures and eliminate all the worry about the side effects that go with various treatments.

One good thing about prostate cancer's timing—coming as it often does, later in life—is that for many men, it may be enough simply to delay the progression of the disease. This isn't exactly prevention—it's not keeping prostate cancer from developing in the first place—but if it means that a man can live *with* his cancer and that it won't progress, this tactic will still save lives. Imagine that you're watching a pretty good program on TV when, suddenly, it's interrupted by a very unwelcome message. That's how, if you'll forgive the TV analogy, prostate cancer blasts into men's lives today. But imagine that you can reduce this disruptive message to a crawl across the bottom of the screen; you can even hit the mute button. It's still there, but it can't hurt you; you're okay. Wouldn't that be wonderful?

Ideally, of course, prevention means forestalling prostate cancer, nipping it before it ever starts. There are two ways to do this: One is to *start* doing something new. The other is to *stop* doing something that you've been doing for years. We'll start with the first.

## Chemoprevention

Cancer has two basic phases: initiation and progression. Chemoprevention—adding a drug or dietary agent to your usual regime—can be used as a weapon for either phase. The idea, as we discussed above, is either to keep cancer from forming or to delay or stop its growth. You may not be familiar with the term, but you're almost certainly well acquainted with the concept. It's what you're doing when you use a fluoride toothpaste to keep cavities at bay. If you have heart disease, you might be using aspirin, cholesterol-lowering drugs, or blood pressure medication as chemoprevention to lower your risk of a stroke or heart attack. It's the chemical idea of "an apple a day," and it has had great success in many areas of medicine. Chemoprevention is still new in prostate cancer, but here are some promising candidates currently under study.

### 5-Alpha Reductase Inhibitors (Finasteride and Dutasteride)

The active form of the male hormone in the prostate is not testosterone but dihydrotestorone, or DHT (see chapter 1 for more details). It is the job of an enzyme called 5-alpha reductase, toiling away in the prostate—like Rumpelstiltskin, transforming straw into gold—to turn testosterone into DHT.

But this process can be stopped short. Two drugs, Proscar (finasteride) and Avodart (dutasteride), can block this enzyme and prevent testosterone from changing into DHT. As a result, the amount of DHT in the bloodstream and in prostate tissue drops. Both of these drugs, called 5-alpha reductase inhibitors, are already in use for another prostate problem. They shrink the prostate, especially the tissue surrounding the urethra, and ease the symptoms of benign prostatic enlargement (BPH). And because testosterone is not affected, impotence is generally not a side effect.

What does this have to do with prostate cancer? For one thing, 5-alpha reductase inhibitors lower a man's levels of PSA. Also, scientists speculate, these drugs might slow down prostate activity in general. Another thought is that, because they alter the prostate's normal hormonal pattern—and prostate cancer is intrinsically linked to hormone activity—prostate cancer might be stopped before the disease gets a foothold. The idea is very similar to the one behind the use of tamoxifen in the prevention of breast cancer.

However, there are a few problems with this thinking. First, it is very possible that testosterone, and not DHT, is the major hormone that feeds prostate cancer. This is based on the fact that the levels of 5-alpha reductase are very low in prostate cancer. Further, when men with advanced prostate cancer are treated with a 5-alpha reductase inhibitor, the effect is marginal at best. This raises questions as to whether these drugs will have any effect in preventing the disease, especially in preventing high-grade, or aggressive, prostate cancer. (Tamoxifen, in contrast, is very active in advanced breast cancer.)

Thus, lowering DHT with a 5-alpha reductase inhibitor may not do much to reduce a man's risk of developing prostate cancer. The National Cancer Institute recently finished a study of nearly nineteen thousand men who were randomly assigned to take either finasteride (5 mg a day) or a placebo for seven years. The men underwent a prostate biopsy if they had an abnormal digital rectal examination or elevated PSA level, and when the study was over, about one-third of the men also underwent biopsies. The study's authors found that there were 25 percent fewer cases of prostate cancer in the men who received finasteride, but there was also a 65 percent *increase* in the number of men who developed high-grade (Gleason 7–10; see chapter 6) disease.

What's going on here? First, let's look at the 25 percent drop in prostate cancer. This may not be as dramatic as it seems. If we look at the men who underwent a biopsy during the study because they developed an elevated PSA or had an abnormal digital rectal examination, there was only a 10 percent decrease in prostate cancer caused by finasteride. The rest of this decrease happened because the men in the finasteride group were less likely to have biopsies at all; 15 percent fewer of these men underwent a biopsy. It may be that they thought they didn't need one, because *5-alpha reductase inhibitors lower PSA by at least half.* The study coordinators knew which men were receiving the finasteride, and simply doubled their PSA levels when they compared them with those from the men who were not receiving the drug. But the men themselves didn't know whether they were receiving the finasteride (this was a single-blind study). Many of them may have rechecked their PSA before undergoing a biopsy, and when they saw how low it was, didn't have the biopsy.

Now, what about the troubling increase in the more aggressive, harder-to-cure, high-grade prostate cancer? Scientists have explored several theories. One is that finasteride simply changed the way the prostate cancer cells looked, making them appear to be high-grade. This was not the case; they really were the aggressive kind of cancer. Another idea is that because finasteride shrinks the prostate, cancer was easier to find in these men with a needle biopsy—that with less tissue there, the odds of finding cancer were higher. This theory, however, didn't hold up in a later study of men who underwent a radical prostatectomy. The high grade cancers remained high grade in the men who took finasteride, and the low-grade cancers did not become high-grade more often in the men who took a placebo. It also appears that PSA testing was more sensitive in detecting high-grade cancers in men on finasteride—and this is most likely the major reason there were more high-grade tumors. And finally, finasteride does not prevent high-grade disease.

Some researchers have suggested that the effect of finasteride is procarcinogenic—cancer-promoting, in other words—and that finasteride actually helps the high-grade cancers grow because more testosterone builds up in the prostate when the 5-alpha reductase enzyme is blocked. That's a possibility. But I believe it's more likely that this is merely a treatment effect and that finasteride simply works better at treating the lower-grade elements of prostate cancer. If it mainly targets the lower Gleason patterns, then the cancers would appear more often to be high-grade.

We'll discuss Gleason grading much more in chapter 6, but briefly, it's a score—two numbers added together to make a total—assigned by the pathologist who looks at the tissue samples taken during a needle biopsy. Prostate cells aren't like checkers, for example, with black ones being normal and red ones being cancer. Instead, they're as varied as marbles. Cancerous cells come in five basic patterns. The pathologist figures out which of these five patterns is most common and which is second most common and then adds them together to create a score. Gleason scores of 6 or lower mean the cancer is considered moderate to low grade; Gleason scores 7 or higher are considered high grade.

If finasteride has a more potent effect on Gleason patterns 1, 2, and 3—leaving only the higher grades behind—this could explain why men who take it are diagnosed with higher-grade cancer. This effect would also be amplified if finasteride does not prevent the high-grade tumors.

At present, there is no general agreement on the use of 5-alpha reductase inhibitors as a means of preventing prostate cancer. But for now, it appears that they do not prevent the high-grade tumors that are the most life-threatening. Until we know more, these drugs shouldn't be used for this purpose. Another study, called Reduction by Dutasteride of Prostate Cancer Events (REDUCE), is testing the effect of dutasteride in eight thousand men over four years. Although dutasteride and finasteride have much in common, they also have some key differences. Finasteride blocks one particular enzyme, which is limited to the prostate. Dutasteride blocks this enzyme and another as well (an enzyme that's also found elsewhere in the body), and it may be that dutasteride is more effective at preventing cancer. If you are taking finasteride or dutasteride for the treatment of BPH and it's working well for you, then you should keep taking it.

### Selenium

Selenium is a mineral found in the soil. It appears in fruits and vegetables, and also in meats and fish. The average American probably eats about 70 mcg (micrograms) of selenium a day. However, this can vary, depending on where we live and, more importantly, where the food we eat has been grown, because some soils are far richer in selenium than others.

In a large study conducted several years ago, people who had been treated for skin cancer were given selenium supplements in hopes of preventing the cancer from coming back. During the course of the study, the researchers noticed that the patients getting selenium developed fewer other cancers—prostate, lung, colon—than patients in the placebo group. The incidence of prostate cancer in these men, in fact, was two-thirds less than that of the men in the placebo group.

Their intriguing results prompted Johns Hopkins researchers to design their own case-control study of selenium's beneficial role in prostate cancer, using the valuable database of the Baltimore Longitudinal Study of Aging (a study begun more than forty years ago and involving about 1,500 men who return every other year for physical examinations and medical tests). In this study, the Hopkins scientists studied fifty-two men with prostate cancer and ninety-six age-matched controls, men of the same age who did not have cancer. Their findings were exciting. For one thing, they discovered that in both of these groups—men who developed prostate cancer and men who did not—the level of selenium in the blood dropped over time. In other words, selenium apparently decreases in everybody with age. "Yet, no other cancer increases more rapidly with age than prostate cancer," notes Johns Hopkins urologist H. Ballentine Carter. "For all we know, selenium levels are playing a role in that." This investigation also confirmed what the skin cancer study had suggested—that selenium seems to protect against prostate cancer. In the Hopkins study, men with the lowest levels of selenium were those most likely to develop prostate cancer, and men with the highest levels of selenium were almost 50 percent less likely to develop it. Other studies have shown that people living in regions of the United States with selenium-rich soil have fewer deaths from many kinds of cancer—including cancer of the lung, colon, esophagus, pancreas, breast, and ovary. One recent study looked at the level of selenium in toenails (the idea being that toenails—like rings on a tree—tell a story of the body's intake of minerals over the last year or so). This study, too, found that men with the highest levels of selenium were significantly less likely to have prostate cancer.

How does it work? It turns out that selenium is an essential component of an antioxidant—glutathione peroxidase, an enzyme like glutathione-S-transferase-$\pi$ that helps the body fight off potentially toxic substances. One of the most exciting things about selenium is that it seems to make a difference in the body within just a few years, which encourages scientists to think that a man can take it later in life and still potentially change the course of prostate cancer.

Some scientists speculate that in the future, when men go to the doctor for a PSA blood test, they will also have their selenium level checked. If it turns out to be low, just taking a daily selenium supplement (already available where most vitamins are sold) for several years or maybe a lifetime may help prevent prostate cancer.

However, to sound the gong for moderation yet again: Too much selenium may do more harm than good. Caution is the message from two recent selenium studies. In one, the effect of selenium was tested in dogs; groups of animals were given different levels of selenium for seven months. DNA damage turned out to be the highest in dogs at either end of the spectrum—those with the lowest and those with the highest levels of selenium. This study suggests that taking more selenium is not the best bet for every man, and that men who participate in similar prevention studies should have their baseline selenium levels tested first to make sure they don't get too much. Similar findings came out of the Nutritional Prevention of Cancer trial. In this large study, adding selenium to the diet reduced the overall incidence of prostate cancer, especially in former smokers and in men with low levels of selenium. But for men who already had high levels of selenium, taking more didn't help; in fact, there was a slightly higher incidence of prostate cancer in this group. Should you take selenium, and how much? See "Now What Do I Do?" below.

### Selenium and Vitamin E

It may be that selenium and vitamin E work better together than either does separately. To investigate this, the National Cancer Institute is sponsoring a twelve-year nationwide trial called the Selenium and Vitamin E Cancer Prevention Trial (SELECT), in which 32,000 men will be given either vitamin E alone, selenium alone, both vitamin E and selenium, or a placebo. The scientists in this study will be looking to see which of these men develop prostate cancer and which of these supplements, if any, seems to have a protective effect. Biopsies will be performed on men who develop an elevated PSA level or cancer that can be felt in a rectal exam. Final results from this study are expected by 2013.

### Vitamin E

Will vitamin E turn out to be the silver lining in the cloud that was the beta-carotene phenomenon? In one study in Finland, more than 29,000 men—all of whom smoked—were given either supplements of vitamin E alone, beta-carotene alone, both compounds, or a placebo for five to eight years. The men in both vitamin E groups (with or without beta-carotene) had a death rate from prostate cancer that was 41 percent lower than that of the other men. (Another benefit of the vitamin E: men taking it seemed to be less troubled by symptoms of BPH.) Another study of male smokers had similar findings—men with low levels of vitamin E in their blood were found to be at higher risk of developing prostate cancer. In laboratory studies, vitamin E—an antioxidant, a free-radical fighter—has been shown to slow down cancer growth; it also may have a boost-

## THE FIZZLE OF BETA-CAROTENE

Identifying beta-carotene as a possible cancer preventer was a milestone in dietary research, and it's important for you to know about it for the simple fact that here was a substance, extracted from vegetables, that sounded good, seemed promising in every way, but shocked everyone when it turned out to be a dud. This has had a profound impact on scientists who study diet and cancer, whose great fear is to end up with "another beta-carotene."

A few years ago, in several case-control studies, scientists noticed that smokers who ate a lot of fruits and vegetables seemed to be protected against lung cancer. What was it about fruits and vegetables that warded off cancer? The scientists homed in on beta-carotene, a nutrient that's abundant in vegetables. They wondered if beta-carotene could be a biomarker—a sort of barometer in the bloodstream—hypothesizing that people with high levels of beta-carotene would have a lower risk of lung cancer. Sure enough, in early studies with lab animals, beta-carotene performed like a champ, seeming to protect against several kinds of cancers.

Suddenly, beta-carotene was the hot new scientific flavor of the month, the focus of three separate studies. But then look what happened: "All of them showed not only that beta-carotene did not do what it was predicted to do and prevent lung cancer development—in two of the trials, it actually made things worse," explains the Johns Hopkins scientist William Nelson. In one study, men who received beta-carotene had an 18 percent *increase* in the incidence of lung cancer. Also, their rate of prostate cancer was 23 percent higher, and the death rate in these men was 15 percent higher than in men who did not receive the beta-carotene.

Beta-carotene turned out to be a cautionary tale that confirmed the perils of leaping before looking—and on the wrong bandwagon, no less. There may be several explanations for these results—whether the men continued smoking, for instance, and how beta-carotene affected their lungs. In any event, the story of beta-carotene highlights yet again the trouble of trying to pinpoint an element of diet and determine whether it has the power to prevent cancer.

ing effect on the body's immune system to help it battle cancer more effectively.

Is vitamin E protective against prostate cancer? Or is it just more protective in smokers than it is in other men? These two trials were limited to men who smoked. Since then, two other major studies have tested vitamin E in nonsmokers, and both failed to show that it helped lower the risk of prostate cancer (or any other cancer, for that matter). Further, scientists are now concerned that high doses of vitamin E—400 international units (IU) a day or more—may have harmful consequences for the heart. One recent meta-analysis found an increased risk of heart failure in people who took these high doses of vitamin E. What does this mean? Until the results from the SELECT trial are known, the safest bet is to *be cautious in taking vitamin E as a means of preventing prostate cancer*. If you take it, you should do so only in the doses that are available in the standard multivitamin—40–60 IU a day.

Note: Too much vitamin E can be dangerous in another way, especially if you are taking aspirin or a blood thinner such as warfarin. Like aspirin and warfarin, vitamin E reduces the blood's ability to clot. Before you jump on the vitamin E (or any) bandwagon, talk to your doctor to make sure this is safe for you. Also, you must stop taking vitamin E before you undergo any surgical procedure to avoid the risk of excess bleeding. (Find this out from your surgeon at least three weeks ahead of time so your blood will be back to normal well before surgery.)

### Nonsteroidal Anti-Inflammatory Drugs (NSAIDs)

In chapter 3, we talked about inflammation's role in the development of prostate cancer. This inflammation is usually so subtle that it causes no symptoms; men don't even know they have it. But within the prostate, it's a different story. Imagine how uncomfortable your face feels when it's sunburned; this is inflammation, and when it's persistent, it can create a situation of chronic stress. Over time, explains the Johns Hopkins epidemiologist Elizabeth Platz, "it may create an environment that is conducive to cancer." This begs the question: If inflammation can cause prostate cancer, could anti-inflammatory agents help prevent it?

Scientists are very interested in finding this answer, and they have a ready-made population in which to start looking—men taking aspirin or other nonsteroidal anti-inflammatory drugs (NSAIDs). These drugs block the cyclooxygenase enzymes, which play a key role in the body's inflammatory response. One large study of these men found that men taking NSAIDs had a 15 percent lower risk of developing prostate cancer than those who weren't taking them.

Platz, with colleagues at Hopkins and at the National Institute of Aging, recently studied 1,244 men participating in the Baltimore Longitudinal Study of Aging. The researchers found that men who used aspirin or other NSAIDs had a 29 percent lower risk of prostate cancer than men who did not use these drugs. This finding was published in the journal *Cancer Epidemiology, Biomarkers & Prevention.* "The lower risk of prostate cancer in the users of aspirin and non-aspirin suggests a modest, but possibly genuine benefit of these anti-inflammatory drugs," Platz says.

But this protection doesn't spring forth overnight, and just taking an aspirin a day for a few weeks won't do it. A large study of seventy thousand men, part of the American Cancer Society's Cancer Prevention Study II Nutritional Cohort, found that an effect could be seen only in men who regularly took thirty pills a month for five years or more. These men showed almost a 20 percent reduction in the development of prostate cancer. Studies on the use of NSAIDs in preventing colon cancer have shown similar results. In one, it took an average of two tablets a day for ten years or longer before doctors could see a noticeable reduction in the formation of polyps.

## Statins

Statins are drugs such as Lipitor, Mevacor, Pravachol, Zocor, Lescol, and Baycol (atorvastatin, lovastatin, pravastatin, simvastatin, fluvastatin, and cerivastatin). They lower cholesterol and reduce the risk of a heart attack or stroke by blocking an enzyme called HMG-coenzyme A (CoA) reductase. Can they also lower the risk of prostate cancer? So far, their effect on cancers, including prostate cancer, has been somewhat inconsistent. But several recent studies suggest that they may reduce the risk of the most deadly kinds of prostate cancer—advanced and metastatic disease.

My colleague, the Johns Hopkins epidemiologist Elizabeth Platz, led a large investigation of nearly 35,000 men as part of the Health Professionals Follow-Up study. The men, ages forty-four to seventy-nine, did not have prostate cancer when the study started in 1990. Ten years later, 2,074 men from the entire study group (those taking statins and those not taking them) had developed prostate cancer. Platz and colleagues found that men who took the cholesterol-lowering drugs had no difference in the risk of early, curable prostate cancer but were 50 to 60 percent less likely to have advanced and metastatic prostate cancer than other men. Also, the longer the men used these drugs, the more their risk for advanced prostate cancer decreased.

Was it the lower cholesterol level that protected these men, or did the protection stem from the drugs that lowered their cholesterol? That's not clear yet, says Platz. But scientists do know that cholesterol isn't just in the arteries—it's in prostate cancer cells, too, and in prostate cell membranes. Getting rid of the cholesterol may interrupt the communication of some proteins that act in prostate cancer. One of these is the interestingly named Hedgehog protein, which is active in high-grade cancers. (This is discussed in chapter 12.) Statins can have side effects in some people, so until more data are available, they are not currently recommended for use as a means of preventing prostate cancer. However, because of the promising results of these studies, they are actively being investigated in this light.

## Zinc

Zinc is an essential element, abundant in a host of foods—red meat, poultry, beans, nuts, and fortified cereals, to name a few. It's so common, in fact, that most of us get all we need just by eating a well-balanced diet. Zinc seems fond of the prostate; it tends to accumulate there in higher quantities than in any other location. Some studies have suggested that zinc might also help protect the prostate from cancer.

There is no good evidence that taking extra zinc increases a man's resistance to prostate cancer, but many men take zinc supplements. Some 10 percent of men who take these supplements get two to three times the U.S. Recommended Daily Allowance (RDA) of 11 mg a day. In this case, once again, more is not better—in fact, there's clearly a point of diminishing returns.

Too much zinc is bad. Recent results from the Health Professionals Follow-Up Study showed that men who take a daily dose of more than 100 mg of supplemental zinc have a higher risk of developing advanced prostate cancer. This is a huge amount of zinc. Where could these men have gotten such high doses? A vitamin store. ProstaPro, for example, contains 65 mg of zinc per tablet, and the suggested dose is two tablets a day. Another supplement, called Maximum Potential for Men, provides 100 mg a day. Many of our patients—men who are trying hard to stay healthy—take several different vitamin supplements every day. Some of these men consume more than 100 mg of zinc a day without even knowing it.

There is no good reason for you to take a zinc supplement. If you do add zinc to your diet, you certainly must not take more than 11 mg daily, the U.S. RDA's suggested dose.

## Dietary Prevention:
## How Food Can Help Your Body Fight Cancer

In chapter 3, we talked about the things that cause prostate cancer, including such environmental factors as food. If "bad" foods can help cause prostate cancer, could it be that "good" foods can help prevent it? Can we use food as preventive medicine? Yes. In fact, many scientists believe this is what rural Asian men do every day and why these men so rarely develop prostate cancer that needs to be treated (see chapter 3).

How can diet help your body fight prostate cancer? There are two main ways. The first is in preventing or delaying onset of the disease. Cancer that is big enough to be diagnosed today probably started growing at least ten years ago (this is discussed in chapter 3). Most men are diagnosed with prostate cancer in their late sixties. This means that even men in their fifties and early sixties should be able to make a significant difference in their body's ability to fight off cancer. The second area of promise is in slowing the growth of cancer that has already begun. Here, diet is one of several avenues being explored to lengthen the life of a man with established or advanced prostate cancer—with the ultimate goal of managing it as a chronic disease, like diabetes or even AIDS, which may not be possible to cure, but which can be controlled for many years.

A recent study from San Francisco is a good example of this new tack in scientific thinking. Men with early, slow-growing, minimal prostate cancer (a very small amount of cancer with a low Gleason score—see chapter 6 for a description) were randomly placed either into a control group or an intervention group for a year. The men in the control group had regular checkups to monitor their cancer, but the men in the experimental group pulled out all the stops in an effort to alter the course of their disease. They embarked on an intensive lifestyle program, including a vegan diet supplemented with soy, fish oil, vitamin E, selenium, and vitamin C. They performed moderate aerobic exercise, learned stress-management techniques, and spent an hour a week in a support group. The doctors who designed this study threw in everything but the proverbial kitchen sink. But the gains, at the end of the year, were modest. Men in the experimental group had a 4 percent decrease in PSA, while men in the control group had a 6 percent increase in PSA. It's hard to know what to make of these results; it may be that the study simply didn't last long enough. Also, changes in PSA level do not necessarily reflect cancer growth. But the study marks an important milestone in our fight against prostate cancer—the idea that diet can be used as a potential weapon.

Another study lasted longer (four years instead of one), and even this might not have been enough time to see the results of eating a cancer-fighting diet. In this study, men who didn't have cancer received intensive training on good eating that promoted eating foods low in fat and high in fiber, and lots of fruits and vegetables, to see if this changed PSA levels or affected the incidence of prostate cancer. The scientists leading the study could detect no difference between these men and those in the control group. But remember, prostate cancer is a disease of a lifetime's worth of incremental building blocks. It may be that four years of healthy living doesn't amass enough positive changes to be detectable on the PSA radar screen.

Compared to research in other aspects of medicine, the idea of altering the course of cancer with diet is still relatively new. In western medicine, doctors have tended to believe in, and search for, the Holy Grail or the magic bullet—that single answer, the one antibiotic to cure the infection, the all-powerful agent to cure cancer. Fortunately, this is changing, and so is the idea of medicinal one-stop shopping. If you were to spend an afternoon in a library reading the medical journals published during the last decade, you would notice that the number of scientific articles pertaining to nutrition, nutritional supplements (vitamins, herbs, and minerals), and disease has skyrocketed in recent years. Now, scientists worldwide are working to isolate specific cancer-fighting substances—some of which we'll discuss in a moment—in the hopes of making nutraceuticals, or drugs extracted from specific nutrients. This is very exciting work.

And yet, to put it in perspective, much of this research is simply confirming something scientists have known for decades, an inescapable finding so basic that it easily could be put into the category called "Duh!" The best way to prevent cancer is to eat more fruits and vegetables, eat less red meat and fewer dairy products, consume fewer calories in general, and burn off a few of those calories with regular exercise. This is why the American Cancer Society, for years, has made the following recommendations: Make sure most of what you eat comes from plants. Eat five or more servings of fruits and vegetables a day and other foods from plant sources, including breads, grains, rice, pasta, or beans, several times a day. Eat foods low in fat, and limit your consumption of meats, particularly meat high in fat. Stay within your healthy weight range (see the body mass index table in chapter 3), and get at least moderate exercise for thirty minutes or more on most days of the week.

An article in the English medical journal *Lancet* doesn't mince words about what needs to happen: "In England, four and a half times as many people die now from cancer as half a century ago. Probably no single factor is more important in determining the outbreak of cancer in the predisposed than high feeding. Many indications point to the gluttonous consumption of meat as likely to be especially harmful. Statistics show that the consumption of meat has reached the amazing total of 131 pounds per head per year, which is more than double what it was half a century ago. No doubt other factors cooperate, among these I should be inclined to name deficient exercise and deficiency in fresh vegetable food." Makes good sense, doesn't it? Apparently not, because this article was written in 1898 as a scathing condemnation of Victorian dietary excess and its negative effect on health. It's a message that many of us still don't want to hear; more than a century later, a wildly popular crash-diet craze in the United States relies heavily on high-fat meats and protein—building a better body with bacon.

## Balance Is the Key

Eating the foods discussed in this chapter makes good sense. Most of them have been put to practical use for centuries in Asia, where clinical prostate cancer is so much rarer than it is in the United States. As we take a look at the most promising of these candidates for prostate cancer prevention, remember one final caveat: *moderation in all things*. The Asian diet isn't all soy, all the time—or all green tea, or all anything in particular. It's composed of a variety of foods, eaten in a balanced way. Because all of this research is still unfolding, take the findings from any of these early studies with—continuing the food metaphor—a big grain of salt. Remember, it is possible to overdose on just about anything. The most harmless substances can make you sick if you eat or drink too much of them. Even water—if you drink huge amounts of it in too short a time—can be harmful, causing dangerous imbalances in the body's electrolytes. This is why you must resist the "more is better" approach: "If 200 mcg of selenium are good for me, then 1,000 must be even more beneficial." Such thinking is dangerous. The body is a delicate thing, and no matter how tough yours may be, you can easily get too much of a good thing and defeat the purpose of trying to stay healthy.

## A Word on Oxidative Damage

Remember the foods in the category "sins of commission"—red meat loaded with animal fat, plus charred meat (see chapter 3)? They're bad, as far as cancer goes, because they hamper the body's ability to fend off oxidative damage. In oxidative damage, cells are injured by free radicals—volatile molecules that cause a buildup of toxic by-products in cells. Normally, free radicals are helpful things, rushing like the local militia to a scene of unrest, fighting bacteria and other foreign invaders. And normally, the body makes substances that are able to control free radicals and limit the damage they cause. The most important of these substances is the enzyme we discussed in the last chapter, glutathione-S-transferase-π (pronounced "pie," called GST-π for short), which cleans up toxins in cells.

The Johns Hopkins oncologist William G. Nelson was the first to figure out GST-π's role in prostate cancer. He showed that in all

---

## THE COMPLICATED BUSINESS OF FOOD RESEARCH

Think for a moment of the many nutrients you ingest every day—hundreds of them, in varying portions. Look at the labels of prepared foods—your morning cereal, a box of cake mix, a package of frozen lasagna, even a slice of bread—and consider just how many different things you're putting into your body with every meal.

Now imagine you're a scientist exploring the link between diet and prostate cancer, trying to figure out exactly what's wrong with the western diet or what's right with the Asian diet. Where do you begin? How many Americans eat one-ingredient meals? In the United States, even a pet goldfish consumes more than a dozen nutrients in a single flake of fish food. But even the simplest meal—a plain potato with no butter, salt, or pepper, for example—raises a host of questions: What is it about that potato that might raise or lower cancer risk? Is it (as many believe) selenium, a nutrient abundant in potatoes and other root vegetables? Or is it something else? Is it something found in all potatoes, or does it vary, depending on the mineral content of the soil in which that particular potato was grown?

Get the picture? Food research is intensely complicated and frustrating because what seems obvious in lab studies—in petri dishes and test tubes—doesn't always pan out when those same tests are attempted in humans. It's also time-consuming. Say the scientist isolates a food or nutrient that actually seems to prevent prostate cancer. What's the dose? How much of it, in other words, does a man need, per day, per week, to achieve the desired effect? Will he have to take it forever? These aren't short-term questions, so it will take several years, at minimum, before we can find the answers.

---

cancers and even in the cells that are not yet cancerous but well on their way (these cells are called PIN, discussed further in chapter 6), GST-$\pi$ is knocked out—it is simply not there to prevent oxidative damage. If cancer is a chain reaction—one genetic mistake, or mutation, that leads to another, and so on—then what happens to this enzyme, he believes, is probably among the very earliest events.

The attack against GST-$\pi$—apparently all that stands in the way of prostate cells and potentially toxic agents—happens first. It's the preemptive strike. A small, smoldering fire in a wastepaper basket doesn't get very far if there's a powerful sprinkler system overhead. The theory is the same here: without this cancer-fighting enzyme— this genetic fire extinguisher—prostate cells are far less able to detoxify carcinogens and are infinitely more vulnerable to prostate cancer. Small fires can become dangerous much more quickly.

Several years ago, Nelson began to wonder whether GST-$\pi$, which can be knocked out by bad environmental agents, can be stimulated by good environmental agents. Is there some dietary equivalent to weight lifting that can build up the wimpy enzyme before it's too late, so it can fend for itself—and perhaps deter prostate cancer? In other words, is it possible to use food or some particular nutrient as preventive medicine?

Nelson, a pioneer in this area, is not alone. All over the world, scientists in many disciplines are studying diet as never before—for the first time, trying to understand exactly how specific foods work in the body, right down to which particular enzymes (like GST-$\pi$) are helped or hurt by what we eat and drink. Where are the smoking guns—the cancer instigators? Again, the basic "omission versus commission" question: is it something we eat too much of or something we routinely omit from our meals?

*How much fat?* If too much animal fat is bad, how much fat is not bad? How much fat is it okay to eat? An American Cancer Society study of more than 400,000 men showed that eating a high-calorie, high-fat diet increases the risk of dying from prostate cancer. In this study, researchers found the risk is lowest when the fat content in the diet is 15 percent or lower—which, in most western countries, is downright hard to achieve (see below). When it's 28 percent or higher, the risk doubles. Results from several other studies give an acceptable fat content that's slightly higher; these studies suggest that no more than 20 percent of your total calories should be in the form of fat.

What does a 20 percent fat diet mean for you? If you weigh about 150 pounds, your caloric intake should be about 2,000 kilocalories (when doctors talk about calories, they really mean kilocalories) a day. There are 9 kilocalories in each gram of fat. Thus, you should have no more than 44 grams of fat a day.

Note: It is not clear whether eating a diet composed of less than 20 percent fat would be even more successful or whether there would be a point of diminishing returns. That's just as well, because in the United States, it is virtually impossible to avoid fat altogether. At almost any restaurant, if you eat a typical menu item—a jumbo beef burrito or a bacon-cheese omelet, for instance—you could blow

---

### FRUITS AND VEGETABLES: WHY EAT "FIVE A DAY"?

What exactly is it about fruits and vegetables that makes the American Cancer Society recommend that we eat at least five servings a day? Well, some of them contain known antioxidants, such as selenium and lycopene. Others—cruciferous vegetables such as broccoli, Brussels sprouts, and cauliflower—contain an ingredient called sulforaphane, which acts by increasing the amount of GST-$\pi$ in cells. The result: Your cells make more of their own natural antioxidants, so they can do a better job of fighting off cancer.

One study suggests that, for prostate cancer at least, vegetables do more than fruits (although fruits are just plain good for you in general, and you still need to eat them, or drink fruit juice, every day). This study, published in the *Journal of the National Cancer Institute*, found no link between fruit intake and prostate cancer risk but confirmed what other studies have shown—that eating a lot of vegetables, particularly the cruciferous kind, lowered the risk.

---

several days' worth of fat content in a single meal. Look at what we Americans like to eat: french fries, fried potato chips, fried chicken (notice a theme here?), multiple-meat pizzas, ice cream—they're all loaded with fat. Even the vegetable offerings at many eateries—such as fried zucchini and onion rings—are not designed with cancer prevention in mind. Your best bet is to check the labels of packaged foods and the fat content of food in restaurants (many big restaurant chains provide this information).

### Soy: Isoflavones, Phytoestrogens, and Genistein

Is soy really a wonder drug? Or does it simply prevent cancer because of all the things soy eaters are not eating instead? (Back to the old "sins of commission" versus "sins of omission" argument.) For example, there aren't many Big Macs in the Asian diet.

Increasingly, scientific evidence suggests that it's more than what soy eaters *don't* eat. In fact, although advertisements proclaim bananas to be "quite possibly nature's most perfect food," the many proponents of soy as a cancer fighter have good reason to disagree. In laboratory studies, an extract of soy has been shown to inhibit the growth of prostate cancer.

What, exactly, is soy? It's soybeans and the many products made from them: tofu (which comes in various forms and textures), soy sauce, soy tempeh (blocks made from fermented soybeans), soy milk, soy flour, and a rapidly expanding host of other products. Phyto-chemicals are chemicals that come from fruits and vegetables (*phyto* means "vegetable matter"). There is a particular class of phyto-chemicals in soy called isoflavones, and the biggest of these—and the one stirring up the most scientific interest—is called genistein.

In the late 1980s, genistein entered the field of potential anti-cancer agents when laboratory studies showed that it could inhibit a key enzyme—the epidermal growth factor tyrosine kinase, which speeds up cell division (thus, it could slow tumor growth). Since then, genistein has also been found to block proliferation of glan-dular cells (such as those found in the prostate) and to thwart a process called angiogenesis. Angiogenesis (which we'll discuss fur-ther in chapter 12) is the laying down of new blood vessels, and this is a major way that cancers spread—paving the road ahead of them-selves. Cancer needs a ready blood supply. If this process is blocked by something called an angiogenesis inhibitor, then the cancer can't go anywhere. It doesn't die, but it doesn't grow, either. Some scien-tists believe that isoflavones such as genistein can prevent tumor pro-motion or progression simply by blocking the formation of new blood supplies. Genistein is also what's called a phytoestrogen; found in some plants, phytoestrogens have the properties of a weak form of estrogen. Genistein has been found to inhibit the growth of breast cancer cells in laboratory studies. Other studies have shown that newborn rats given genistein had a lower incidence of breast cancer, and that genistein can also restrain the growth of prostate cancer cells and lower PSA levels.

For most Asians, soy is a mealtime staple. For most Americans—although this is slowly changing—it's barely a blip on the dietary radar. Consider these statistics: Most American men eat only 1 to 3 mg of isoflavones a day. In contrast, the average Japanese man con-sumes an estimated 12 mg a day. The blood levels of isoflavones may be at least seven times higher in Japanese men than in men on the typical western diet—and maybe much higher.

*Et tu, tofu?* Remember our dietary mantra. The key to all of this, even soy, is *moderation in all things*. This was suggested yet again by the unexpected results of one long-term study, the thirty-five-year longitudinal Honolulu-Asia Aging study, of the effects of different foods on rates of disease, aging, and death. In this study, 3,734 surviving participants over age seventy answered questions about their eating and drinking habits, including their consumption of rice, fish, meat, soy products, milk, green tea, and coffee.

Surprisingly, the researchers found that elderly Japanese American men who ate tofu regularly during midlife showed more cognitive decline in their later years than those who didn't eat as much. The increased rates of cognitive decline were "roughly of the magnitude as would be caused by a four-year difference in age," said the Honolulu researchers, who reported their findings in the *Journal of the American College of Nutrition*. Only tofu, they found, could be linked to this decline: 96 percent of the men who "almost never" ate tofu had normal cognitive function (based on screening tests, adjusted for age and education)—compared to 80.7 percent of the men who ate tofu more than four times a week.

These results have engendered much speculation as to how it could be that tofu might have an adverse effect on the aging brain. One theory is that tofu is high in glutamate, a neurotransmitter (a chemical messenger in the brain), and elevated levels of glutamate can cause free-radical damage to brain nerve cells, called neurons. However, as with any study of diet, it's tough to be certain. For example, researchers noted, it may be that the men who ate large quantities of tofu were from poorer families, and the lower cognitive ability was due to inadequate nourishment in childhood. In any event, we can be sure that many scientists will be seeking answers here. What does this mean for you? Again, moderation.

## Carotenoids: Vitamin A and Lycopene

There are two main types of vitamin A. One, called preformed vitamin A, comes from animals. This is the kind of vitamin A that most Americans get. The other is a carotenoid—a pigment found in green and yellow vegetables. Guess which kind is found most in the Asian diet? Yes, the carotenoid. It's hard to know what to make of vitamin A (see The Fizzle of Beta-Carotene above), because there is conflicting evidence. Although one group of researchers, in laboratory experiments with mice, found that vitamin A could reduce the incidence of prostate cancer, other studies suggest that not only does vitamin A *not* protect against prostate cancer, it might even increase a man's risk of getting it.

And yet, vitamin A is known to help cell differentiation. Cell differentiation is discussed more in chapter 6, but the idea here is that normal tissue and even slow-growing and "incidental" cancers are well differentiated. Well-differentiated cells, as seen under the microscope, have distinct, clearly defined borders and clear centers, and their growth is relatively slow and orderly. Poorly differentiated cells are murkier, not so well defined, and as cancer progresses, they seem to melt together into aggressive, malignant blobs. In the Gleason scoring system, well-differentiated cells are given a low score, and the more dangerous, poorly differentiated cells are given a high score (it's the opposite of when you were in school; in prostate cancer, low scores are better). The advice here is to keep eating carrots and other vegetables—which we know are good for you, even if we haven't yet pinpointed the exact reason *why* they are.

Today, the most exciting member of the group of carotenoids (although this one can't be converted to vitamin A) is another antioxidant—a free radical fighter that combats oxidative damage—called lycopene. In laboratory studies, lycopene has been shown to slow the growth of endometrial cancer cells, certain breast cancer cells, and some forms of lung cancer and leukemia.

Lycopene, found in tomatoes, pink grapefruits, watermelons, and berries (but not strawberries), entered the world of potential prostate cancer preventers a few years ago, as scientists studied results of a food frequency questionnaire (an analysis of diet). Of the men who had a lower incidence of prostate cancer, the common theme seemed to be food that contained cooked tomatoes—tomato sauce, like what tops pizza or spaghetti. The scientists zeroed in on lycopene as the likely reason for this decrease in cancer. However, although this idea is very popular—a great excuse to eat pizza and spaghetti—there may be more secret cancer-fighting agents lurking in tomatoes. In a study using rats, eating tomato powder—not just lycopene by itself—helped prevent prostate cancer from developing. Note: Cooking appears to release more of the lycopene in tomatoes, so cooked tomato-based pasta sauces and soups may be especially beneficial. And, because lycopene is fat soluble, it is best absorbed by the body when it's eaten along with some fat. Hello, olive oil! Rich in healthful monosaturated fats (see chapter 3), olive oil is the perfect choice for cooking tomatoes.

In a recent study, thirty-two men with localized prostate cancer (for more on what this means, see chapter 6) ate pasta dishes with tomato sauce for three weeks before their scheduled radical prostatectomy. When the prostate tissue was examined after surgery, pathologists found that DNA damage in prostate tissue—oxidative damage—was decreased significantly. Much evidence suggests that lycopene, and tomato sauce in general, can help protect the body against prostate cancer, although more studies are needed to prove this and to answer other questions. For example: Do men with prostate cancer have less lycopene in their prostates than men who don't have it? (The prostate seems to like lycopene. For one thing, lycopene—unlike many substances, including some medications—is actually absorbed by the prostate; for another, levels of lycopene are higher there than anywhere else in the body.) Are there lower levels among people who are going to get prostate cancer? (This could be tested in a study such as the Baltimore Longitudinal Study of Aging, which has decades' worth of data already stockpiled, monitoring the levels of lycopene in the blood samples of men as they age.) What do lycopene supplements actually do in men? One problem with studying any potential preventive treatment in prostate cancer is that such outcomes can take years. On the plus side for lycopene is the simple fact that—unlike many substances, including some antibiotics—it does manage to reach the prostate. In any event, it certainly won't hurt you to eat more tomato sauce.

### Green Tea

In Asia, many people drink more green tea than they do water—and many scientists believe the tea (like the other two commonly consumed nonherbal teas, black and oolong) has healthful, healing properties. Scientific evidence suggests that tea may help prevent cancer of the esophagus and maybe other cancers as well, including cancer of the pancreas, colon, and liver. It also may be beneficial to the heart.

The key is in the brewing. Interestingly, green, black, and oolong tea are all harvested from the same plant. The difference is in what happens to the plant next. If it's processed by heating the leaves right away, the leaves stay green and produce green tea. If the leaves are heated a bit later, the result is oolong tea; heating the leaves even later than this produces black tea. Despite their differences in taste and appearance, black and green teas (iced or hot) contain many of the same chemicals—including polyphenols, chemicals that are known to have cancer-fighting properties. Both black and green teas (less is known about oolong) are antioxidants. How much of a prostate cancer–fighter is green tea? Nobody knows yet. However, results from studies involving other types of cancer are encouraging: In one National Cancer Institute study in China, 900 patients with esophageal cancer were compared with 1,500 healthy people. Looking at the patients who didn't smoke or drink alcohol, the study found that green tea drinkers were about 60 percent less likely to develop cancer than others. In another study, of 14,000 older Americans in California, the risk of developing pancreatic cancer decreased in those who drank tea, and in an eight-year study of 35,000 postmenopausal women in Iowa, women who drank at least two cups of tea a day were much less likely—some 40 to 70 percent—to develop cancer of the digestive system or urinary tract than women who drank little or no tea.

Some components of green and brown teas, including catechin (pronounced "ca-TEAK-en"), epigallocatechin gallate (EGCG), and epicatechin, are being studied now. They are known to be biologically active, but the big question remains whether the consumption of large amounts of green tea is the reason that people in Asia—who also consume a lot of soy and eat more vegetables and less red meat—get prostate cancer less often. Nobody knows yet.

Note: In addition to all the good things it has, tea also has caffeine, which can make some people feel jittery or anxious. If you have heart problems—irregular heartbeats or high blood pressure—drinking a lot of tea may not be good for you. Tea can also heighten symptoms of gastroesophageal ulcers, colitis, and Crohn's disease, and—because it is rich in oxalates, a common ingredient of kidney stones, and potassium, which is sometimes difficult for people with kidney disease to process—may also increase the risk of kidney disease.

## DON'T OVERDO IT, ESPECIALLY WITH HERBAL REMEDIES

**H**erbs are natural. They're nature's healers—and that's a good thing, right? Well . . . the message we've been sending all along certainly applies here, too: *moderation is the key to any dietary agent.* Herbs can make you feel better; they can also make you sick. Even though they're natural, a single herbal remedy may contain thousands of active chemicals, and you can have a reaction to herbs just as you can to other drugs or foods.

A few examples:

• Long-term use of comfrey (*Symphytum officinale*) can cause significant liver damage.
• Ginkgo biloba, feverfew, and vitamin K should not be taken by people who are also taking blood thinners such as Coumadin (warfarin). Also, ginkgo biloba can react with MAO inhibitors (found in many antidepressants).
• Saint-John's-wort can also interfere with MAO inhibitors, can interact with chemicals found in certain types of cheese, red wine, and cured meats, and can make your skin more sensitive to sunlight (and thus, more likely to burn).
• Ginseng and ephedra can raise blood pressure and should not be taken by people with high blood pressure, diabetes, heart disease, or a blood-clotting disorder.

Closer to home, just a few years ago, many people sang the praises of—and gambled their health on—an herbal compound called PC-SPES, used to slow the progress of advanced prostate cancer. Unfortunately, it turned out that this natural drug had been significantly doctored up—with a synthetic estrogen called diethylstilbestrol (DES), plus an antianxiety drug, plus an anticoagulant to reduce the risk of clots that accompanies estrogen treatment. Similarly, there is a suggestion that some of the herbal compounds currently being advertised as treatments of erectile dysfunction contain small amounts of Viagra-like drugs.

The main thing you should know about herbal remedies is this: *caveat emptor*, or buyer beware. The U.S. Food and Drug Administration (FDA) makes sure that any drug sold in this country is safe and that it lives up to the manufacturer's claims. It takes its job very seriously. In fact, a common criticism of this agency is that its exacting standards often require manufacturers to perform years of testing before a drug can be made available to patients who need it. *But the FDA doesn't apply these same rigorous testing policies to herbs or the labels on herbal products.* Many people don't realize this; they are too trusting and think "It must be safe, or they couldn't sell it at the health-food store," or "It's natural. How could it hurt you?" Wrong. Because of the 1994 Dietary Supplement Health and Education Act, dietary supplements—a murky category that includes vitamins, minerals, herbal remedies, amino acids, and other herbal derivatives—are not only exempt from most federal regulation, manufactuers of them don't even have to file reports when someone has an adverse reaction to one of their products. How responsible is that?

Further, even though the law requires that an herbal remedy's label tell you how much each dose contains, these are often inaccurate. If this is true of a remedy you try, at best you'll be spending your money for a product whose benefit you're not fully receiving. At worst, you could get sick or even cause permanent damage to your liver or kidneys.

Your best bet is to buy herbs—even herbal teas—from a reputable company. Your odds of getting a contaminated product or substandard quality—such as some Asian herbals found by California investigators in 1998, which were tainted with lead, arsenic, or mercury—are much greater if you buy herbs or teas packaged in loose form, without manufacturer's packaging or detailed labels. And make sure your entire knowledge of the herb's benefits is greater than just the list of claims on the box or bottle. Even if the label says it's clinically proven, it may be referring to study results involving another brand—and there may be a difference in quality and effectiveness. Try to choose brands with the words "standardized extracts" on the label.

If you start to have any side effects, such as dizziness or nausea, or symptoms of allergic reaction, stop taking the drug, and talk to your doctor. If you develop more urgent symptoms, especially heart palpitations or trouble breathing, call your doctor or seek medical help right away. And finally, don't forget to mention any herbal supplements you're taking when your doctor asks you to list all of your medications.

## Red Wine

As we've said, if you like red wine, you're in luck: a large study in King County, Washington, found that men who drank red wine were less likely to develop prostate cancer. Drinking alcoholic beverages—even white wine—didn't seem to have this protective effect. No, it was definitely red wine; further, a man's relative risk of developing prostate cancer decreased by 6 percent with each additional glass of red wine he drank per week. Men who drank four or more glasses of red wine a week had a 50 percent reduction in relative risk. The study was carefully designed to avoid screening bias—say, for example, men who drink red wine are less likely to go to the doctor, and thus are less likely to have their cancer detected; then, their lack of detected cancer wouldn't have anything to do with their choice of beverage. Even more exciting, the researchers were able to show a 60 percent reduction in the diagnosis of Gleason 8 disease, which is more aggressive and more difficult to cure.

What's the secret ingredient? It may be something called resveratrol, a polyphenol that is concentrated in grape skins. It's made in response to a fungus that gathers on the skin of grapes—which means that there's more of it found in red wines from rainier years. Resveratrol appears to be an antioxidant and anti-inflammatory agent that also reduces cell proliferation (which means that it also slows down the growth of cancerous cells). It also inhibits angiogenesis (the making of new blood vessels, which allows cancer to spread). It's also antiandrogenic (it interferes with male hormone action). The researchers speculate that this may help explain why France has half as much prostate cancer as the United States and why Italy has 20 percent fewer cases.

## Pomegranate Juice

The most famous pomegranate in literature is eaten by a girl named Persephone in a Greek myth that explains why plants become dormant in the winter and come back to life again in the spring. The pomegranate has recently entered the literature of prostate cancer, and it's a major antioxidant. Native to Persia, this fruit is rich in polyphenols and cancer-fighting compounds called tannins, and it has a higher antioxidant activity than red wine or green tea. In a laboratory study from the University of Washington, pomegranate juice appeared not only to kill experimental tumors but to interrupt cancer-forming pathways—suggesting that it might be helpful in preventing cancer or perhaps in keeping it dormant. A preliminary study of forty-eight men with rising PSA levels suggested that drinking 8 ounces of pomegranate juice daily increased the time it took for PSA to rise.

## Cruciferous Vegetables

You know they're good for you. Broccoli, cauliflower, cabbage, Brussels sprouts, bok choy, kale—they're cruciferous vegetables, and they're rich in many things that your body needs to stay well. One of them is a protective compound called sulforaphane, which is known to increase GST-$\pi$—which, in turn, is the prostate's prime defender against oxidative damage and, ultimately, cancer. Several epidemiological studies have suggested that the more cruciferous vegetables a man eats, the lower his risk of prostate cancer. In one study, men who ate five or more servings of cruciferous vegetables a week eight years ago had a 10 to 20 percent lower risk of developing prostate cancer. This is very interesting because it suggests that eating these vegetables may be most effective as a preemptive strike early in the cancer-forming process.

## Now What Do I Do?

If you want to lower your risk of developing prostate cancer and dying from it, the first thing you should do is *eat fewer calories* or else exercise more, so you can maintain a healthy weight. Remember, as we talked about in chapter 3, the fat from red meat and dairy products fuels the enzyme that is most active in prostate cancer. Thus, *try to keep the amount of fat you get from red meat and dairy products to a minimum.*

*Watch your calcium intake.* Don't take supplemental doses far above the Recommended Daily Allowance (RDA). Some calcium is okay, but too much may not be. The risk of prostate cancer increases substantially only when men get more than the U.S. RDA of 1,000 to 1,500 mg of calcium a day. But a calcium intake at or lower than 1,500 mg daily may be helpful in preventing colon cancer and osteoporosis in older men.

*Eat more fish.* Evidence from two large studies suggests that fish help protect against prostate cancer because they have "good" fat—particularly omega-3 fatty acids.

Try to incorporate *cooked tomatoes*—cooked with olive oil, which also has beneficial fat—and *cruciferous vegetables* into many of your weekly meals.

*Eat more soy.* It doesn't have to be tofu; you can use soy sauce or drink soy milk (which comes in vanilla and chocolate flavors) or have frozen soy "ice cream."

Top off your meal with *green or black tea* or a glass of *red wine*.

The good thing about many of the foods we've discussed here is that they have very low toxicity. Eating more soy is not going to hurt you. It may help in terms of preventing cancer, and if eating more soy means that you eat less red meat and high-fat foods, it will benefit your cardiovascular system, too.

Now, for chemoprevention: until we know more about the effects of *5-alpha reductase inhibitors*, we cannot recommend them as a tool for preventing prostate cancer. If you are on a statin or NSAID for other reasons, you should keep taking it, under your doctor's care. But because these drugs can have side effects, you should not start taking them purely with the hope of preventing prostate cancer.

*Selenium:* How much selenium is good and how much is too much? The Institute of Medicine, part of the National Academy of Sciences, recommends 55 mcg per day; this is the amount that's present in many multivitamins designed for men. Before you take more than this, you should have your selenium level tested (it's a blood test; you can do it when you have your PSA test) to see whether you have a deficiency.

*Vitamin E:* The Institute of Medicine recommends 15 mg, or 22 IU, per day. Because of concerns raised in recent studies—the cardiovascular side effects in men taking 400 IU per day or more—you shouldn't add more vitamin E to your diet than 40 to 60 IU a day. This is the amount found in many multivitamins designed for men. Note: As noted above, vitamin E can increase the risk of excess bleeding. Before you begin this supplement, talk to your doctor. Also, it is essential that you stop taking vitamin E well in advance of any type of surgery. Once the SELECT trial is completed, we will know more about the safety and success of vitamin E (400 IU daily) and selenium (200 mcg daily) together.

What about other vitamins and supplements? *Moderation in all things.* Sobering evidence from a report by the Institute of Medicine warns the health conscious against taking megadoses of vitamins and dietary supplements. Not only does a jumbo-sized portion of selenium, for example, *not* provide jumbo-sized cancer protection, it can make you sick. The consequences of selenium toxicity, or poisoning, to the body include loss of hair and even fingernails. There is no evidence to suggest that megadoses of anything, even dietary antioxidants, can prevent chronic diseases.

*Other advice:* Eat an apple a day. Better yet, an apple, an orange, a bowl of vegetable soup, tomatoes, broccoli, and maybe some corn on the cob. Try nature's packaging of phytochemicals instead of the health-food store's. Findings from a Cornell University study published in *Nature* suggest that simply eating an apple gives your body far more antioxidant and cancer-fighting help than taking megadoses of vitamins.

Think about it: When a scientist isolates a single chemical from a piece of fruit, or a vegetable and a laboratory churns out huge doses of the compound, and you buy it, you're gambling that the scientist got it right. There may be hundreds of phytochemicals that were overlooked—and maybe one of these is the magic ingredient. Nobody knows yet. The best way to hedge your bets is to diversify: eat the real thing, if you can. In a study funded by the New York Apple Research and Development Program and the New York Apple Association, scientists found higher free radical–scavenging ability in apples with the skin than in those without the skin. And a single fresh apple packed a wallop of antioxidants—equal to 1,500 mg of vitamin C.

Finally, eating all the broccoli in the world—though it may make a difference in the long run—doesn't take away your risk of having prostate cancer right now. If you are age forty or older, have a family history of prostate cancer, or are African American, you need more than a good diet can guarantee. You need a yearly rectal exam and PSA test. Which brings us to chapter 5: Do I Have Prostate Cancer? Screening and Detection.

# 5

# DO I HAVE PROSTATE CANCER? SCREENING AND DETECTION

## ▶▶▶ READ THIS FIRST

At its earliest stages, prostate cancer is silent. There are no early warning signals—no symptoms at all, in fact, until the cancer grows outside the prostate and progresses to the point where it's rarely curable. Thus, if a man wants to maximize his odds of surviving prostate cancer, he needs to find out he has it when the disease is easiest to cure. The best way to detect prostate cancer early is through regular screening.

Although scientists are working hard to prevent prostate cancer, we're not there yet. So we're doing the next best thing—reducing deaths from prostate cancer through what's called secondary prevention. This means diagnosing the disease when it's at a curable stage and going after it with curative therapy.

The last two decades have seen a revolution in prostate cancer detection and treatment. Today, with the one-two punch of prostate-specific antigen (PSA) testing and the digital rectal examination of the prostate, most men are diagnosed at a curable stage, and the last decade has seen thousands of lives saved by this effective screening combination.

### Prostate Cancer Screening: What Should I Do?

Have a digital rectal exam and PSA test at age forty.
If your PSA level is lower than 0.6 ng/ml, have your next examinations at age forty-five.
If your PSA level is greater than 0.6 ng/ml, begin screening every two years.
If your rectal exam shows a suspicious lump or hard spot, have a biopsy *even if your PSA level is low.*

If the rectal exam is negative, the next step depends on your PSA level: You should have a biopsy if your PSA level is

- Greater than 2.5 ng/ml and you are age forty to forty-nine
- Greater than 3.0 ng/ml and you are age fifty to fifty-nine
- Greater than 4.0 ng/ml and you are sixty or older
- Lower than the above ranges (between 1 and 4), but has increased by more than 0.2 to 0.4 ng/ml per year over the last two years
- Greater than 4.0 but has increased by more than 0.75 ng/ml per year

These recommendations do not include free PSA. Should you have your free PSA tested? The free PSA test works best in men with PSA levels between 4 and 10, and less well in men with PSA levels of 2.5 to 4.0, and not well in men with lower PSA levels. It may come down to what bothers you most—the thought of missing cancer at the earliest possible diagnosis or having an unnecessary biopsy because of a false alarm.

You can relax until the next rectal exam and PSA test if your PSA level is:

- Less than 2.5 ng/ml and you are age forty to forty-nine
- Less than 3.0 ng/ml and you are age fifty to fifty-nine
- Less than 4.0 ng/ml and you are age sixty or older

And if your PSA velocity is:

- Lower than 0.2 to 0.4 ng/ml per year and your PSA level is between 1 and 4 ng/ml.

- Lower than 0.75 ng/ml per year and your PSA level is greater than 4 ng/ml.

Remember, these recommendations refer to total PSA alone, not to free PSA. If you are worried about having cancer and your free PSA is less than 25 percent, you should undergo a biopsy even if your total PSA is within the above ranges. And finally, all of these recommendations may change if one of the promising new approaches to testing comes into widespread use.

## Why You Should Be Tested

Tomorrow, we may be able to prevent prostate cancer. Today, the best we can do is work to catch the disease early—at a point where the tumor is curable in men who are going to live long enough to need to be cured (more on this below). Over the last decade, thousands of lives have been saved by the highly effective one-two punch of the PSA blood test and the digital rectal examination. ("Digital" here doesn't mean some high-tech test; indeed, it's just the opposite. It simply means that this exam is performed using the doctor's finger, or digit).

Scientists have learned an awful lot about PSA over the last two and a half decades. (PSA stands for prostate-specific antigen, an enzyme made by the prostate that can be checked in a simple blood test). Despite this, it's still a pretty new diagnostic tool. Until the late 1980s, the test was virtually unheard of by patients and was used by doctors mainly to monitor already diagnosed prostate cancers. But the 1990s were, in effect, the "PSA decade." We learned that simply checking a man's blood regularly and watching for a rise in his levels of PSA can predict cancer years before it can be diagnosed by any other means. Any recurrence of PSA after treatment for prostate cancer—even more specifically, how soon it comes back and how fast it rises—can give important clues about the nature of the cancer (whether it's aggressive or mild-mannered, for instance, and how best to attack it). Despite all these advances, there are still some basic questions about PSA—which, by the way, still rattles or just plain stumps many physicians who discourage use of the test because they are unsure how to interpret the results, or because they cling to the persistent but obsolete belief that prostate cancer screening will never work.

This is the problem: Prostate cancer is easiest to cure early on, before it spreads outside the prostate. But unfortunately, it hardly ever produces symptoms until it spreads outside the prostate. Thus, if a man wants to maximize his odds of having prostate cancer detected when it's most curable, he needs to catch it early, and the best way to do that is with regular screening.

It's a simple idea—and one that's been proven to save lives. And yet, the PSA test didn't just spring forth out of the laboratory and into the pantheon of trusted tests for cancer. Many doctors in the 1980s and well into the 1990s were concerned that the test would open a diagnostic can of worms by finding cancer in every man—and then what would happen? This is because, at autopsy, about 30 to 40 percent of men are found to have a small amount of prostate cancer that doesn't do a whole lot—that just seems to percolate in the prostate but not spread. This cancer never causes symptoms, is very slow-growing, and may never need treatment. Would the PSA test, then, do more harm than good? Would it take these heretofore happy men, put the fear of cancer in them, force them to choose a course of treatment—which, nearly two decades ago, often had unpleasant side effects and did not always cure the cancer—and otherwise generally ruin their lives? Fortunately, as it turns out, the answer is no. Over the years, we have learned enough about PSA to identify these men with slow-growing, indolent cancer—"good" cancer, if there is such a thing—and manage their disease without subjecting them to premature, aggressive treatment.

In the early days of PSA screening, there was also great concern, and for good reason, that the test was not cancer-specific, but merely prostate-specific. And because not every man with an elevated PSA level had cancer, this screening forced some men to undergo further tests, such as a needle biopsy, that were not necessary. This, too, has proven largely unfounded. For perspective, let's look at the accuracy of mammography. Which test do you think is more of a bull's-eye for cancer? Say a fifty-year-old woman learns that her mammogram is positive, and on the same day her fifty-year-old husband finds out he has a PSA level greater than 4 ng/ml. Which spouse is more likely to harbor cancer? It's the husband. In the United States, the odds that a woman with a positive mammogram will have cancer vary with her age. The likelihood of having cancer is 19 percent for women over age seventy, 17 percent for women in their sixties, 9 percent for women in their fifties, 4 percent for women in their forties, and 3 percent for women in their thirties. For a man in his fifties with a PSA greater than 4, the likelihood of having prostate cancer is 25 percent.

One of the most powerful arguments against PSA testing was the widely held belief that "there is no evidence that treatment of localized prostate cancer saves lives." However, there was no evidence that it *didn't* save lives, either. Fortunately, today we do have evidence (we'll discuss this more in chapter 7). For years, men in Sweden were never treated for prostate cancer. They were just followed expectantly, a form of treatment that's also called watchful waiting. In Sweden, 50 percent more men died of prostate cancer than women died of breast cancer. Then, scientists in Scandinavia carried out a large study in which men with prostate cancer were randomly assigned either to undergo radical prostatectomy or to have watchful waiting. The results, published in the *New England Journal of Medicine*, came faster than anyone expected, and they were dramatic: Within ten years, the scientists were able to show that radical prostatectomy reduced the progression of cancer to metastasis, reduced death from prostate cancer by 40 percent, and decreased death from all causes by 26 percent. As a result, we can now say with certainty that finding and treating localized prostate cancer—cancer that is confined to the prostate and has not yet spread—in the man who is otherwise healthy and who will live long enough to need to be cured can significantly reduce his chances of dying of prostate cancer.

## But What About Screening?

In the world of prostate cancer, the introduction of PSA testing in the late 1980s was the equivalent of an earthquake. The number of new cases diagnosed increased sharply—by a staggering 83 percent—between 1988 and 1992. Was there a sudden epidemic of prostate cancer? No, the number of men with the disease was the same then as it is now. It's just that, for the first time, we could catch it earlier, in men who had not yet developed symptoms. And there were a lot of them—ticking time bombs, in effect. After this "bubble" of not yet symptomatic men was diagnosed, the number of new cases has fallen steadily. Today, the number of new cases is still somewhat greater than it was in the days before PSA testing, as one would expect after a new diagnostic tool is introduced. (The same is true for the incidence of breast cancer after the introduction of mammography.)

By and large, the cancers diagnosed with PSA testing have proven to be significant, not harmless. In the United States between 1991 and 2001, the death rate from prostate cancer dropped by 27 percent. Even more exciting: There has been a decrease in the detection of advanced cancers at the rate of 18 percent a year since 1991—and today, fortunately, only about 5 percent of men are diagnosed with prostate cancer that has metastasized. This is a dramatic improvement from the pre-PSA era: In 1988, 20 percent of American men had metastatic disease by the time it was diagnosed. In 1995, the American Cancer Society estimated that 35,000 men died of prostate cancer; by the early 2000s, the number was down to 29,000. In short, what was supposed to happen has happened. In 1997, researchers at the National Cancer Institute found the number of men between the ages of sixty and seventy-nine who died from prostate cancer was lower than in any year since 1950. This study's senior author, for years an outspoken critic of PSA testing, told *The New York Times*, "We are starting to have evidence that there may be a positive to prostate cancer screening and treatment."

Clearly, we're doing something right. What is it? Back in the 1980s, men were not diagnosed with cancer until they had symptoms—or, if they were lucky, a cancer that was large enough to be felt. Back then, few men—only 7 percent—underwent surgery, and radiation treatment was too underpowered to provide a cure. By 1990, with the advent of a better, safer surgical procedure (see chapter 8) and an increase in the number of men being diagnosed with localized disease, 35 percent of men chose surgery. Critics originally pointed to this rise in radical prostatectomy as a troubling trend. However, it may well prove that this, too, is something we were doing right. For the first time, men with prostate cancer were being treated aggressively, by surgeons aiming for a cure, in large numbers.

So why are fewer men dying from prostate cancer? The answer may be the fortunate combination of early diagnosis plus better treatment. In the Scandinavian study we talked about earlier, at ten years after diagnosis, 5 percent fewer men died of prostate cancer in the surgery group than in the watchful waiting group. In 1993, 100,000 men underwent surgery for prostate cancer in the United States. If the numbers are about the same, and surgery reduced prostate cancer deaths by 5 percent, this may explain much of the improvement that we have seen over the last decade.

Regardless of the cause, the most important message here is that we are on a winning streak. In the United States, fewer men are dying from prostate cancer. The disease is being diagnosed earlier, and treated at a more curable stage.

## How Do You Know If You Have Prostate Cancer?

### No Early Warning Signs

If prostate cancer started where benign prostatic hyperplasia (BPH) does—right by the urethra—then the disease would almost announce itself: "Hey! Something's wrong; I'm having trouble urinating! I need to get this checked out!" But it doesn't. Instead, the disease begins in a different part of the prostate, relatively far away from the urethra, in the peripheral zone (see fig. 1.3 in chapter 1) and grows silently for years. As a result, there really aren't any clear-cut, telltale symptoms of prostate cancer—signs that men notice and worry about, signs that make a doctor say, "Aha! This must be prostate cancer!"

### Every Single Symptom of Prostate Cancer Can Be Attributed to Another Cause

Say a tumor becomes large enough to encroach on the urethra and block the urinary tract. It produces classic symptoms of BPH: frequent or urgent urination, hesitancy, interrupted or weakened flow, dribbling, trouble urinating at all, or even blood in the urine. In the past, valuable time was wasted as these BPH-like symptoms were pursued while the real trouble remained hidden. (Fortunately, this is changing as more doctors are using the PSA test.) A less common symptom is the development of impotence or of less rigid erections, which can happen with advanced tumors as cancer invades the nerves involved in erection. But this, too, is accepted as something else—a normal sign of aging (and the subject of Viagra ads, which

---

### SYMPTOMS IN MEN WITH ADVANCED PROSTATE CANCER

- BPH-like symptoms: trouble urinating, frequent or urgent urination, interrupted or weakened flow, hesitancy, dribbling
- Less rigid erections or impotence
- A decrease in the amount of fluid ejaculated
- Blood in the urine or ejaculate
- Severe pain in the back, pelvis, hips, or thighs

---

describe erectile dysfunction as a commonplace problem in men of a certain age), but certainly not a cause for alarm. Similarly, a decrease in the amount of fluid ejaculated, a problem that results when the ejaculatory ducts become blocked by the tumor (this blockage can also cause blood in the semen), can be written off as normal aging. Still other manifestations, such as severe pain in the back, pelvis, hips, or thighs (which can develop as the cancer begins to attack the bone), also might be mistaken for other problems, such as arthritis or fibromyalgia.

Obviously, if you have any of these symptoms, see a urologist right away—even if you think it's "just" BPH or prostatitis. As we have seen, prostate cancer is an excellent impersonator. But better yet, don't wait until you have any symptoms to get tested for prostate cancer. Men can have palpable cancer—a tumor big enough to be felt during a rectal exam—and never even feel a twinge or experience the slightest change to suggest that something is wrong. Look at it this way: If you haven't had a PSA test and a digital rectal exam, how do you know that you're *not* harboring a potentially lethal cancer?

### Why You Need the Rectal Exam

Why do men over forty need a yearly rectal exam? Why not get the most painless test—PSA—by itself and then have a rectal exam if the blood test suggests cancer? *Because the PSA test is not foolproof.* About 25 percent of men with prostate cancer have a low PSA level, one that doesn't get flagged as suspicious. For this and other reasons (including the way some tumors make PSA), the PSA test does not detect every cancer early. Then again, neither does the digital rectal exam: In more than half of men with prostate cancer, the tumor is growing in an inopportune spot just out of finger's reach, where it simply cannot be felt by a doctor. In other men, the cancer is multifocal—there are several patches of cancer, not just one—and the prostate feels uniformly firm. It's a deceptive feeling, but the doctor's finger doesn't have a microscope on it and doesn't always know when it's being fooled. A firm prostate doesn't necessarily mean cancer; although most normal prostates feel soft, some don't—so this alone might not call attention to itself as something that warrants further investigation. Similarly, not all prostates feel smooth: in some men, the balance between muscular (stromal) and the smoother glandular (epithelial) tissue tilts toward muscle; these men have small, dense prostates. Finally, the cancer may simply be too small to feel yet, even though it's growing and dangerous.

### THE RECTAL EXAM: AN INSIDER'S GUIDE

This is the test that men dread. In fact, some men hate the idea of a rectal examination so much that they jeopardize their health by avoiding it like the plague. The rectal exam is certainly not fun; in fact, it's downright awkward and uncomfortable. But it shouldn't hurt, it's generally brief, and—most important of all—this little exam can provide essential information that simply can't be gotten any other way. (Note: If what you feel during the exam goes beyond the obvious discomfort of having someone's finger in your rectum and is clearly pain, this could be an important signal of another problem, such as prostatitis or inflammation. If the exam is excruciating, don't be stoic—tell your doctor.)

Unfortunately, many men hate this test for another reason—their doctor's bedside manner, or lack of it. Many doctors are not as thoughtful as they should be; they fail to position the patient correctly and then perform a hasty, rough examination. From a medical standpoint alone, this is a mistake: A soft touch can detect areas of suspicious firmness much better than a rough hand. Worse, because some men learn—from their doctor's brutish technique—to perceive the exam as dehumanizing or just generally unpleasant, they put off going to the doctor because they don't want to deal with someone who is rude, gruff, disrespectful, or uncommunicative. This is a terrible shame. Good doctors know how to make their patients feel at ease. They talk to their patients and treat them with respect. If your doctor's unfortunate bedside manner is keeping you away from this or any other exam, find another doctor. There are plenty of good ones out there.

Now, from your standpoint, what can you do to make the rectal examination as painless and productive as possible? First and foremost is how you "assume the position": the best way for the doctor to feel the prostate is for the patient to bend over the edge of the examining table. (Some doctors perform the examination by having the patient lie on his side. This is not as good. At best, the doctor can feel only the lower edge of the prostate.) For most men, the worst part of the exam is the introduction of the doctor's finger through the anal sphincter and past the muscles in the pelvic floor. Although the examining finger is gloved and well lubricated, if these muscles are tense (a very normal reaction, especially in men who are undergoing this exam for the first time), the doctor must exert more pressure—which adds to the discomfort, which then makes the man even more tense.

How can you relax these muscles? Don't even try; let your position do it for you. First, don't rest your elbows on the examining table—even though it feels more comfortable. Instead, put all your weight on your upper torso: Bend your knees so that your feet are just barely touching the floor. Your feet should not be supporting any weight. This way, your buttocks muscles will be completely relaxed, permitting the doctor's finger to be introduced easily—and ideally slowly, giving the muscles a chance to relax ahead of time.

To understand what the doctor is looking for, feel your hand. The normal prostate usually feels like the soft tissue in your palm—the fleshy part at the base of your thumb. Now, slide your fingers around to the other side, and feel the knuckle of your thumb. This is how cancer often feels—like a knot or hard lump.

Also, the PSA test may spot *different* cancers than the digital rectal exam—another reason doctors can't rely on an either-or approach for early detection. (It's like using breast exams and mammograms together to find breast cancer in women.) This was confirmed in one study of 2,634 men; investigators found that the PSA test and the digital rectal exam were nearly equal in cancer-detecting ability, but that they didn't always find the same tumors—that if only one technique had been used, some cancers would have been missed. Together, these two tests make a formidable team.

*If you are an American man, you should begin testing for prostate cancer at age forty.* With PSA tests, earlier is better; younger men don't have BPH to muddy the waters, so this makes the PSA test more accurate. If you are African American or you have a strong family history of

---

### BEFORE THE PSA TEST

- Don't ejaculate for at least two days before you have your blood drawn (this can raise your PSA level).
- Be sure to have this test *before* your digital rectal exam (the physical exam can raise PSA levels, too).
- Remind your doctor if you are taking Proscar (finasteride) or Avodart (dutasteride) for BPH, or Propecia (finasteride) for hair loss; all three of these drugs lower PSA. To correct for this, if you have been on one of these drugs for a short time, your PSA level should be multiplied by 2.0. If you have been taking it for five years or longer, your PSA level should be multiplied by 2.5. Fortunately, these drugs do not affect free PSA measurements. Also, report any history of prior prostate surgery. A transurethral resection (TUR) for BPH can lower your PSA level to less than 1 ng/ml, giving the false impression that everything is okay. If your PSA begins to increase steadily, even if this increase is very small, you should see a urologist.
- If the PSA reading indicates a borderline elevation or a significant increase since the last reading, repeat the test in the same laboratory. In 25 percent of such cases, the reading will be back down to its former level. If there is a clear-cut elevation, ask your doctor about prescribing antibiotics to rule out a possible infection. (Often, men receive ciprofloxacin (Cipro) or levofloxacin (Levaquin) for three to four weeks and have the PSA measured again.) If it is elevated again, you should have a biopsy.

---

prostate cancer, it's all the more important to begin testing at age forty, because in high-risk men—this means you—these cancers are diagnosed at an earlier age. As for the rectal examination, just bite the bullet. The digital rectal exam can tell an astute clinician many things about prostate cancer—whether it encompasses part of one lobe, an entire lobe, or both lobes of the prostate; whether it has spread outside the prostate, into the pelvic side wall or seminal vesicles. (For a description of the prostate's anatomy, see chapter 1.) But as good as this exam can be, the digital rectal exam is not an ironclad guarantee that cancer will be found in its earliest stages. Frankly, the digital rectal exam is only as good as the doctor performing it. It is a subjective test. In this area, urologists probably have some advantage over general practitioners simply because diagnosing prostate cancer is a major part of this specialty. In some cases, a general practitioner has felt a suspicious area on a rectal exam but has not pursued it because the PSA level was in the normal range (less than 4 ng/ml)—not realizing that one-quarter of men with prostate cancer have a low PSA level.

## Why You Need the PSA Test

No other cancer is diagnosed strictly by trying to feel it. Why? Just think how much a cancer must grow—how many times those early cancer cells must divide, what a tremendous head start this gives the tumor—before it becomes big enough to be felt. This is why, for years, doctors searched for a man's version of the Pap smear—an early-warning cancer detector that could spot a tumor long before it is clinically evident.

In this area, no development has been more promising than the PSA test. PSA is an enzyme that's made by the prostate in large amounts. It is secreted through the prostate's network of ducts, and it forms a major part of the ejaculate (for more information, see chapter 1). Although the enzyme PSA is made only by the prostate, it doesn't just stay in the prostate; it leaks into the bloodstream, and can be detected in a simple blood test.

The PSA test is not new. In years past, however, its purpose was limited; it functioned mainly as a means of monitoring the progression of already diagnosed prostate cancer. Could it do more? Could it detect cancer that had not yet been diagnosed? The answer, doctors found in the late 1980s, is yes—that elevated levels of PSA can indeed point to the presence of cancer, that PSA testing leads to the detection of prostate cancer at an early stage, and that PSA screening reduces the number of men who are diagnosed with metastatic disease.

However, although our knowledge of PSA has grown exponentially over the last decade, the basic PSA test is not a magic wand, pointing with resolute certainty toward prostate cancer—and that's the problem. Doctors are still figuring out how best to use the test and how to make sense of the information it provides. An American man's lifetime risk of death from prostate cancer is 3 percent, but his lifetime risk of being diagnosed with prostate cancer is 17 percent. Inevitably, until we have surefire markers that can accurately identify which men have life-threatening cancers, screening is going to result in the overdiagnosis and overtreatment of some men. And because many older men are being screened as often as younger ones, it is unlikely that screening and treatment of prostate cancer will extend every man's life.

Remember, PSA is *prostate-specific*, not *cancer-specific*. This is why a blood test alone isn't enough, why a digital rectal exam is also a must. *Having a high PSA level does not necessarily mean you have prostate cancer*—many men with high PSA levels don't. And *you can have prostate cancer and still have a low PSA level.* Fifteen percent of men who turn out to have prostate cancer have a very low PSA level, less than 4 ng/ml. About 25 percent of men with a PSA level between 4 and 10 ng/ml turn out to have cancer. In men with a PSA level over 10 ng/ml, about 65 percent are found to have cancer. Finally, many conditions can cause PSA to rise (see My PSA Is Elevated: What Else Could It Be?, below).

---

### MY PSA IS ELEVATED: WHAT ELSE COULD IT BE?

Just as having a low PSA doesn't mean that you *don't* have prostate cancer, having a high PSA doesn't automatically mean that you *do*. If your PSA is high, you have some form of prostate disease—trauma, enlargement, infection, or cancer—and you need to see a urologist to figure out which one it is.

For example, trauma, even a particularly vigorous rectal exam, can make a man's PSA levels shoot up temporarily. (To illustrate how complicated PSA is, consider this. In one study, French scientists found that the rise in PSA after a rectal exam is mainly in free PSA; still, the number went up, and the result could be misleading.) This means that, ideally, your blood should be drawn before you have a rectal exam or any other procedure, such as cystoscopy, prostate biopsy, or TUR, which could affect the prostate and falsely elevate PSA. For this reason, it makes sense to wait six or eight weeks after you have a needle biopsy before having your PSA taken if you are planning to use the results to make treatment decisions. And even then, it can still be higher than it was before your biopsy—so if this happens, don't panic, thinking your PSA is shooting up uncontrollably.

BPH itself can elevate PSA. A mild case of prostatitis can raise PSA, too, and an acute infection, such as bacterial prostatitis, can cause it to skyrocket. Because of this, many physicians treat an abrupt rise in a patient's yearly PSA test with antibiotics for several weeks, followed by another PSA test, just to rule out infection as a possible cause (and to avoid an unnecessary biopsy). If the trouble is indeed prostatitis and the episode is severe enough, it may take four to six weeks of antibiotics for the PSA to return to its normal, or baseline, levels—although in some men, the baseline level moves up to a new plateau and falls no further.

Sexual activity can elevate PSA as well: PSA levels can increase by as much as 41 percent in less than an hour after ejaculation. (Thus, it is wise to abstain from sex for two days before you are due to have your PSA tested.)

An episode of urinary retention (from BPH or urinary tract infection) can also cause an abrupt elevation in PSA, which takes as long as a week to return to normal. In rare cases, BPH can block blood supply to areas of the prostate. This is called a prostate infarction, and the cutoff of blood is much like that in a myocardial infarction, or heart attack. An episode of prostate infarction can trigger urinary retention and cause a temporary jump in PSA, sometimes to startling levels—as high as 100 or 200 ng/ml. One study by Michigan scientists found that infarcts can elevate not only levels of PSA but also of acid phosphatase (another enzyme made by the prostate; see chapter 6), and that "infarcts may be responsible for some otherwise unexplained levels" of both of these enzymes in the blood.

Finally, a mistake in the medical laboratory can cause a wrong PSA reading and create needless anxiety in the process. This happens more often than you might think. For all of these reasons, no treatment decision should be made on a lone PSA reading. (For more on confirming the diagnosis of prostate cancer, see chapter 6.)

Note: One activity that *does not* raise PSA levels is bicycling. In one study, published in the *Archives of Family Medicine*, scientists studied twenty men, aged twenty-seven to fifty-four, who were members of a cycling club. They found that even long-distance cycling (although it did seem to cause numbness in the perineum, the area between the scrotum and rectum) did not raise blood levels of PSA. A larger study, of 260 men who competed in a four-day race, found no significant change in PSA levels. (However, four of these men already had PSA levels higher than 4 ng/ml, and these levels did increase slightly after the race.)

Gram for gram, cancerous tissue results in PSA levels in the blood that are about ten times higher than levels in benign tissue. This is because normally, PSA is secreted and disposed of through tiny ducts in the prostate. But prostate cancer doesn't have a working ductal system; its ducts are "blind"—dead-end streets. So instead of draining into the urethra, PSA builds up, leaks out of the prostate, and shows up in the bloodstream. That's why it has proven to be such a good marker for cancer.

## New Approaches to PSA Testing

And yet, there is room for improvement. As good as the PSA test is, many scientists are working to make it more meaningful and specific. Some of the most promising approaches are discussed below.

### Bound and Free PSA

Chemically speaking, a PSA molecule is like a tiny pair of sharp scissors (the main function of PSA is to break down coagulaged semen after intercourse, see chapter 1). Now imagine millions of these tiny scissors clanking around in the bloodstream, each pointed blade slicing tissue to ribbons. If PSA circulated in the blood in its native form, it could be devastating to everything it touched. But the body is smarter than that. Normally, PSA is packed in a protective case—a chemical straitjacket that keeps it from harming innocent tissue. In this form, PSA is bound—tied to other proteins and rendered harmless. But sometimes, PSA inactivates itself. Imagine a pair of scissors with one broken blade. These scissors don't fit in the case anymore, but they don't need it; they are chemically passive. This form of PSA is called free. It circulates freely in the bloodstream on its own.

In a regular, or total PSA, blood test, both of these forms are lumped together—the dangerous scissors in the case and the scissors with the broken blade. But in recent years, scientists have developed assays sensitive enough to isolate and quantify both bound and free forms of the PSA molecule. The goal is to characterize these forms of PSA in the blood, measure each part, and determine what these levels mean over time—so we can chart the course of normal and abnormal growth of the prostate. This separation of PSA into bound and free forms can help men in two important ways: It can make the PSA test more specific, for one thing. It can also help determine how aggressive a man's cancer is.

*A More Specific Test: The Free PSA Test*

As we'll discuss later in this chapter, an elevated PSA level does not automatically mean that you have prostate cancer. What it means is that you have prostate trouble—which could mean cancer, enlargement, infection, or even recent trauma—and you need to see a urologist to figure out exactly what's going on in there. The most common reason for a higher-than-normal PSA level is BPH. It is common for a man's PSA to be as high as 10 percent of his prostate weight; for example, if a man has an enlarged prostate that weighs 60 grams, he may well have a PSA of 6—but not have cancer.

*Free PSA Comes Almost Exclusively from BPH Tissue*

An easy way to remember this is "The higher the *free* PSA, the more likely that you are *free* of cancer." Men with prostate cancer are more likely to have low levels of free PSA (also known as percent-free PSA). Thus, if a man has an elevated PSA and most of it is free, then it's probably coming from BPH; if it's mostly bound, then the PSA elevation is probably coming from cancer. This is where measuring free PSA is especially useful.

Can the free PSA test reduce your risk of an unnecessary biopsy? Probably. Can overreliance on the free PSA test mean that your prostate cancer might be missed? Possibly. In one study, researchers used a free PSA cutoff of 19 percent in men with total PSA levels between 3 and 4 and detected 90 percent of all cancers. Another study, of men with PSA levels between 2.6 and 4, had a higher cutoff—27 percent free PSA—but also detected 90 percent of cancers. This study found that 18 percent of unnecessary biopsies could be avoided by using this cutoff. Note: Again, because men with low free PSA levels are more likely to have aggressive cancers and more advanced disease found at the time of radical prostatectomy, even if the needle biopsy is inconclusive or shows little cancer, if the percent-free PSA is lower than 15 percent, a man is likely to be harboring more tumor than a man with a higher level of free PSA.

Another study of men with higher PSA levels (between 4 and 10) found that using the free PSA test—and performing biopsies only on men with less than 25 percent free PSA—could diagnose 95 percent of the cancers and reduce unnecessary biopsies by 20 percent. However, some scientists, worried about diagnosing that remaining 5 percent of cancers, object to this cutoff number, because it means that some cancers will be missed.

## Complexed PSA

This test, called cPSA, is another way of looking at the separation of bound and free PSA. It's like taking the same picture using a different lens, measuring how much of a man's PSA is bound—because in men with prostate cancer, a greater fraction of their total PSA is bound. In one study of men with PSA levels between 2.5 and 4.0, cPSA as a single test proved better than the regular PSA test and comparable to percent-free PSA for detecting cancer. The potential advantage is that this measurement involves only one blood test and thus is more cost-effective. However, it does not tell us the percent-free PSA level, which is useful in estimating the aggressiveness of the cancer.

### Should You Get It?

There are several points to consider. One drawback to the free PSA test is that it's twice as expensive, because two blood tests must be measured—the total amount and the free amount, from which the percent-free number is calculated. Although many doctors are overlooking the additional costs involved in this, free PSA testing has not yet become widespread. Some urologists, guided by free PSA measurements, recommend biopsy only when the percentage of free to total PSA is lower than 25 percent. This is good in that it reduces the number of unnecessary biopsies, but it also means that about 5 to 10 percent of cancers may be missed. It may come down to what bothers you most—the thought of missing cancer at the earliest possible diagnosis or having an unnecessary biopsy because of a false alarm.

However, there are two situations in which percent-free PSA can be particularly useful. Say a man has had multiple biopsies because his total PSA is higher than normal. Every biopsy is negative, yet the worry remains. Here, if the free PSA is high, the man and his doctor can relax. If it's very low, it means he will need further biopsies. The second situation is the man with a strong family history of prostate cancer who worries that he is headed down the same pathway as his father, brother, or other male relatives—even though his PSA is low for his age. Here again, knowing the free PSA percentage can be re-assuring. If it's high, this man can relax. If it's very low, this is a good reason to have a biopsy.

### How Aggressive Is the Cancer?

A doctor can't determine from looking at the total PSA level in a man with prostate cancer the source of the PSA elevation. For example, in many men with small amounts of early-stage cancer, most of the PSA is actually coming from noncancerous tissue in the epithelium. How-ever, *if the free PSA is less than 15 percent, it's more likely that most, if not all, of that PSA is coming from cancer, that the cancer is significant in size, and that it will prove aggressive.* The differences in PSA illustrate once again that not all prostate cancers are created equal. Some are very slow-growing and never need treatment. Others can be fatal within a matter of years after they are diagnosed. So for scientists, just as im-portant as finding cancer early is knowing which kind of cancer—the "good" or the "bad"—we're dealing with. Research at Johns Hopkins has established the guidelines on which men can afford to watch and wait (see chapters 6 and 7). We are also working to pinpoint the men at the other end of the spectrum—those with aggressive cancers that will almost certainly be lethal if not treated immediately. New evi-dence shows that free PSA can predict which tumors will be aggres-sive—and need to be treated as soon as possible—several years before total, or regular PSA tests can even spot cancer. In one Johns Hopkins study, researchers made use of the massive database of the Baltimore Longitudinal Study of Aging. The study, led by the urolo-gist H. Ballentine Carter, compared blood samples from men who de-veloped prostate cancer with those from men who did not and found that *fifteen years before cancer was diagnosed,* all of the men who turned out to have aggressive prostate tumors had levels of free PSA that were lower than 15 percent. Men with slower-growing, nonaggres-sive cancer all had free PSA levels greater than 15 percent. This land-mark study suggests that percent-free PSA may be an excellent predictor of aggressive tumors that will need to be treated.

## PSA Velocity

Another promising diagnostic approach using PSA testing is to look at PSA velocity—its rate of change from year to year. The supposition is this: if cells double at a much faster rate in prostate cancer than in BPH, and if prostate cancer produces more PSA than BPH does, it's likely that PSA's yearly rate of change will be much greater in a man with prostate cancer than in a man with BPH.

However, for this technique to be accurate, at least three PSA measurements should be obtained during a two-year period—the tests should be taken at least eighteen months apart. It is not helpful for a man to have two PSA tests in a short span of time—a couple of months apart, for example—because there is a natural fluctuation in PSA readings that may be as much as 15 to 30 percent. Say you have a PSA test result of 4.1; two months later, your next PSA test is 4.7. This could be a normal variation, yet it could well spark a panic if you believed you had cancer and it was growing fast.

In one study, using data from the Baltimore Longitudinal Study of Aging, investigators looked at three groups of men—those with BPH, those with prostate cancer, and a control group of men with no prostate disease. Studying twenty years' worth of stored blood samples, investigators found that PSA velocity, for those who know how to read it properly, is a veritable crystal ball at predicting prostate cancer. The men who turned out to develop prostate cancer had "significantly greater rates of change in PSA levels than those without prostate cancer up to ten years before diagnosis." In other words, by tracking changes in PSA levels, they were able to detect prostate cancer years before it could be diagnosed by other means. For example, at five years before diagnosis—when PSA levels weren't appreciably different between men with BPH and men with prostate cancer— there was already a big difference in PSA velocity in men who turned out to have prostate cancer versus men who had BPH and the control group.

PSA velocity is highly valuable in detecting prostate cancer and in distinguishing it from BPH early—particularly now, when an increasing number of men are returning to their doctor every year for a digital rectal examination and PSA test. But the whole idea here with PSA velocity is that it's a fluid continuum, not a cut-and-dried, one-shot reading. It's like having a prostate barometer—your doctor doesn't have to wait for the PSA level to reach a magic number (currently, it's 4 ng/ml). With PSA velocity, what matters is a significant change over time, and this varies, depending on the level of PSA. *For men with PSAs greater than 4, an average, consistent increase of more than 0.75 ng/ml over the course of three tests is considered significant.* Say over eighteen months a man's PSA level went up from 4.0 to 4.6 to 5.8. Clearly, something's going on here. With PSA velocity, we can make a more accurate diagnosis of prostate cancer at even lower levels than the raw cutoff of 4. Because we now realize that men with PSA levels as low as 1.0 may have cancer, new guidelines have been established for PSA velocity in men with PSA levels between 1 and 4. Work by Carter and the Baltimore Longitudinal Study of Aging suggests that any consistent increase is alarming, even an increase as small as 0.2–0.4 ng/ml a year. *If you have a PSA level between 1 and 4 and it is consistently rising faster than 0.2–0.4 ng/ml a year, you should get a biopsy.* Also, PSA velocity is more specific. If doctors use the PSA level of 4 as a cutoff point, about 40 percent of men who have only BPH undergo unnecessary biopsies. But with PSA velocity, this number is reduced; only 10 percent of men with BPH undergo an unnecessary biopsy.

A major change in PSA can also be a sign that something is very wrong—that there is significant cancer, and that it may be difficult to cure. Two large studies of men who received radical prostatectomy or radiation therapy found that men who had a PSA velocity of 2 ng/ml within the year before diagnosis were much more likely to have an aggressive form of cancer and more likely to die from prostate cancer within ten years. Thus, if you have a sudden jump in your PSA and it is confirmed in a repeat measurement at the same laboratory, you may have significant disease that needs treatment immediately and that may require more than surgery or radiation therapy to cure. (For more on this, see chapter 10.)

Although PSA velocity is a big improvement over looking at a raw PSA score and trying to figure out what it means, even this isn't a perfect system. Paradoxically, in men who already have prostate cancer, following changes in PSA is less helpful over time. About 25 percent of men with prostate cancers *that are growing* do not have a big increase in their PSA levels. Thus, just because your PSA isn't

---

### MY PSA IS LOW. AM I OKAY?

Taking a 5-alpha reductase inhibitor, such as Proscar (finasteride) or Avodart (dutasteride), to treat BPH can artificially lower the PSA reading by as much as half. The drug Propecia, used to deter hair loss, is a low-dose form of finasteride and can lower PSA as well. To account for this, if you have been taking one of these drugs for a short period of time, your PSA should be doubled. If you have been taking it for five years or longer, your PSA should be multiplied by 2.5. (Fortunately, these drugs do not appear to affect percent-free PSA.)

Obesity can artificially lower PSA, too. Scientists are concerned that this could prevent prostate cancer from being detected as early as possible. As we discussed in chapter 3, men who have a significant weight gain in the twenty-five years before prostate cancer is diagnosed are more likely to develop a rising PSA after radical prostatectomy, which means that some prostate cancer cells have remained behind. Is this because their cancer was spurred on by hormones related to obesity? Or was their diagnosis delayed because their PSA was deceptively low?

If you have had a surgical procedure to treat BPH (such as a TUR), your PSA should fall to around 1.0 ng/ml and stay there. If your PSA is higher than that, even though it's still considered low, this is not normal and should be investigated.

---

high, and just because your PSA isn't going up, that doesn't mean you don't have cancer and that it isn't dangerous.

### Age-Specific PSA

As a man ages, his prostate gets bigger. So why should the PSA cutoff point be the same for a forty-year-old man as for an eighty-year-old man (who probably has a higher PSA level anyway due to BPH)? It doesn't make sense; the younger man almost certainly has a much smaller prostate. Studies show that using a cutoff of 2.5 ng/ml in men under age fifty will enable doctors to catch about 20 percent more cancers—but require only 5 percent more biopsies. Because detecting prostate cancer early is more important in these younger men whose lives are likely to be cut short by malignancy, this is a good rationale for using a lower cutoff for these men. Some scientists have suggested using a higher cutoff for men over age sixty, because so many older men have enlarged prostates. However, in doing this, some significant, curable cancers will almost certainly be missed. Therefore, we do not recommend raising the PSA bar over 4 ng/ml for anyone.

## PSA Density

This technique begins with a theory—that most men in the age group for prostate cancer also have at least some BPH, which can elevate the PSA concentration and make diagnosis more difficult. One way to distinguish between BPH and cancer, some doctors believe, is PSA density—the blood PSA score divided by the volume of the prostate, as determined by transrectal ultrasound. Basically, if you have benign disease, your PSA should be approximately 10 percent, and no higher than 15 percent, of the weight of your prostate (which translates to a PSA density of 0.1 to 0.15). For example, if you have a PSA of 8 ng/ml and your prostate weighs 80 grams, most of the PSA is probably coming from BPH. But if your prostate weighs only 30 or 40 grams, your PSA level is too high to be explained by BPH alone.

The next question you might have is, "How do we weigh my prostate?" Well, there's the problem. It's impossible to estimate a man's prostate size without an invasive procedure such as transrectal ultrasound. Therefore, PSA density has not proven to be of widespread value in screening for prostate cancer. For men who—because of an abnormal PSA or rectal exam—do undergo ultrasound-guided biopsy, PSA density can be helpful in determining how much cancer is in the prostate. It can also be useful in men who have had repeated negative biopsies to determine whether they need to go further in searching for cancer. In men without cancer, because most of the PSA is coming from BPH, some investigators have suggested using the weight of the transition zone to calculate density rather than total prostate weight.

## PSA Thresholds

First, of course, there was the number 4. When PSA testing first came out, the general consensus was that a PSA greater than 4 ng/ml was considered abnormal. Then we learned about age-specific PSA and

TABLE 5.1

**HOW MANY MEN MY AGE HAVE MY PSA LEVEL?**

| Age | 50–59 | 60–69 | 70 or above | Total |
|---|---|---|---|---|
| **PSA Level** | | | | |
| 2.5 or lower | 88% | 75% | 61% | 78% |
| 2.6–4.0 | 8% | 14% | 18% | 12% |
| 4.1–9.9 | 3% | 9% | 16% | 8% |
| 10 or higher | 1% | 2% | 5% | 2% |

Adapted from the *Journal of the American Medical Association*

the need to lower the threshold to 2.5 for men in their forties. At that point, some experts suggested that 2.5 should be used for everyone. That way, they argued, we wouldn't miss anybody by delaying biopsies until the PSA rises above 4 ng/ml. Far better, they said, to strike cancer sooner, while men have lower PSA levels. They do have a point. But the counterargument to this, of course, is that prostate cancers detected at lower PSA levels are more likely to be small in volume and low grade, and thus more likely to represent clinically insignificant disease—and may not need to be treated right away, if ever. True, any approach to prostate cancer screening that finds more cancers without telling us how dangerous they are will only increase overdiagnosis and overtreatment. In an article published in the *Journal of the National Cancer Institute*, some scientists have estimated that if the threshold for biopsies were lowered to 2.5 ng/ml in the United States, this would double the number of men defined as abnormal—up to six million. This could be disastrous. The scientists wrote, "Until there is evidence that screening is effective, increasing the number of men recommended for prostate biopsy—and the number potentially diagnosed and treated unsuccessfully—would be a mistake."

And then, in the midst of this 2.5 vs. 4.0 debate, a bombshell exploded. In a study published in the *New England Journal of Medicine*, based on biopsies of three thousand men with PSAs lower than 4 ng/ml, investigators found that 15 percent of these men had cancer. And of the men diagnosed with cancer, 15 percent had Gleason scores of 7 or higher. Now, this study left a number of unanswered questions—specifically, how many of these men had small-volume cancers—but it removed all complacency with using PSA thresholds as a means to distinguish men with and without cancer. (For some final thoughts on this, see the summary at the end of this chapter.)

Realistically, the only PSA threshold that we can use to rule out cancer entirely is 1.0 ng/ml. Although some men with a PSA this low may harbor prostate cancer, it is unlikely to be the life-threatening, high-grade kind. What matters more is *what happens to this PSA level—whether it rises over time, and how fast.*

## BPH Makes It More Confusing

The presence of BPH clouds the crystal ball of PSA, making a man's levels harder to interpret—causing higher PSA levels that usually have nothing to do with cancer. Because of this, the PSA test is better at finding cancer in men who don't have BPH; these men generally have lower PSA levels anyway, are younger, and have more to gain from an early diagnosis of cancer. It may be that we should rethink the emphasis on absolute PSA thresholds, explore in depth the patterns of increase in PSA when it is less than 4 ng/ml, and identify any factors that can help us predict life-threatening disease at a time when the disease is most curable. As the Johns Hopkins urologist H. Ballentine Carter discovered, men with PSAs between 1 and 4 who had a PSA velocity greater than 0.2–0.4 ng/ml per year were more likely to die of their prostate cancer.

TABLE 5.2

**WILL MY BIOPSY SHOW CANCER?**
**WHAT ABOUT HIGH-GRADE DISEASE?**

| PSA | Odds that the biopsy will be positive for cancer | Odds of high-grade disease (Gleason 7–10) |
|---|---|---|
| Less than 0.5 | 7 percent | 0.8 percent |
| 0.6–1.0 | 10 percent | 1.0 percent |
| 1.1–2.0 | 21 percent | 2.6 percent |
| 2.1–3.0 | 27 percent | 5.7 percent |
| 3.1–4.0 | 30 percent | 9.4 percent |
| 4.1–10 | 23–38 percent | 5–15 percent |
| >10 | 65 percent | — |

Data adapted from *New England Journal of Medicine*

## PSA and Race

There is no question that black men without cancer have higher PSA levels than their counterparts of other races. For example, in one retrospective study conducted by Chicago researchers, the average PSA level of black men was slightly higher than that of white men and Hispanic men. Black men had higher PSA density levels as well. This might suggest that there should be a higher PSA cutoff for African Americans. However, the other side of the coin is that black men also have a greater risk of developing cancer (see chapter 3), and when they are tested with the same PSA cutoff level as white men, are more likely to be harboring a cancer. In one study using a PSA cutoff of 4 ng/ml, 38 percent of white men were found to have cancer, but 52 percent of black men turned out to have cancer.

More research is needed to determine the guidelines for PSA testing in black men. However, because African American men are more likely to develop the disease—and to have a more advanced, lethal form of it—they need to be followed carefully. It may be that combining PSA with additional tests, such as free PSA, will prove to be most useful for these men.

## Investigational Blood Tests

The more we know about PSA and its subtleties, the more we're learning about the chemistry of the prostate and the many biochemical signals it sends out all the time. If we can only figure out how to read them! Several sophisticated tests looking at other prostate cancer markers in the blood are currently being investigated.

### EPCA-2 (Early Prostate Cancer Antigen-2)

This new marker for prostate cancer detection was discovered by Robert Getzenberg, the director of research at Johns Hopkins' Brady Urological Institute. The discovery of EPCA-2 comes after decades of work by Getzenberg's predecessor, Donald S. Coffey, who noticed something striking about the nuclei of cancer cells: they're funny-looking and misshapen. Coffey then characterized the structural proteins that caused this mess within cancer cells, and when Getzenberg was a predoctoral fellow with Coffey, they identified EPCA-2. Recently, in an exciting study, Getzenberg and colleagues were able to show that EPCA-2 was *far more specific than any other marker identified so far—even PSA*—in distinguishing men with prostate cancer from other men. Further, this test was able to tell which men had organ-confined cancer and which men had cancer that had spread beyond the prostate.

These findings are remarkable, and if they hold up when the marker is tested in a larger group of prostate cancer patients, they may revolutionize the approach to screening for prostate cancer. At the very least, EPCA-2 could help determine which men with abnormal PSA levels have prostate cancer. But it's possible that EPCA-2 may even replace PSA one day as the screening test of choice.

### Antibody Signatures

We make antibodies to every virus, bit of bacteria, and toxin—anything that our body's immune system recognizes as foreign or potentially harmful—that comes down the pike. Scientists have known for years that we make antibodies to cancer, too; specifically, men with prostate cancer make antibodies to fight proteins in their own tumors. Investigators at the University of Michigan recently looked for antibodies to a set of twenty-two proteins in the blood of men with and without prostate cancer. In preliminary studies, their antibody tests could detect 83 percent of the cancers and could distinguish cancer from normal tissue in 88 percent of these men—far surpassing the diagnostic ability of PSA. This technique will require more work before it is validated and ready for clinical use, but it looks very promising.

### Molecular Derivatives of PSA

PSA begins as a larger molecule called pro-PSA, which is then broken down by a related enzyme called hK2 to form active PSA, which can then be broken down into BPSA. BPSA is a particular form of free PSA produced by BPH in the prostate's transition zone, a thin ring of tissue that surrounds the urethra. (You may remember from chapter 1 that this area is not involved in cancer, which strikes the prostate's peripheral zone instead.) BPSA is not so much a marker for prostate cancer as a marker for BPH. BPSA may help distinguish benign from malignant disease when measured against levels of pro-PSA in men who have a low free PSA level. Next, *hK2:* PSA is in a family of proteolytic (protein-cutting) enzymes called kallikreins. One of PSA's cousins—like PSA, it's expressed by the prostate, can be measured in the blood, and responds to hormones—is called human kallikrein-2 (hK2). The enzyme hK2 is expressed more in poorly differentiated—more aggressive and advanced—cancers and may be helpful in assessing a man's cancer. And what about pro-PSA? One study, looking at the percentage of total PSA that was pro-PSA (confusingly, this is called percent p-PSA), found that this marker may be most useful in men with PSA levels in the range of 2 to 4 ng/ml.

### Serum (Blood) Proteomic Patterns

Each organ or tissue makes its own mark on the bloodstream by adding to, taking away from, or changing some of the circulating proteins, or peptides (small proteins). The pattern of these proteins, called the serum proteome, may show that something is wrong in a particular organ or tissue. A new technique, with the acronym SELD-TOF (for surface-enhanced laser desorption ionization time-of-flight) mass spectroscopy, has been developed to identify these protein patterns. In this technique, researchers analyze blood from patients with various disorders, including prostate cancer. They're looking for telltale patterns instead of specific markers, and they don't even bother to identify the specific proteins involved—all that matters is that they turn up recognizable footprints. This technique is still very new, but intriguing evidence from early studies suggests that it can identify men with prostate cancer and women with ovarian cancer.

### A Urine Test for Prostate Cancer?

A completely different approach to diagnosing prostate cancer is in the works. It's based on the molecular detection of prostate cancer cells in the urine after a needle biopsy of the prostate or after prostatic massage. (Prostatic massage, currently used as a way to test for prostatitis, is done during a digital rectal exam. A doctor vigorously massages or presses on the prostate to express, or force, fluid out of the prostate and into the urethra.) So far, three cancer-specific markers are being studied as potential urine test candidates.

### DD3

This gene, discovered at the Brady Urological Institute at Johns Hopkins, is one of the most prostate cancer–specific genes known, making it a promising marker for the early diagnosis of prostate cancer. A commercial test, called uPM3 or PCA3, has been developed, with claims that it has as high as 81 percent accuracy.

### AMACR

This gene, discussed in chapter 3, is involved in fatty acid metabolism and is also highly expressed in prostate cancer. In a small study, the Johns Hopkins urologist Christian Pavlovich was able to predict prostate cancer correctly in 87 percent of patients by locating this gene.

### GST-π

This is the gene that normally protects against oxidative damage and is one of the first genes to be methylated, or chemically knocked out, when prostate cancer develops (see chapter 3). Methylated GST-π is another relatively specific marker for prostate cancer that can be identified in the urine.

## Who Needs Screening?

The most important thing to think about here is that in its earliest, most curable stages, prostate cancer produces no symptoms. This means that most men with curable prostate cancer feel perfectly fine. Men who do not feel fine—who have symptoms of prostate cancer— probably do not have curable disease. And this leads to the philosophy of screening: men who can expect to live ten to twenty more years and who don't want to die from prostate cancer should be screened. This is especially true for the men who are at highest risk

## ON THE HORIZON: BRAINY COMPUTERS
## HELP PREDICT CANCER RISK

Alan Partin, the director of the Brady Urological Institute at Johns Hopkins, loves statistics, facts, and figures—rearranging them, making sense out of them, and using what he's come up with to help patients. A prime example is the Partin Tables he developed, which filled a great need by correlating three facts about a man's disease—PSA level, Gleason score, and clinical stage—and accurately estimating the extent of a man's prostate cancer to help him make an educated decision about treatment (see chapter 6).

Now, instead of just three pieces of information, Partin is taking many more, feeding them into a sophisticated neural network—a "thinking" computer program he has helped develop—and asking new questions, such as, What will the results of this man's biopsy be? What will be the pathologic stage of his tumor? Will he have positive lymph nodes?

"Neural networks are not new," says Partin, "but they're fairly new to medicine. The stock market uses them all the time. They watch trends; the network tells them what's going to happen in the next quarter, so they know which stock to buy. Factories use them to measure the temperature of water, steam coming out of the pipes, the noise level in the building—about fifteen or twenty variables that they continuously monitor—and they know two days before the machine's going to go down, because they've seen the pattern before. The neural network says, 'You're going to be in trouble; you'd better stop the line and fix something.'"

Neural networks recognize patterns. Their answers are educated guesses. The neural networks—so called because they function like artificial brains and have the ability to learn from their mistakes—can look at a complex series of results and determine a pattern—the possibility of cure, perhaps, or the likelihood that cancer will be aggressive.

In addition to more obvious pieces of information, such as PSA, PSA velocity, free PSA, age, race, and other markers, neural networks can help make sense of many other confounding variables. For example, some men with prostate cancer have low testosterone levels, because the cancer suppresses testosterone production (see chapter 3). Recently, we have learned that severely overweight men have lower PSAs, which may delay the diagnosis of cancer. In a large group of men with prostate cancer, most of these variables would be minor factors—bit players on the stage. But in individual men, some of these may be essential in pinpointing cancer risk.

of developing the disease—African Americans and men with a strong family history of the disease.

Now, what does that mean? Simply that if a man's age or health suggests that he won't live longer than ten years, there is no reason to make an early diagnosis of prostate cancer. If a man who is very old or very ill has early, localized prostate cancer now, it is unlikely that he will live long enough for the cancer to become a problem. If the cancer progresses, there are many ways to control the disease and keep symptoms at bay for years. Creating anxiety about what to do—what treatment decisions to make—is not helpful for these men. One of the major missing pieces here, especially as the average life span lengthens—is determining how long a man is going to live. One urologist has said that he would not perform a PSA test on a man older than eighty unless he was brought to the office by both of his parents. But we desperately need an accurate way to distinguish the eighty-year-old man who will live to be one hundred from his counterpart who may die the next year.

Obviously, nobody wants to die from prostate cancer—or heart disease, or any ailment, for that matter. For many men, however, this is much more than an abstract concept, it is a great fear. These men have seen death from prostate cancer, watched the suffering of their father, brother, or friend, and prayed it wouldn't happen to them, too. But other men don't understand this. They know only what they read in the newspapers and hear on television—that the treatment of prostate cancer is associated with a lot of side effects and is a thing to be avoided at all costs. Frankly, if you have not seen a family member or friend die of prostate cancer, it's hard to imagine it. The disease progresses relentlessly, subjecting your loved one to a variety of uncomfortable and dehumanizing experiences, including hormonal therapy, and ultimately culminating in death from metastases to bone, which are agonizing to experience and tough even to witness. Because prostate cancer rarely interferes with any normal bodily functions, patients die a painful death, with their body's defenses usually broken down to the point at which they succumb to pneumonia. Watching this terrible thing happen to someone you love makes you feel helpless and angry. You think, "With all of the wonders of modern medicine, shouldn't we be able to do something? Shouldn't we be past suffering like this by now?" We aren't past it yet, although scientists are working furiously, and this may change someday soon. This is the side of prostate cancer that you rarely hear about. It's the side of prostate cancer that critics of screening avoid talking about. Instead, they emphasize the side effects of treatment.

The thing is, today—thank goodness—all forms of treatment for prostate cancer have fewer side effects, especially if men are diagnosed when they are young. As we discussed earlier in this chapter, there is accumulating evidence that screening and effective treatment have reduced the number of men who are diagnosed with advanced disease and have improved the survival rate of those who have prostate cancer. The number of American deaths from the disease are falling. In 1995, 35,000 men died of prostate cancer in the United States; in 2006, the number was 27,400. Thus, the man who's going to live long enough to need to be cured should have the opportunity to be cured. Screening is the first step.

### You Should Start Screening at Age Forty

When prostate cancer is discovered in younger men, it is more likely to be curable. Recognizing this fact, the Johns Hopkins urologist H. Ballentine Carter and colleagues began looking for a way to improve prostate cancer screening.

They used an approach that has worked well to answer questions such as when to start screening and how often to screen for cervical and breast cancer— a highly sophisticated computer model, called a Markov model, which mathematically simulates the progression of a disease in a group of people. "Basically, it takes a hypothetical population of individuals and walks them through life," Carter explains, with some men developing prostate cancer, some dying of prostate cancer, and some never getting the disease and eventually dying of other causes—just like in real life. Setting up the model was the hard part. But then, the researchers used it to test various screening strategies to see how they affected the death rate from prostate cancer and how many PSA tests and biopsies were needed to detect each cancer.

The results, published in the *Journal of the American Medical Association*, were unexpected: For men who are not at higher risk of developing prostate cancer, beginning screening at age fifty was not the best strategy. Instead, they found a more effective strategy was to give PSA tests at age forty and at age forty-five, and then at age fifty (or earlier, if PSA was 2 ng/ml or above), start testing every other year instead of every year. "That was the only strategy that did three things: it reduced the death rate of prostate cancer, reduced the overall number of PSA tests, and reduced the overall number of prostate biopsies for each cancer detected," says Carter.

But many scientists, including Carter, are very troubled by the recent finding that 15 percent of men with a PSA level lower than 4 ng/ml have cancer, and 15 percent of these men with cancer have high-grade cancer. Because of this, *there is no safe, absolute cutoff above a PSA level of 1.0 ng/ml* at which a man can rest assured that he is not at risk of harboring a high-grade cancer. Thus, what probably is going to matter the most in the future is your PSA history. Getting your first PSA test and digital rectal examination at age forty, when you are unlikely to have BPH, will give you a valuable baseline for every other PSA measurement you'll ever need; the results of these baseline PSA tests have been shown to predict a man's risk of being diagnosed with prostate cancer over the next twenty-five years. After this, depending on the baseline level—specifically, on whether you are above or below the 50th percentile for your age—all you need to do is take a repeat PSA test every two to five years. Men in their forties who have a PSA level greater than 0.6 ng/ml are in this group, as are men in their fifties who have a PSA level greater than 0.7 ng/ml. (In a study of a larger group of men led by William Catalona of Northwestern University, scientists found the comparable numbers to be 0.7 for men in their forties and 0.9 for men in their fifties). If you are in this group, you should have your PSA measured every two years. If your PSA is below this percentile, you may be able to wait as long as five years for the next test.

From this baseline, your doctor will calculate your yearly rate of increase in PSA. If you have a low PSA level (between 1 and 4 ng/ml), any increase is alarming. In a study using data from the Baltimore Longitudinal Study of Aging, Carter and colleagues found that PSA increases greater than 0.2–0.4 ng/ml per year were predictors of death from prostate cancer. Currently, change in PSA over time is the most valuable tool we have for interpreting PSA and for predicting prostate cancer, including whether it is life-threatening.

---

## WHY SHOULD I BEGIN IN MY FORTIES?

Three reasons: First, many men whose prostate cancers go unde-
tected before they're in their fifties eventually die of the disease. Most
of these men have no particular reason to worry about prostate cancer—
they don't have a strong family history, and they're not African American.
But it is very likely that most of the men between ages fifty and sixty-four
who die of prostate cancer could have been been saved if the disease
had been caught when they were in their forties.

Second, younger men are more likely than older men to have curable
disease and to have fewer side effects from treatment.

And finally, PSA is a better, more specific test in younger men who—
unlike older men—don't tend to have BPH, which can falsely raise the
PSA level.

---

### What If You Don't Have a Baseline?

What if this is your first PSA test? If you are in your fifties or sixties
and have never had a PSA test, if your level is greater than 3.0 ng/ml,
and you are otherwise healthy and can expect to live at least another
fifteen to twenty years, you should have a biopsy. Similarly, you
should undergo a biopsy if you are in your forties, and your PSA is 2.5
ng/ml or higher. If your PSA level is higher than 4 ng/ml, and your
biopsy finds no cancer, you should continue to have your PSA level
rechecked at regular intervals, and your PSA should not rise more than
0.75 ng/ml each year.

## When Should You Stop Screening?

The upper age limit for enrollment in most current screening trials
is seventy-four years. Organizations that have endorsed screening
have generally recommended it only for men with a life expectancy
of at least ten more years. Since most men who are diagnosed with
prostate cancer without regular screening rarely die of the disease before fifteen years without treatment, and because, through the use of
screening, that number can be extended by five or ten more years, it
may be that screening could be discontinued earlier in life—at age
seventy, perhaps—for men who have been screened and who have

## PROSTATE CANCER RUNS IN MY FAMILY: SHOULD I THINK ABOUT GENETIC TESTING?

At the moment, that's all you can do—think about genetic testing, because it isn't available yet. However, it may be soon. This means, theoretically, that the 3 or 4 percent of men who inherit a defective gene involved in prostate cancer can have their blood drawn, and find out whether they're at extra risk for developing prostate cancer.

Right? Well, the answer is maybe. Today, we have identified and characterized three genes that are responsible for the development of prostate cancer in small clusters of families. We believe that there probably will be a large number of genes that will turn out to be responsible for the disease that runs in families, but we do not know whether there will be common ones, such as the BRCA-1 and BRCA-2 genes found in families prone to breast cancer.

Then, once a blood test is developed, what will happen? Men with prostate cancer who have a strong family history can be tested to see whether they have one of the mutated genes. If you test positive, after a lot of counseling about the consequences of testing, other family members can be tested to determine whether they, too, carry the gene and are at high risk.

In chapter 3, we talked about how cancer starts—the "domino effect," or chain reaction caused when a single gene goes bad, then causes another to mutate, until finally the result is cancer. Some men are born with the genetic deck stacked against them. But this doesn't mean a man with this sword hanging over him can't delay cancer indefinitely—for example, by changing his diet. And it definitely doesn't mean that a man with an inherited gene linked to prostate cancer should start making out his will, or take up hang gliding or bungee jumping. Actually, the more we can learn about how these genes go astray, the better the news will be for everybody. We believe that once we identify these genes, we will know more about what causes prostate cancer and may be able to restore the genetic balance through diet or medication and—this is the key—*prevent cancer*. Remember, half of what causes prostate cancer is genetic; the other half is environmental. If you are in a high-risk family, you now have a heads-up—a warning that your father and grandfather never received.

Thankfully, we are talking about a disease that can be cured if it's caught early enough. Many families with inherited illnesses—Huntington's disease, for instance—would give their eyeteeth to face an enemy that can be beaten. And this brings us to one of the great ethical issues of genetic testing. For some families, the counseling and preparation process in genetic testing is extensive. This is because, sadly, some diseases are so horrible and so dreaded that finding the gene is sometimes accompanied by suicide.

But prostate cancer is not such a disease. Not only is it curable if caught early, there are many good treatments that can prolong life, and the next decade will see a virtual explosion—not only of new drugs but of new approaches aimed at turning incurable prostate cancer into a chronic illness, such as diabetes, which might not be eradicated, but can be stopped. The bottom line: there is much hope here, more than ever before.

Although there is no genetic testing available yet, we know that one of the most powerful predictors of prostate cancer risk is a strong family history. If you have two or more relatives who developed prostate cancer, especially if they developed it at a younger age, you are a prime candidate for careful screening. Your best bet for now is to do everything you can to stay ahead of the game. Start screening at age forty, change your diet (for more on food, see chapter 4), and keep learning as much as you can about this disease.

maintained PSA levels consistent with a low risk of developing prostate cancer. In other words, if your PSA track record is good, you can probably retire from PSA screening at around age seventy. In his research, the Johns Hopkins urologist Carter showed that if PSA testing were discontinued at age sixty-five in men who had PSA levels below 0.5–1.0 ng/ml, it would be unlikely that prostate cancer would be missed later in life.

# 6

# DIAGNOSIS AND STAGING

## ▶▶▶ READ THIS FIRST

Do you have prostate cancer? Maybe your prostate-specific antigen (PSA) level was high, or it's higher than it was last year and the year before that. Maybe your doctor felt something suspicious during the rectal exam. What happens now? The next step is to determine whether you have cancer, and the only way to do that is with a biopsy.

But before we go on, we should note that *if it is cancer, there is no need to panic and make any hasty decisions.* If you do have cancer, it didn't start today, this month, or even this year; it's been in there a long time—most likely at least ten years, growing very slowly. Taking a few more weeks to be absolutely certain of the diagnosis, to determine the extent of the disease, to decide on the right treatment, and to find the best doctor to administer that treatment won't mean that you'll miss your window of opportunity to be cured. Instead, taking a few weeks to be sure you have enough information to make the right decision may be the best investment in your health, and your life, that you'll ever make.

Once you have all of this information, it's time for some hard decision-making. It's time to ask yourself, What are my options? And what should I do? For most men, the diagnosis of prostate cancer is un-expected—like a sudden punch in the stomach. As with any other unex-pected calamity in your life, you've got to face it square on and collect all the facts. At your fingertips are three facts you will probably come to know as well as your Social Security number—your PSA, Gleason score, and clinical stage. With just these three facts, almost immediately you will have a good idea of where you stand. The cancer either appears to be clinically localized to the prostate—the most common scenario in the United States today because of improved diagnostic testing—or the can-cer has spread locally, but does not appear to be present at distant sites; or rarely, less than 10 percent of the time, the cancer has been caught later and has spread to either the lymph nodes or bone. Once you know where you stand, your next move is to examine the options for treatment and find the one that you feel is best for you. *Whatever the finding, don't become discouraged. There is more hope now than ever.*

## Diagnosis and Staging

Do you have prostate cancer? Maybe your PSA level was high, or it's higher than it was last year and the year before that. Maybe your doctor felt something suspicious during the rectal exam. What happens now? The next step is to determine whether you have cancer, and the only way to do that is with a biopsy.

But before we go on, we should note several things: First of all, the chances are good that the biopsy will be negative. Only 15 percent of men with a PSA level lower than 4 ng/ml and 25 percent of men with a PSA level between 4 and 10 ng/ml will turn out to have cancer. And even if it is cancer, there is no need to panic and make any hasty decisions. Nothing has to happen today. If you have cancer, it didn't start today, this month, or even this year; it's been in there a long time—most likely at least ten years, growing very slowly. Taking a few more weeks to be absolutely certain of the diagnosis, to determine the extent of the disease, to decide on the right treatment, and to find the best doctor to administer that treatment won't mean that you'll miss your window of opportunity to be cured. Instead, taking a few weeks to be sure you make the right decisions may be the best investment in your health, and your life, that you'll ever make.

Now, how do you make any wise investment? By learning as much as you can before you commit to a plan of action. So let's move ahead with this crash course on biopsy.

## Biopsy

Until the early 1990s, biopsy of the prostate was done "blind"—doctors couldn't see what they were doing—and often, the biopsy wasn't actually taken from the part of the prostate doctors thought they were reaching. Today, using transrectal ultrasound as a guide, urologists can see what they're doing in real time, as they're doing it. So a biopsy of the prostate is more accurate than ever—and, because the needle is smaller, it's less painful, and complications are minimal.

Imagine the prostate as a large strawberry—except this strawberry has just a few seeds, maybe seven little black dots in all. These seeds are tumors, and seven is the average number of separate cancers found in a radical prostatectomy specimen. The development of several cancerous spots happens because prostate cancer is multifocal. It causes what scientists call a field change, in which the entire prostate undergoes a transformation. Multiple tumors pop up like dandelions, all at about the same time. Each spot can be millimeters in size.

This is the challenge facing urologists, for whom the prostate biopsy is a critical scouting mission. Our tactical weapon in this search for cancer is a spring-loaded biopsy gun, a tiny device attached to the ultrasound machine. It's a sophisticated needle, hollow in the center, designed to capture tiny cores, or glands, of tissue—each about a millimeter thick—which pathologists will then analyze under a microscope.

Before the biopsy, you will be asked to have an enema and take some antibiotics to minimize the risk of infection. (For more information, see Before and After the Biopsy below.) The biopsy is done with you wide awake, lying on your side. The urologist inserts the ultrasound probe through the rectum and uses the ultrasound image to direct the needle to strategic sites in the prostate.

Although needle biopsies are much better than they used to be, they still aren't perfect and don't always provide definitive answers. Sometimes what's under the microscope is almost impossible to label definitively as cancer. Just as often, the needle misses the cancer—because it's just plain tricky to hit a tiny seed inside a strawberry, especially one you can't see.

Thus, we hedge our bets. It used to be that urologists took four measly samples of tissue, one from each quadrant of the prostate. Then, the number increased to six (one from the top, middle, and bottom of the gland on the right and left sides). Now it's clear that taking ten or twelve samples is better still. We have also become much more strategic in where we fish for cancer. We know, for instance, where the cancer is most likely to be hiding—in the prostate's peripheral zone, extending along its sides like a shallow horseshoe (see fig. 6.1). We also know that it's likely to spread laterally—like a thin sheet—and that it's easy to stick the needle in too deep and overshoot the target area. Urologists are learning to guide the needle so it catches the edge of the prostate, rather than sampling tissue from the center, for a higher yield of cancer cells. In a Johns Hopkins study, the urologist H. Ballentine Carter found that if only six biopsies are taken in the usual way (from the top, bottom, left, and right sides), 25 percent of prostate cancers are missed. However, if six samples are taken from the area where the cancer most probably is—right along the edges of the peripheral zone—only 12 percent of cancers are missed. But the odds of finding cancer are even better if more samples—twelve to fourteen—are taken. And men with very large prostates (especially men with benign enlargement, or BPH) should have still more samples taken. If, say, instead of a large strawberry, you were trying to pinpoint tiny cancers in an orange, it just makes sense that you're in for a tougher job, unless you sample a greater portion of tissue.

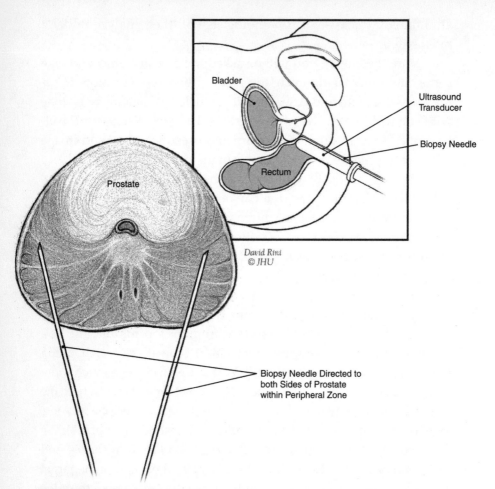

Bladder

Ultrasound
Transducer

Biopsy Needle

Rectum

Prostate

*David Rini*
*© JHU*

Biopsy Needle Directed to
both Sides of Prostate
within Peripheral Zone

**FIGURE 6.1   Fishing for Cancer**

Cancer is most likely to be hiding in the prostate's peripheral zone, extending along its sides like a shallow horseshoe. Because prostate cancer tends to spread laterally—like a thin sheet—it's easy to stick the needle in too deep and overshoot the target area. Urologists are learning to guide the needle so it catches the edge of the prostate, rather than sampling tissue from the center, for a higher yield of cancer cells.

"Breast or lung cancer makes a solid nodule, just like a fist, that you usually can detect by palpation or imaging," says the Johns Hopkins pathologist Jonathan Epstein (see Biopsy: Why You Should Get a Second Opinion below). But prostate cancer tends to infiltrate normal tissue, meandering around normal cells. Or, as the Johns Hopkins scientist Don Coffey explains, it spreads out like a hand whose

## TRANSRECTAL ULTRASOUND:
## BEAUTIFUL PICTURES, LIMITED VALUE BY ITSELF

Like sonar on a submarine, ultrasound creates pictures using sound waves. Transrectal ultrasound can sometimes detect differences between cancerous and normal tissue in the prostate by means of a probe inserted in the rectum (that's what *transrectal* means—literally, "through the rectum"). This probe—in effect a big microphone—is a dramatic improvement over what we had years ago—a lower-frequency, lower-resolution technique in which sound waves had to travel all the way through the abdomen to reach the prostate.

A decade ago, many doctors believed transrectal ultrasound could be a "male mammogram," another means of screening for and detecting prostate cancer early. That hasn't happened. Transrectal ultrasound is neither quick nor cheap, and the results often depend on the skill of the doctor using the ultrasound equipment. But the biggest drawback is that even though ultrasound can produce spectacular images of the prostate, they are often misleading.

*Hit or Miss:* Originally, imaging specialists believed cancers could be distinguished from surrounding tissue because they lacked internal echoes—thus, the sound waves would bounce differently, in distinct patterns. Unfortunately, however, this has not turned out to be a dependable system: just as prostate cancer can feel different to a doctor's finger, based on many factors (see chapter 5), it can also sound different from man to man. Transrectal ultrasound misses about half of prostate cancers greater than 1 centimeter in size because they sound just like regular prostate tissue. And, because some normal tissue sounds just like cancer, ultrasound also mistakes many benign lesions for cancer. *Thus, most cancers are not seen on ultrasound, and most lesions that are seen on ultrasound are not cancer.* The main role for transrectal ultrasound is in guiding the needle biopsy to make sure that the prostate is systematically sampled. Ultrasound can also be useful in determine the weight of a man's prostate, which can, in turn, determine PSA density.

*The Bottom Line on Ultrasound:* It can neither diagnose cancer nor rule it out. Beware of the doctor who wants to do an ultrasound "just to see if there's cancer there" because, again, ultrasound is not a diagnostic technique. Its only purpose is in helping the urologist aim the biopsy needle.

fingers flow into nearby tissue "like a river flooding a valley." This means that there can be a significant amount of cancer—even if it's not in the form of an obvious lump that's easy to feel or see on ultrasound.

## BEFORE AND AFTER THE BIOPSY: WHAT TO DO AND WHAT TO EXPECT

The specifics (such as how long before the procedure you should stop taking aspirin) vary from hospital to hospital, but here are some basic guidelines.

### Before

- No dietary restrictions. Eat breakfast or lunch before you go to the hospital. Drink plenty of fluids—juice, coffee, or water.
- Give yourself an enema (such as Fleet) the morning of the biopsy.
- Continue taking your regularly scheduled medications, but *do not take* aspirin, arthritis medication, high doses of vitamin E, Motrin (ibuprofen), or any blood-thinning medications, such as Coumadin (warfarin) or heparin. If you have pain, take Tylenol (acetaminophen). *Your biopsy will likely be canceled* if you take any pain medication other than Tylenol.
- If you are taking a daily dose of aspirin, *stop taking it ten days before the biopsy.* If you have taken any aspirin within one week of the biopsy, it is safest to reschedule the procedure.
- Do not urinate or empty your bladder just before the procedure. Your bladder should be partially full (this makes it easier for the ultrasound to get a good image).
- Take antibiotics ahead of time. You should receive antibiotic tablets to minimize the risk of infection. The most common antibiotic used for this is a fluoroquinolone, such as Levaquin (levofloxacin) or Cipro (ciprofloxacin). If you have ever had ciprofloxacin—for example, if your doctor suspected that you had an infection in your prostate—you may be resistant to it. Make sure the doctor performing the biopsy knows this, and ask for a different antibiotic, such as Augmentin (amoxicillin and clavulanate potassium). If you are allergic to ciprofloxacin, you should take Augmentin. Also, if you have problems with the valves in your heart or you must take antibiotics before dental work, remind your doctor. In this case, Omnipen (ampicillin) and Garamycin (gentamicin) would be more appropriate. Antibiotics should be taken

the day before the biopsy, on the day of the biopsy, and for two days afterward.

### During

- The biopsy will take about thirty minutes.
- You will be asked to lie on your side. The procedure itself is uncomfortable but usually not painful.

### Afterward

- Your urine will probably be tinged with blood; you may even pass a few blood clots during urination and see blood when you have a bowel movement. This is normal; do not be alarmed. The bleeding should stop the same day or the next morning.
- Force fluids—basically, this means drink a lot—the rest of the day. This is to dilute your urine to prevent the formation of blood clots in the bladder.
- Do not drink any alcoholic beverages for twenty-four hours after the biopsy.
- Resume any prescription medications except blood-thinning agents such as Coumadin (warfarin) or heparin. (Don't start taking these again until your urologist gives you the go-ahead.)
- Do not do any heavy lifting or straining for five days after the biopsy.
- You may see blood in your ejaculate for several months after the biopsy; this is normal.

### Call Your Doctor Immediately If . . .

- You have fever or chills.
- Your bladder feels very full and you are unable to urinate (this is serious; if necessary, go directly to the emergency room).
- Rectal bleeding (usually with a bowel movement) lasts for more than two to three days or is significant.
- Blood in the urine persists for more than five days.

## What Complications Can I Expect from My Biopsy?

Prostate biopsy is an invasive procedure—a minor one, but invasive all the same, and there is a minor risk of complications. These include the following:

## Pain

Although nobody would describe a biopsy as fun, for most men the experience is more in the category of discomfort than significant pain. However, in some men, particularly those who have ten, twelve, or more tissue samples taken, the biopsy can really hurt. What's hurting is not, as you may think, the rectum (there are no pain fibers in the tissue lining the rectum); the pain is from the needle traveling through the prostate itself. How can you make the biopsy less painful? Explore the options with your urologist. One choice is what's called conscious sedation. This is what doctors use in procedures such as colonoscopy. Patients feel no pain and remain conscious throughout the procedure—but don't remember anything that happened during it. (So be aware that even though you may carry on a full conversation with your urologist during the biopsy, afterward you will almost certainly ask the same questions all over again, because you won't remember asking them the first time.) Note: Sedation of any kind increases the cost of a procedure and also introduces the rare but serious risk that there will be complications from the sedation itself. A safer, cheaper solution is the use of a prostatic block—a local anesthetic, similar to the kind your dentist uses to numb your gums before you have a cavity filled. This block is injected into the tissues surrounding the seminal vesicles on both sides of the prostate (this area is called the pelvic plexus). The same nerves that are responsible for erections (these are the neurovascular bundles and are discussed in detail in chapter 8) also carry pain fibers that run to the prostate. Simply blocking these fibers can reduce pain markedly. Alternatively, some urologists believe that the procedure is less painful if an anesthetic jelly is used to lubricate the probe.

## Infection

Despite the fact that the biopsy is taken through the rectum, infection is hardly ever a problem, if its risk is kept to a minimum—if a cleansing enema is given beforehand and antibiotics are given both before and after the biopsy. In most patients, this means getting an oral dose of an antibiotic (in the category of fluoroquinolones) an hour or so before the biopsy and then taking it for two to three days afterward. In some men, however, this may not be enough. If you have a chronic illness such as diabetes, for instance, you may be more susceptible to infection and may need a longer course of antibiotics. Also, if for some reason the trauma to the rectum is greater than usual, infection can develop. This is terribly important: *If you have any fever after the biopsy, contact your urologist immediately.* In very rare cases, infection can be fatal. In the vast majority of men, however, infection never happens, and complications are minimal.

### Bleeding

The urethra, the tube that carries urine from the bladder out of the body, runs right through the prostate (see fig. 1.2). It is very common, therefore, for a man who has had his prostate biopsied to notice a little bit of blood in his urine immediately after the procedure. You also may notice traces of blood in the ejaculate, sometimes for several months afterward. Don't let this scare you. The prostate is like a sponge, riddled with tiny ducts, and any bleeding caused by the biopsy can seep into its many nooks and crannies. This blood turns brown with age, and although it's unpleasant, it is no cause for concern, and it absolutely does not signal some turn for the worse in your cancer. It's just old, dried-up blood.

Now, there's a different type of bleeding that can occur during the biopsy, and although this, too, is rare, it can also be serious and require immediate attention. If a man has large hemorrhoids and the biopsy needle inadvertently punctures one of these veins, this can cause significant rectal bleeding and may necessitate another procedure on the spot—sewing up or tying off the broken vein to stop the bleeding.

### Impotence

A much rarer complication after biopsy is erectile dysfunction. Some men have reported that their erections after their biopsy are not as strong as they were before the procedure; rarely, a man will even experience impotence. If this happens, it is most likely because the biopsy needle hit too close to one of the neurovascular bundles (for more on these, see chapter 8), and *this is a temporary problem.* It's temporary because the nerves are still there and still intact, and there should be a full recovery of sexual function once the bruised nerve heals. Again, this is extremely rare—and most important, you should never let the fear of temporary impotence keep you away from a biopsy. Urologists don't schedule biopsies lightly, and you wouldn't be getting one if your doctor didn't think you needed it.

## If I Have Cancer, Will the Biopsy Spread It?

This is an excellent question and a very common fear. It just makes sense, doesn't it, that if you poke a hole in a wall that's holding back cancer, the cancer might escape. Doctors have worried about this, too, in many forms of cancer. But the good news is that there is no evidence this has ever happened or that it could ever happen. Think about it: almost every cancer you can think of—breast, colon, lung, prostate—is diagnosed by biopsy. If the biopsy itself could spread cancer, then the whole concept of early diagnosis and treatment wouldn't work. But many thousands of people—all of whom had initial biopsies to confirm what they had—have been cured of cancer.

### But What If Some Cancer Cells Escape into My Bloodstream?

Well, they may. In fact, the more we learn about cancer in the prostate and elsewhere, the more we understand that the circulation of cancer cells in the blood is probably a fairly common event, even in cancers that are curable. And it's not unreasonable to assume that a few more cancer cells may find their way to the bloodstream when the tumor is manipulated, as it is during a biopsy. The key is the stage of your cancer. When cancer is confined to the prostate, even if a few cells escape into the blood, they won't survive. This is because they haven't yet gotten the hang of living outside the area where they developed. But over time, cancer cells change. They get more aggressive with age, and they become, in many ways, "smarter." They not only move to distant sites but have the wherewithal to thrive in these new locations as well. So there are two different issues: One is the presence of cancer cells in the blood; the other is the survival of these cells in distant locations. Prostate cancer cells are simply unable to live outside their normal environment until they develop this ability, called metastatic capability.

## They Didn't Find Cancer: Am I Off the Hook?

Perhaps the most troublesome thing about prostate biopsies—already a troublesome subject—is figuring out what to do if the cells aren't cancer. Does that mean there's no cancer there—and if so, then why did your PSA level go up, or what was that hard lump your urologist felt during the rectal exam? If something suspicious prompted the biopsy in the first place, that something is still there. Each needle biopsy samples only one-thousandth of the prostate; if there is no nodule to aim at, it's easy to see how a tumor could be missed, even if twelve cores are taken. If something was palpable during the rectal exam, then you should probably get a repeat biopsy immediately. One explanation for a no-show of cancer is that if a doctor can feel a tumor, that means it's hard—and sometimes, when a needle hits this hard tissue head-on, it just glances off the edge of it without actually penetrating the tumor and taking a sample of it.

Similarly, if your PSA level is significantly higher than it should be for your age or if it's been going up more rapidly than it should, or if your free PSA is low (see chapter 5 for PSA guidelines), it's possible that the needle biopsy simply missed the cancer. In this case, you should have another biopsy. It's not uncommon for a needle biopsy to be negative *even though cancer is present*. This is called a false negative, and it can give both the urologist and the patient "a false optimism that the cancer isn't there," says the Johns Hopkins pathologist Jonathan Epstein. Imagine the difficulty of trying to capture this elusive tissue in a biopsy using only a tiny needle. In some cases, it's like looking *with* a needle in a haystack.

### How Helpful Are Repeat Biopsies?

There is definitely a point of diminishing returns. In a large study from Europe, men with PSA levels between 4 and 10 ng/ml underwent eight-core biopsies, and if cancer was not found but still suspected, they had repeat biopsies. On the first attempt, cancer was present in 22 percent of the men; in 10 percent on the second attempt, and in 5 and 4 percent, respectively, on the third and fourth attempts. Looking at the cancers discovered on the first and second biopsies, the pathologists found the tumors to be similar in volume, grade, and extent. But the cancers detected on the third and fourth go-rounds had a lower stage, grade, and cancer volume—cancers that may not have cried out for urgent detection. The men who underwent third and fourth biopsies had slightly more complications as well. Thus, the researchers felt that a second biopsy was justified in all cases when the initial biopsy was negative. But, they felt, third and fourth biopsies should be done sparingly—only in men in whom there is a high suspicion of cancer.

Another point about a repeat biopsy: more samples should be taken, and the search for elusive cancer should broaden to include out-of-the-way locations, such as the transition zone, where BPH occurs, and up near the top of the prostate (in the anterior or lateral part; see fig. 1.3), where a needle would not normally go.

## New Tests on the Way

Remember the field change we talked about earlier? In prostate cancer, the tissue isn't divided up into areas that are either "normal" or "cancer," with both sides clearly marked to show which is which. We know that in a cancerous prostate, the whole gland changes. So then, if all of the tissue is at unrest, maybe there is no "normal"—even in tissue that doesn't look cancerous. Exploring this idea, the Johns Hopkins scientists Robert Getzenberg and Donald Coffey discovered a nuclear matrix protein, called EPCA (for early prostate cancer antigen; confusingly, this protein is different from EPCA-2, which we discussed in chapter 5). EPCA shows up in both normal and abnormal prostate tissue in men with prostate cancer, which makes it a very good marker for this field effect. This test may help identify cancer in men with biopsies that appear falsely negative.

Also on the horizon is a computerized approach to evaluating the nucleis of biopsied prostate cells. This technique, called quantitative nuclear grade (QNG), was pioneered by the Johns Hopkins urologists Robert Veltri and Alan Partin. The idea, again, is to detect abnormalities in the normal-looking biopsy tissue from men who may well have prostate cancer. If these tests pan out, they may not only save men further biopsies but give peace of mind to men who don't have cancer, and may help men who do have cancer to get treatment sooner.

## Interpreting the Biopsy Findings

Is a biopsy ever just negative? Yes, often the pathologist will state that no cancer is seen, that everything that was biopsied was benign. That is what's called a negative biopsy (although you should still seek a second opinion; see below). However, there are two other diagnoses that sound like cancer is not present, but which can be misleading. The first is a word that pathologists love, atypical. *Atypical* means that the cells can't definitely be called cancerous, but then again, cancer can't be ruled out with certainty. In other words, *atypical* means "maybe." It also means two other things: It means you should have your slides reviewed by a pathologist who is an expert in prostate cancer to be sure that cancer isn't present. And if the pathologist concurs that it is atypical, you need a repeat biopsy.

### What If It's PIN?

The other diagnosis is PIN. As any pathologist will tell you, diagnosing prostate cancer is like trying not to fail a particularly tough multiple-choice test—the kind with bewildering answer options like "All of the above" and "Other." Which brings us to another wrinkle in the ambiguous world of needle biopsies—PIN, or prostatic intraepithelial neoplasia. For lack of a better description, PIN cells are funny-looking prostate cells. They're not cancerous, but they're not benign, either. They're other. They're abnormal, and they're strongly linked to prostate cancer.

Like cancer itself, PIN has its own distinct patterns—mild (PIN1), moderate (PIN2), and severe (PIN3). It's generally believed that mild PIN is insignificant and doesn't require further evaluation. But many pathologists now group together moderate and severe PIN (PIN2 and 3) as high-grade PIN and believe that these cells should be taken very seriously. Some even call these premalignant cells, although again, technically, it's not clear that the cells themselves actually go on to become cancerous. High-grade PIN cells are suspicious characters, often considered guilty by association—harbingers of cancer. "We'll often find high-grade PIN next to cancer," explains the Johns Hopkins pathologist Jonathan Epstein, whose work over the last decade has helped define these cells and who probably knows more about PIN than anyone.

### Not as Sharp a Pointer as It Used to Be

In fact, PIN is so often found along with cancer that, just a few years ago, we believed that if PIN was found on a needle biopsy, a man needed another biopsy because the cancer was just missed—that the needle had found Tweedledee, but somehow missed Tweedledum. Today, this happens less frequently, because we sample more tissue. Previously, we used to take only four or six sample cores, and in doing so probably *did* miss the cancer that was just sitting there, right alongside the PIN cells. Today, however, because we frequently take twelve samples—which means our biopsies are much more accurate—the associated cancer is often picked up with the PIN. If it isn't, and PIN is found alone, we usually don't advise an immediate repeat biopsy. Evidence from a large, Hopkins-led study of thousands of men with prostate cancer shows that when men with high-grade PIN undergo a repeat biopsy, they are no more likely to have cancer than other men, unless there is a lot of PIN. The determining factor, Epstein believes, may be the number of cores that contain high-grade PIN. In a recent study, he found that if PIN was found in three to four cores, 40 to 75 percent of men were eventually diagnosed with cancer. If you have high-grade PIN in three to four cores, your doctor may want you to have another biopsy.

### Can PIN Be "Nipped in the Bud"?

Here's a new idea: Recognizing that PIN is abnormal and although not harmful by itself, that it may either lead to something worse (cancer) or that it marks a bad trend in the prostate, what if we treat it? Some scientists are trying this. New studies suggest that treatment with an antiestrogen drug called toremifene (Fareston), which currently is being used to treat metastatic breast cancer, may be helpful.

In a very preliminary study of men diagnosed with PIN who later underwent another biopsy, toremifene appeared to reduce the number who went on to develop prostate cancer. The drug appears to work best at very low doses, but this is all so new that there are many things we don't yet know. For instance, how long should a man be treated? And does this indeed prevent cancer, or does it just delay it? This is an intriguing new line of research.

## Making Sense of the Gleason Score

Under a microscope, prostate cancer is a mess. Imagine some work of modern art, a painting with countless shades of gray—some nearly white, some nearly black, most subtle variations of shades in the middle. This is prostate cancer—a hodgepodge, a mixed-up batch of cells that range all the way from the almost normal-looking to cells that are so poorly differentiated and obviously diseased that they could never be considered normal.

The concept here is known as heterogeneity, and it's one of the most frustrating aspects in determining how serious a man's prostate cancer is. A pathologist looks at cores of tissue taken in a needle biopsy, and cells from one part of the prostate may look one way, and those from another part may look completely different. So vexing is this, in fact, that for years, pathologists felt that it was impossible to classify, or grade, prostate cancer cells at all.

Then Donald F. Gleason did what nobody else was able to do: he made sense out of these cells. For years, Gleason, the reference pathologist for the Veterans Administration Cooperative Group, studied thousands of prostate cancer biopsies. Gradually, he was able to identify five specific patterns of cancer cell architecture that could be seen under a low-powered microscope. These patterns are called grades and are numbered from 1 to 5. He then found that if he added the number of the most common pattern to the number of the second most common pattern, he came up with a score, and this score proved more accurate at classifying prostate cancer than just picking one pattern alone. Now the Gleason scoring system is accepted universally as the best way to assess the aggressiveness of prostate cancer cells.

The lowest possible Gleason score is $1 + 1 = 2$; the highest is $5 + 5 = 10$. However, although in theory this creates nine distinct risk groups, in practice it works a little differently. Today, hardly any men with Gleason scores of 2, 3, and 4 cancers—the least aggressive and least likely to metastasize—are diagnosed by biopsy. These tumors are most often found in the transition zone, the home of BPH. They're usually found when tissue samples from a transurethral resection of the prostate (TUR) are sent to a pathologist for routine testing; they're generally considered harmless and usually are managed with watchful waiting. These are the slow-growing incidental cancers (discussed in chapter 3) that show up in as many as half of all men by age eighty. These, too, are the cancers that critics of PSA testing worried would be found by regular screening for prostate cancer, leading to unnecessary treatment in men with cancer that would never become a threat.

But again, these very low grade tumors are also the ones we hardly ever see on needle biopsy: fewer than 2 percent of men who have a needle biopsy turn out to have a Gleason score of 2, 3, or 4 cancer. Fortunately, there is good news on the other side of the Gleason scale. We only see high-grade Gleason tumors—Gleason 8, 9, and 10—in about 8 percent of all biopsies. The vast majority of men diagnosed with prostate cancer fall right in the middle of the Gleason scoring system— Gleason 5, 6, and 7. Gleason 5 and 6 tumors are much alike; they behave similarly and are both relatively slow-growing—the kind of cancers that can be cured. To get a Gleason 7, one part of the equation is a 3 and the other is a 4, which means the cancer is more aggressive. However, Gleason 7 is still different from Gleason 8. Furthermore, there is a difference between Gleason 3 + 4, in which most of the tumor is Gleason grade 3, and Gleason 4 + 3, in which most of the tumor is Gleason 4. It is now known that tumors with more Gleason 4 behave more aggressively. (Thus, when talking about Gleason 7, it's important to know which tumor grade is predominant.)

The Gleason grade ranks cell differentiation (fig. 6.2). Basically, the pathologist determines how clear-cut the cancer cells' structure and edges are? The architecture of normal, well-differentiated cells involves distinct, clearly defined borders. Well-differentiated cells have clear centers. "They're like little round doughnuts," says the Johns Hopkins pathologist Jonathan Epstein. When cancer cells become poorly differentiated, they seem to melt together into malignant clumps. These cancers are the most aggressive. They run rampant,

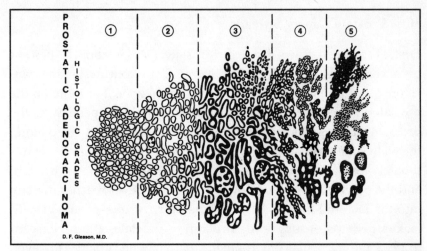

**FIGURE 6.2    The Many Faces of Prostate Cancer: The Gleason Scoring System**

This is prostate cancer—a hodgepodge, a mixed-up batch of cells that range all the way from the almost normal-looking (pattern 1) to cells that are so poorly differentiated and obviously diseased that they could never be considered normal (pattern 5). The Gleason system of evaluating prostate cancer is based on these five specific patterns of cancer cell architecture, called grades. Pathologists add the number of the most common pattern to the number of the second most common pattern and use this score—such as $3 + 3 = 6$ or $3 + 4 = 7$— to assess the aggressiveness of prostate cancer cells.

sweeping through nearby tissue and launching missiles into distant sites in the body, no longer respecting boundaries—their own or those of other cells. The results are often devastating. Without treatment, the fastest, most out-of-control cancer cells can kill a man within several years of their initial clinical presentation. Well-differentiated cancers, in contrast, tend to progress very slowly.

Cancers with a high Gleason score are more likely to be margin-positive (to have cancer that has penetrated the prostate wall to a point where it can't all be removed in surgery; more on this in chapter 7), more likely to have spread to the seminal vesicles, and more likely to defy treatment than cancers with a lower score. With a high Gleason score, there's also a higher likelihood of cancer spreading to the lymph nodes. Therefore, if a man has a high Gleason score, there is a greater probability that his cancer has spread beyond the prostate wall.

### How Prostate Cancer Spreads

First, of course, it grows inside the prostate. (Most—about 72 percent of cancers—begin in the peripheral zone, 20 percent start in the transition zone, and 8 percent start in the central zone. For more on the prostate's zones, see chapter 1.) It reaches, and then penetrates, the prostate wall, also called the capsule. Then it starts to creep along the wall of the prostate, heading north toward the seminal vesicles, ultimately extending in advanced cases into the bladder, the urethra, and the pelvic side walls. (However, it hardly ever reaches directly into the rectum.) Biologically, for whatever reason—certain growth factors, perhaps, or supporting structures—prostate cancer cells seem to need the particular environment that spawned them. However, once the tumor has matured enough to live on its own beyond the prostate—that is, once it can grow around the seminal vesicles—it is also more likely to have spread to distant sites. That's why the finding of cancer cells around the seminal vesicles is so important. It is a sign that this cancer can survive outside the environment of the prostate. When doctors speak of distant metastases of prostate cancer, they generally mean it has hitched a ride via the bloodstream or lymph system to the lymph nodes (channels that run throughout the body), the bones—the spine, ribs, or pelvic bones—or the lungs.

Note: Prostate cancers don't always spread in an orderly fashion, like a marching band in a parade, from point A to point B to point C—from the prostate to the seminal vesicles to the lymph nodes and beyond. Sometimes, especially when there is high-grade disease, even though the cancer is still confined within the prostate, a few cells can invade blood vessels or the lymph system. If the cells have become sophisticated enough to survive on their own, outside the main tumor, they can spread the cancer to a distant site. This is why, even though a cancer may be confined within the prostate with no obvious cells outside the organ, distant metastases can still develop.

## What About Perineural Invasion?

As cancers grow, they compress normal tissue, looking for elbow room—spaces with less resistance, where they can spread. It so happens that nerves are usually surrounded by some empty space. For cancer, this is the real estate equivalent of a nice suburban lot with a big backyard; plenty of elbow room. Thus, it's not uncommon to find prostate cancer in the spaces around the nerves; this is called perineural invasion. Because the nerves are most common close to the surface of the prostate, the finding of perineural invasion on a biopsy suggests that the cancer is close to the edge of the prostate and may well have penetrated the capsule. However—this is important to keep in mind—*cancer that has penetrated the capsule can still be cured.* Which makes this a paradoxical finding—because, although men with perineural invasion are more likely to have capsular penetration than men without it, perineural invasion has no long-term impact on whether a man can be cured. For this reason, some noted pathologists have suggested that it should not even be commented on when found in a biopsy, because it's not worth worrying about.

## Rare Forms of Prostate Cancer

Almost all—95 percent—cancers of the prostate are of a type called adenocarcinoma. These are cancers that form in the tiny glands within the prostate. (For an illustration of the prostate, see chapter 1.) But there are some rare exceptions. One of these is small-cell carcinoma. This form of cancer develops in different cells, called neuroendocrine cells, in the prostate. Small-cell carcinoma of the prostate is very similar to small-cell carcinoma of the lung. It grows rapidly and is very difficult to cure. The main treatment is chemotherapy. (This is discussed in chapter 12.) It is rare for small-cell carcinoma to be diagnosed initially; usually, it's found in patients who were initially diagnosed with "regular" prostate cancer, an adenocarcinoma, that was not controlled by surgery, radiation, or chemotherapy. In these men, cancer typically comes back as a large pelvic mass or as metastases to such organs as the liver. The tip-off to this diagnosis is that small-cell carcinoma does not make PSA. Thus, if a man has a large, local cancer and a low PSA level, he should be evaluated for small-cell carcinoma.

Another rare form of prostate cancer is transitional-cell carcinoma. (Note: This is different from cancer that is found in the prostate's transition zone.) This cancer arises from the prostatic ducts and the prostatic urethra, the stretch of urethra that runs through the prostate. It is the same kind of cancer seen in men with bladder cancer—which means that if this diagnosis is made, a man should be checked for bladder cancer as well—and the treatment is often directed at removing both the prostate and bladder.

Finally, sarcoma of the prostate is very rare. These tumors arise from the stroma, the smooth muscle and connective tissue within the prostate, and they can be very large at the time of diagnosis. Treatment, as with "regular" prostate cancer, is based on the extent of the tumor.

---

### BIOPSY: WHY YOU SHOULD GET A SECOND OPINION

You're a pathologist staring at cancer cells under a microscope. Just a few tiny cores of tissue, and a man's life may depend on what you have to say about it. You make the call: your word is a huge part of the treatment decision-making. So think, think—what about those funny-looking cells over there? Is it cancer?

A prostate biopsy can be a pathologist's worst nightmare. "Of all biopsies, prostate biopsies are probably the hardest" explains the Johns Hopkins pathologist Jonathan Epstein, who is world-renowned for his expertise and accuracy in judging prostate cells, and who has probably examined more prostate tissue than any other pathologist. "You're dealing with such a limited amount of tissue, and cancers tend to creep around the benign gland," rather than forming a solid mass. Imagine a Tootsie Roll, wrapped in paper. The cancer is like the paper, a veneer over an expanse of healthy tissue. And the veneer is often maddeningly ambiguous. So not only can the hollow-core biopsy needle overshoot and miss the cancer, the cancer cells it does get don't always match the pictures in the textbooks.

One result of this is the biopsy labeled atypical—a diagnosis that appears in about 5 percent of biopsies at most institutions, says Epstein. "Basically, what that means is that a pathologist will see something that he thinks could be cancer, but is not comfortable calling cancer." For many patients, the next step is having a repeat biopsy—and the value of this is often questionable, he says. "The problem is, in about 20 percent of cases, the biopsy can miss cancer—so even if it's negative, it doesn't mean the patient doesn't have cancer; in fact, the cancer can be extensive. We've seen some missed entirely. They were called totally benign, yet they were cancer." So instead of having a repeat biopsy, the next step should be getting a second opinion on the "atypical" diagnosis.

Another problem Epstein has found is that many pathologists seem just as likely to overdiagnose cancer. "There are many mimickers of prostate cancer under the microscope, and people not as familiar with prostate biopsies can diagnose cancer when it's not." About 1.5% percent—six to eight men—of the patients who come to the Brady Urological Institute each year with a diagnosis of prostate cancer are found to have been misdiagnosed. "We switch the diagnosis. We say, 'This is not cancer; this is benign.'"

Perhaps the best option in the case of tricky diagnoses, says Epstein, is to have the slides sent to an expert. "About 70 to 80 percent of the time, it can be resolved as being definitively benign or definitely cancer." But even biopsies that seem straightforward deserve another look. "We recommend getting a second opinion before anybody undergoes any form of treatment," says Epstein. "It's just as important as getting a second opinion for surgery or radiation. You could have the best surgeon in the world, but if you don't have the right pathology, you could have the wrong thing done for you."

On this point, Epstein is blunt: "We have done numerous studies showing the reproducibility of Gleason scores" at academic medical centers and in the general pathology community, looking at the Gleason grade based on a biopsy and then comparing it to the actual specimen removed during surgery. Although the "before" and "after" Gleason grades are usually in excellent agreement at academic medical centers, "by and large, the Gleason grading that's performed in the community is disappointing. All across the map, it doesn't correlate with what you see in a radical prostatectomy. People are having decisions made—surgery or radiation, or watchful waiting—based in part on a Gleason grade, when it's not accurate."

Beware the Low-Grade Gleason Score: Particularly erroneous, Epstein has found, are biopsies given low Gleason scores. "From the standpoint of patient care, the low-grade Gleason (a score of 2, 3, or 4) doesn't exist, and it gives a false sense of optimism. Even if I call something a 2 + 2 = 4 in a biopsy, when the prostate is removed in a radical prostatectomy, it will turn out to be Gleason 5, 6, or higher." Low-grade Gleason tumors do exist, Epstein says, "but where they exist is in the central transition zone of the prostate, not in the peripheral zone where you do biopsies. A low Gleason score is the kind of thing that shows up more in a transurethral resection of the prostate" (TUR), a procedure used to treat BPH, in which tiny bits of tissue from the center of the prostate are chipped away and removed through the urethra. "If a tiny focus of low-grade cancer shows up on a TUR, it's not as worrisome as a tiny bit of intermediate tumor found on a biopsy. A low-grade Gleason score is valid on a TUR, but not on a needle biopsy."

## The Diagnosis Is Cancer: What Next?

Do you need further tests? Probably not, if you have localized prostate cancer. At this point, you and your doctor have the main information you need to determine the extent of your cancer and to decide on a course of treatment. The Gleason score tells you the kind of cancer cells you have. The next step is to estimate the extent—how far these cells may have spread. This is called determining the clinical stage of the cancer (or staging the cancer). Is cancer confined to the prostate? Or has it spread, and if it has, how far?

## The Stages of Prostate Cancer

The staging of prostate cancer used to be based on the Whitmore-Jewett staging system, which had four basic categories, ranging from cancer too small to be felt to cancer that had metastasized to the lymph nodes and bone. However, it became clear that more refinements were needed for localized cancer categories, and for this reason, the International Union Against Cancer and the American Joint Committee on Cancer have promoted the use of the TNM system. Here, T represents the local extent of the tumor, N indicates the presence of metastases to the lymph nodes, and M indicates distant metastases. The T stage

TABLE 6.1

### TNM STAGING SYSTEM

| Stage | Description |
| --- | --- |
| T1a | Not palpable in a rectal exam; found incidentally, when benign tissue is removed by a TUR; 5 percent or less of the removed tissue is cancerous. |
| T1b | Not palpable; found incidentally, but greater than 5 percent of the tissue removed by the TUR is cancerous. |
| T1c | Not palpable; identified by needle biopsy because of elevated PSA level. |
| T2a | Palpable; involves less than half of one lobe of the prostate. |
| T2b | Palpable; involves more than half of one lobe, but not both lobes. |
| T2c | Palpable; involves both lobes. |
| T3, T4 | Palpable; penetrates the wall of the prostate and/or involves the seminal vesicles. |
| N+ | Has spread to the lymph nodes. |
| M+ | Has spread to bone. |

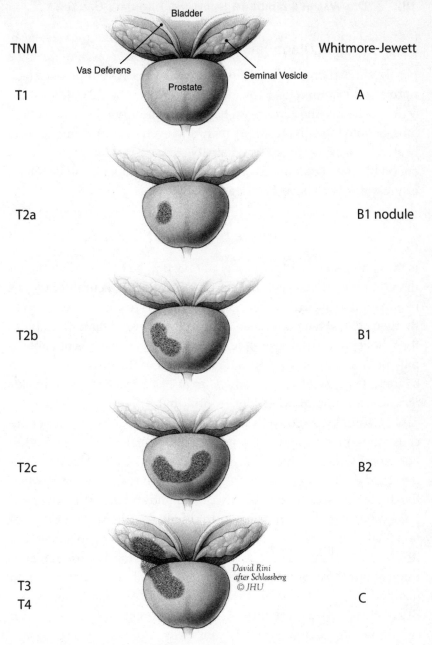

TNM

T1

T2a

T2b

T2c

T3
T4

Whitmore-Jewett

A

B1 nodule

B1

B2

C

Bladder

Vas Deferens

Prostate

Seminal Vesicle

David Rini
after Schlossberg
© JHU

**FIGURE 6.3  The Stages of Prostate Cancer**

This illustration, using both the TNM and the Whitmore-Jewett staging systems, shows prostate cancer in all its stages, ranging from cancer that's too small to be felt to cancer that has spread to the seminal vesicles.

is divided into eight categories, depending on whether the cancer can be felt (an area of firmness is often referred to as a nodule) during a rectal examination—and if so, how extensive it is. If your prostate feels normal on examination, you have T1 disease; the T2 category describes whether the cancer can be felt in half of one lobe, one entire lobe, or both lobes. Note: Many men, and even some doctors, confuse bilateral biopsies with bilateral palpable disease. If your cancer is present on biopsy in both lobes of the prostate but nothing can be felt on examination, you have T1 disease.

## Where Do I Stand?

Is the cancer so small that it may not need to be treated? Is it bigger than that but still localized within the prostate and curable? Or has it spread to a distant site, and the best hope is to control the cancer? By themselves, the various tests you've had aren't enough to paint the whole picture. For example, the digital rectal exam is not able to pick up microscopic cancer that has spread to the prostate wall and beyond. Because of this, *the digital rectal exam tends to underestimate the stage of cancer*. Studies have found that a significant number of cancers initially staged as T2b end up being classified as higher because the cancer has invaded the seminal vesicles or lymph nodes. For cancer with an initial clinical evaluation of T2c, this degree of understaging ranges as high as 38 percent. One reason for this is that the digital rectal exam is subjective; it depends on the experience and perceptiveness of the doctor performing it. Another is that the digital rectal exam can give information only about the prostate gland itself—and not even all of it, at that. And it certainly can't tell anything about the nearby pelvic lymph nodes or bones. Also, if a man has had other surgery on the prostate—a TUR, for instance, for BPH—this can cause the prostate to feel different on an exam, and it can throw off the digital rectal exam.

### What About PSA?

We know a high PSA level can signal the presence of cancer. But can PSA be more specific—can it tell the stage of a man's tumor? Yes, it can. As always, though, PSA is tricky. As a tumor gets bigger, the PSA level generally goes up. However, as the tumor grows, it tends to be overrun by more malignant, poorly differentiated cancer cells that have a higher Gleason score. These poorly differentiated cancer cells are different from normal prostate cells, and as a consequence, they make less PSA. In fact, these cancer cells elevate PSA less per gram of tissue than well-differentiated cancer cells—which means that as cancers grow, the PSA level doesn't go up in a directly corresponding way. That's why PSA levels can be normal even when cancer has spread to the seminal vesicles or pelvic lymph nodes, or it can be higher than expected in men with cancer that's confined to the prostate. *PSA levels do not accurately estimate the growth of cancer.* Thus, *the true meaning of a PSA level can't be interpreted without knowing the Gleason score.*

By itself, the tests you have had are pieces to a puzzle. Scientists at Johns Hopkins have found a more accurate way to estimate the exact extent of prostate cancer using a special table that puts these pieces together—correlating clinical stage, Gleason score, and PSA level, based on information from thousands of men. The result is called an estimated pathologic stage.

The best way to predict a cancer's curability is to remove it and have a pathologist examine every bit of it. This is called the pathologic stage. The information you're working with before treatment—the clinical stage—is an estimate, what a doctor believes a man's prostate cancer to be, based on the rectal exam, PSA level, transrectal ultrasound, and needle biopsy. However, pathologic stage is much more certain for predicting the likelihood of cure, because a pathologist has been able to examine actual prostate tissue and, often, tissue from the lymph nodes—not just make guesses about it based on a few cells and test results.

## The 2007 Partin Tables

My colleague at Johns Hopkins, Alan Partin, and I developed the Partin Tables after he studied the course of prostate cancer in hundreds of my radical prostatectomy patients over the years. They're designed to help men and their doctors predict the definitive pathological stage before treatment so they can determine the best course of action. The latest Partin Tables are based on the results of 5,734 men who underwent surgery at the Johns Hopkins Hospital between 2000 and 2005. It is important to use these tables, because they reflect the improvement in cancer control that has come with increasingly earlier diagnosis. The several tables can predict the likelihood of a man's having organ-confined disease, capsular penetration (cancer that has reached the prostate wall), cancer in the seminal vesicles, and cancer in the lymph nodes with 95 percent accuracy. (These are the numbers in parentheses in the table; they indicate that only 5 percent of the patients will fall on either side of those limits.)

These tables are the next best thing to "virtual surgery"—they help predict what would be found if the prostate were removed surgically and examined by a pathologist. This provides an excellent way to predict the chances of cure—the chances that treatment will eliminate the disease forever and that no cancer cells have escaped the prostate. (For more on the chances of cure with each pathologic stage, see below.)

If the tumor is found to be confined to the prostate or even if the tumor has penetrated the capsule of the prostate but the surgeon can obtain a clear margin, then the chances for cure are very good. (The surgical margin is the edge of the removed tumor; a clear margin means there aren't any cancer cells on the edges—an excellent sign the surgeon got it all.)

How can this be? Isn't there a distinction? Not as much as you might think, and it has to do with the behavior of prostate cancer cells before cancer becomes advanced. For a long time, prostate cancer cells are a bit like hothouse flowers that need the shelter of the greenhouse and can't survive in the harsher world outside. Even though these cancer cells have escaped the prostate, they're still right next to it, and when they are removed surgically with a clear margin, the results are excellent—cancer is cured. Now, if the cancer has made it to the nearby seminal vesicles, it is likely that some cancer cells have escaped the local area—the prostate and its immediate vicinity—and it is possible that these cells may be tough enough to survive on their own at a distant site. However, about 40 percent of men who have seminal vesicle involvement will have an undetectable PSA level (in surgeons' terms, an undetectable PSA level equals cure) ten years after radical prostatectomy. Finally, if cancer has spread to the lymph nodes, it is very unlikely that the PSA level will be low ten years later. But there still may be a role for radical prostatectomy in some men (see below).

## How to Use the Tables

To figure out where you fit into these tables, start by plugging in your PSA level. For example, if a man has a PSA level between 2.6 and 4 ng/ml and a normal-feeling prostate (T1c disease) with a Gleason score of 6, there is an excellent chance that the cancer will be confined to the surgical specimen—what would be removed in a radical prostatectomy, if the man chooses this avenue of treatment. The chances of organ-confined disease are 88 percent and of capsular penetration are 11 percent. These men have a 90 to 99 percent chance of having an undetectable PSA ten years later if their surgical margin is negative. There is a very low probability (1 percent) that the cancer has escaped to the seminal vesicles and no chance that it has spread to the lymph nodes. This is clearly a curable cancer.

Conversely, the higher the PSA level, more poorly differentiated the cancer cells, and the more advanced the clinical stage, the lower the likelihood of cure. For example, if a man has a PSA level of 14 ng/ml, palpable cancer involving both lobes of the prostate (T2c), and Gleason 8 disease, the probability that the cancer will be confined to the surgical specimen is 45 percent and the likelihood that it will involve the lymph nodes or seminal vesicles is 54 percent. In this scenario, it is likely that micrometastasis to distant sites has occurred.

One final comment: The PSA values in these tables are static; they do not reflect rapid changes in PSA levels from one year to another. As we discussed in chapter 5, if your PSA went up by more than 2 ng/ml in the year before your cancer was diagnosed, your disease may be more aggressive than these tables suggest.

### The Han Tables

Ten years after the Partin Tables were developed, we went on to the next logical extension. Although we can learn much about the likelihood of cure from studying radical prostatectomy specimens, the proof is in the actual number of men with these various findings who have an undetectable PSA level ten years later. These tables, developed by Misop Han, Alan Partin, and me, are based on more than two thousand consecutive men who underwent radical prostatectomy between 1982 and 1999 and estimate the likelihood that a man's PSA level will be undetectable ten years after surgery. Because men in recent years have better results, these tables have been corrected to reflect the improvement in survival that comes from diagnosing cancer earlier.

---

### *TABLE 6.2: THE 2007 PARTIN TABLES*

Scientists at Johns Hopkins have found a more accurate way to estimate the exact extent of prostate cancer using a special table that puts these pieces together—correlating clinical stage, Gleason score, and PSA level—based on information from thousands of men. The Partin Tables are designed to help men and their doctors predict the definitive pathological stage before treatment, and then—based on this more accurate information—determine the best course of action. These updated tables are based on the outcome of 5,734 men who underwent radical prostatectomy at the Johns Hopkins Hospital between the years 2000 and 2005. The average age of these men was fifty-seven. These tables predict a man's likelihood of having organ-confined disease, capsular penetration (cancer that has reached the prostate wall), cancer in the seminal vesicles, and cancer in the lymph nodes with 95 percent accuracy. (These are the numbers in parentheses in the table; they indicate that only 5 percent of the patients will fall on either side of those limits.)

## 2007 PARTIN TABLES

### TABLE 3

### PREDICTING PATHOLOGIC STAGE OF PROSTATE CANCER BASED ON CLINICAL STAGE (TNM), PSA, AND GLEASON SCORE
### CLINICAL STAGE T1C (NONPALPABLE, PSA ELEVATED)

| PSA Range (ng/ml) | Pathologic Stage | Gleason Score | | | |
|---|---|---|---|---|---|
| | | 5 – 6 | 3 + 4 = 7 | 4 + 3 = 7 | 8 – 10 |
| 0–2.5 | Organ confined | 93 (95–91) | 82 (87–76) | 73 (80–64) | 77 (85–65) |
| | Extraprostatic extension | 6 (8–5) | 14 (18–10) | 20 (28–14) | 16 (24–11) |
| | Seminal vesicle (+) | 0 (1–0) | 2 (5–0) | 2 (5–0) | 3 (8–0) |
| | Lymph node (+) | 0 (1–0) | 2 (6–0) | 4 (12–1) | 3 (12–1) |
| 2.6–4.0 | Organ confined | 88 (90–86) | 72 (76–67) | 61 (68–54) | 66 (74–57) |
| | Extraprostatic extension | 11 (13–10) | 23 (27–19) | 33 (39–27) | 26 (34–19) |
| | Seminal vesicle (+) | 1 (1–0) | 4 (7–2) | 5 (8–2) | 7 (13–3) |
| | Lymph node (+) | 0 (0–0) | 1 (1–0) | 1 (3–0) | 1 (3–0) |
| 4.1–6.0 | Organ confined | 83 (85–81) | 63 (67–59) | 51 (56–45) | 55 (64–46) |
| | Extraprostatic extension | 16 (17–14) | 30 (33–26) | 40 (45–34) | 32 (40–25) |
| | Seminal vesicle (+) | 1 (1–1) | 6 (8–4) | 7 (10–4) | 10 (15–6) |
| | Lymph node (+) | 0 (0–0) | 2 (3–1) | 3 (6–1) | 3 (6–1) |
| 6.1–10.0 | Organ confined | 81 (83–79) | 59 (64–54) | 47 (53–41) | 51 (59–41) |
| | Extraprostatic extension | 18 (19–16) | 32 (36–27) | 42 (47–36) | 34 (42–26) |
| | Seminal vesicle (+) | 1 (2–1) | 8 (11–6) | 8 (12–5) | 12 (19–8) |
| | Lymph node (+) | 0 (0–0) | 1 (3–1) | 3 (5–1) | 3 (5–1) |
| >10.0 | Organ confined | 70 (74–66) | 42 (48–37) | 30 (36–25) | 34 (42–26) |
| | Extraprostatic extension | 27 (30–23) | 40 (45–35) | 48 (55–40) | 39 (48–31) |
| | Seminal vesicle (+) | 2 (3–2) | 12 (16–8) | 11 (17–7) | 17 (25–10) |
| | Lymph node (+) | 1 (1–0) | 6 (9–3) | 10 (17–5) | 9 (17–4) |

## CLINICAL STAGE T2A (PALPABLE < ½ OF ONE LOBE)

| PSA Range (ng/ml) | Pathologic Stage | Gleason Score | | | |
|---|---|---|---|---|---|
| | | 5 – 6 | 3 + 4 = 7 | 4 + 3 = 7 | 8 – 10 |
| 0–2.5 | Organ confined | 88 (90–84) | 70 (77–63) | 58 (67–48) | 63 (74–51) |
| | Extraprostatic extension | 12 (15–9) | 24 (30–18) | 32 (41–24) | 26 (36–18) |
| | Seminal vesicle (+) | 0 (1–0) | 2 (6–0) | 3 (7–0) | 4 (10–0) |
| | Lymph node (+) | 0 (1–0) | 3 (9–1) | 7 (17–1) | 6 (16–1) |
| 2.6–4.0 | Organ confined | 79 (82–75) | 57 (63–51) | 45 (52–38) | 50 (59–40) |
| | Extraprostatic extension | 20 (24–17) | 37 (42–31) | 48 (55–40) | 40 (50–30) |
| | Seminal vesicle (+) | 1 (1–0) | 5 (9–3) | 5 (10–3) | 8 (15–4) |
| | Lymph node (+) | 0 (0–0) | 1 (2–0) | 2 (5–0) | 2 (4–0) |
| 4.1–6.0 | Organ confined | 71 (75–67) | 47 (52–41) | 34 (41–28) | 39 (48–31) |
| | Extraprostatic extension | 27 (31–23) | 44 (49–39) | 54 (60–47) | 46 (54–37) |
| | Seminal vesicle (+) | 1 (2–1) | 7 (10–4) | 7 (11–4) | 11 (17–6) |
| | Lymph node (+) | 0 (1–0) | 2 (4–1) | 5 (8–2) | 4 (9–2) |
| 6.1–10.0 | Organ confined | 68 (72–64) | 43 (48–38) | 31 (37–26) | 36 (44–27) |
| | Extraprostatic extension | 29 (33–26) | 46 (51–41) | 56 (62–49) | 47 (56–37) |
| | Seminal vesicle (+) | 2 (3–1) | 9 (13–6) | 9 (14–5) | 13 (20–8) |
| | Lymph node (+) | 0 (1–0) | 2 (4–1) | 4 (8–2) | 4 (8–1) |
| >10.0 | Organ confined | 54 (60–49) | 28 (33–23) | 18 (23–14) | 21 (28–15) |
| | Extraprostatic extension | 41 (46–35) | 52 (59–46) | 57 (66–48) | 49 (59–39) |
| | Seminal vesicle (+) | 3 (5–2) | 12 (18–7) | 11 (17–6) | 17 (25–9) |
| | Lymph node (+) | 1 (3–0) | 7 (14–3) | 13 (24–6) | 12 (22–5) |

## CLINICAL STAGE T2B (PALPABLE ≥ ½ OF ONE LOBE) OR T2C (PALPABLE ON BOTH LOBES)

| PSA Range (ng/ml) | Pathologic Stage | Gleason Score | | | | |
|---|---|---|---|---|---|---|
| | | 5 – 6 | 3 + 4 = 7 | 4 + 3 = 7 | 8 – 10 | |
| 0–2.5 | Organ confined | 84 (89–78) | 59 (70–47) | 44 (58–31) | 49 (65–32) | |
| | Extraprostatic extension | 14 (19–9) | 24 (33–16) | 29 (42–19) | 24 (36–14) | |
| | Seminal vesicle (+) | 1 (3–0) | 6 (14–0) | 6 (14–0) | 8 (21–0) | |
| | Lymph node (+) | 1 (3–0) | 10 (25–2) | 19 (40–4) | 17 (42–3) | |
| 2.6–4.0 | Organ confined | 74 (80–68) | 47 (56–39) | 36 (45–27) | 39 (50–28) | |
| | Extraprostatic extension | 23 (29–18) | 37 (45–28) | 46 (55–36) | 37 (48–27) | |
| | Seminal vesicle (+) | 2 (5–2) | 13 (21–7) | 13 (22–7) | 19 (32–9) | |
| | Lymph node (+) | 0 (1–0) | 3 (7–0) | 5 (14–0) | 4 (13–0) | |
| 4.1–6.0 | Organ confined | 66 (72–59) | 36 (43–29) | 25 (32–19) | 27 (37–19) | |
| | Extraprostatic extension | 30 (36–24) | 41 (47–33) | 47 (55–38) | 38 (48–28) | |
| | Seminal vesicle (+) | 4 (6–2) | 16 (23–10) | 15 (23–9) | 22 (33–13) | |
| | Lymph node (+) | 1 (2–0) | 7 (12–3) | 13 (21–6) | 11 (23–4) | |
| 6.1–10.0 | Organ confined | 62 (68–55) | 32 (38–26) | 22 (29–17) | 24 (33–17) | |
| | Extraprostatic extension | 32 (38–26) | 41 (49–33) | 47 (56–38) | 38 (48–29) | |
| | Seminal vesicle (+) | 5 (8–3) | 20 (28–13) | 19 (28–11) | 27 (39–16) | |
| | Lymph node (+) | 1 (2–0) | 6 (11–3) | 11 (19–5) | 10 (20–3) | |
| >10.0 | Organ confined | 46 (83–39) | 18 (24–13) | 11 (15–7) | 12 (18–7) | |
| | Extraprostatic extension | 41 (50–34) | 40 (51–31) | 40 (52–30) | 33 (46–22) | |
| | Seminal vesicle (+) | 7 (12–4) | 23 (33–15) | 19 (29–10) | 28 (42–16) | |
| | Lymph node (+) | 5 (8–2) | 18 (30–9) | 29 (44–15) | 26 (44–12) | |

## TABLE 6.3: THE HAN TABLES

Once again, taking the same information that we used in the Partin Tables—our old friends PSA, Gleason score, and clinical stage—these tables go a step further. They predict the likelihood that a man will have an undetectable PSA level ten years after surgery and therefore give a very clear picture of the probability of cure. Note: Like the Partin Tables, these tables can predict with 95 percent accuracy.

*How to Use These Tables:* Find your biopsy Gleason score (from the left column) and your PSA level (from the top row), obtained before surgery. The intersection of the two is your probability of having an undetectable PSA level (less than 0.2 ng/ml) ten years after surgery. In the parentheses next to each percentage is the 95 percent confidence interval. A broader range means that this percentage is less certain than a narrower range.

### PERCENTAGE OF MEN WITH UNDETECTABLE PSA AT 10 YEARS FOLLOWING RADICAL RETROPUBIC PROSTATECTOMY FOR *STAGE T1C DISEASE*

| T1c cancer | PSA 0–4 | PSA 4.1–10 | PSA 10.1–20 | PSA Greater Than 20 |
|---|---|---|---|---|
| Biopsy Gleason score 5: | 99% (95–100) | 97 (91–99) | 94 (80–98) | 87 (59–96) |
| Biopsy Gleason score 6: | 97 (91–99) | 95 (83–98) | 90 (69–97) | 81 (47–94) |
| Biopsy Gleason score 3 + 4: | 95 (83–98) | 91 (72–97) | 84 (54–95 | 73 (33–91) |
| Biopsy Gleason score 4 + 3: | 89 (67–97) | 83 (53–95) | 74 (36–92) | 62 (18–88) |
| Biopsy Gleason score 8–10: | 79 (40–94) | 71 (30–91) | 61 (18–87) | 50 (06–84) |

### PERCENTAGE OF MEN WITH UNDETECTABLE PSA AT 10 YEARS FOLLOWING RADICAL RETROPUBIC PROSTATECTOMY FOR *STAGE T2A DISEASE*:

| T2a cancer | PSA 0–4 | PSA 4.1–10 | PSA 10.1–20 | PSA Greater Than 20 |
|---|---|---|---|---|
| Biopsy Gleason score 5: | 98% (94–100) | 96 (88–99) | 92 (74–98) | 83 (50–95) |
| Biopsy Gleason score 6: | 97 (89–99) | 93 (79–98) | 87 (61–96) | 75 (37–92) |
| Biopsy Gleason score 3 + 4: | 93 (78–98) | 88 (64–96) | 79 (44–93) | 65 (22–89) |
| Biopsy Gleason score 4 + 3: | 86 (58–96) | 78 (43–93) | 67 (26–89 | 53 (10–84) |
| Biopsy Gleason score 8–10 | 72 (30–92) | 63 (20–88) | 63 (20–88) | 39 (03–78) |

## PERCENTAGE OF MEN WITH UNDETECTABLE PSA AT 10 YEARS FOLLOWING RADICAL RETROPUBIC PROSTATECTOMY FOR *STAGE T2B/C DISEASE*

| T2b cancer | PSA 0–4 | PSA 4.1–10 | PSA 10.1–20 | PSA Greater Than 20 |
|---|---|---|---|---|
| Biopsy Gleason score 5: | 98% (92–99) | 95 (83–99) | 89 (66–97) | 77 (38–93) |
| Biopsy Gleason score 6: | 95 (85–99) | 91 (72–97) | 83 (51–95) | 68 (25–90) |
| Biopsy Gleason score 3 + 4: | 90 (71–97) | 84 (54–95) | 73 (33–91) | 57 (13–85) |
| Biopsy Gleason score 4 + 3: | 81 (48–94) | 72 (32–91) | 59 (15–86) | 43 (04–80) |
| Biopsy Gleason score 8–10: | 65 (19–89) | 54 (11–84) | 41 (04–78) | 28 (01–72) |

## What Do I Do with All This Information?

First of all, know that although these figures are as accurate as we can make them, *they are just statistics.* There are no absolutes; every man's situation is different. Thus, factors beyond cold, hard numbers can be terribly important in determining the best course of action. For some men over sixty, expectant management may be a good choice (for a discussion, see chapter 7). What if you're in a situation where cure is unlikely but possible? For a man in good health who otherwise could expect to live at least ten to fifteen more years, *the side effects of radical prostatectomy are low enough that it's worth it to attempt a cure.* For older men or men with other health problems (because radical prostatectomy, a major operation, does take a certain physical toll) who are more likely to have severe side effects from surgery and less likely to receive the same benefit, radiation is probably a better choice.

So take this information as your starting point. Consider carefully your overall health and potential longevity. Then you and your doctor can decide whether it's reasonable to select curative forms of therapy or simply to adopt a policy of expectant management, in which the tumor is treated only after there is evidence of progression.

And finally, *whatever your finding, don't get discouraged.* Even cancer in the highest stages can be controlled and kept at bay indefinitely, sometimes for many years. There is always hope. Even men with cancer in their lymph nodes can live for many years clinically disease-free (without any symptoms). There is much more about this in later chapters.

## Factors That May Affect Your Outlook

### Age

Age is one of the most important considerations in making a decision about treatment, and it's also one of the hardest. For most of us, on the scale of unpleasant things to do, estimating how many more years we have left to live would rank right up there with having a root canal. But now is the time for you to make an honest appraisal of your general health. If you appear to have localized cancer but you've got some other medical problems—say you've had a heart attack or you have trouble breathing—then it may be necessary only to keep an eye on the tumor, a treatment that's called expectant management. You might also opt for one of the less strenuous forms of treatment. On the other hand, if your family has a history of longevity (if your parents lived into their eighties or nineties), your blood pressure is low, you don't have diabetes, you don't smoke, and you have no history of heart disease, then you may live long enough to *need* to be cured, and your cancer may be aggressive enough that it requires aggressive therapy.

We used to believe that prostate cancer was an "old man's disease"—rather doddering, slow to progress, and more harmless than cancer in younger men. We don't believe that anymore. Research has shown that in older men, prostate cancer is often more aggressive than it is in younger men, and it's often diagnosed at a later stage. In a recent study of 341 men under age fifty who underwent a radical prostatectomy at Johns Hopkins, we found that these men were more likely to be diagnosed with organ-confined disease and that they were more likely to remain cancer-free than older men. The urologists Alan Partin and H. Ballentine Carter looked at men with stage T1c disease and found that the older the patients, the more likely they were to have Gleason scores of 7 or higher.

Now, why is this? Simply because the cancer has been there longer. As prostate tumors grow, they become more heterogeneous and poorly differentiated. They accumulate more mutations and become more aggressive. Prostate cancer generally is a slow grower. In its early stages, it can take months or even years for a tumor to double in size. Before a tumor ever gets big enough for a doctor to feel—about 1 cubic centimeter in volume—it has to double at least thirty times. But after this, it takes only about ten more doublings for prostate cancer to become fatal—when it reaches 1 kilogram in volume. Each time the tumor doubles, there are more mutations. The cancer begins to grow faster; it becomes more aggressive, and the cells learn how to live outside the comfortable environment of the prostate. *So in some older men, it may be wise to undertake aggressive therapy if it is likely that they will be living for many more years.*

## Race

As we discussed in chapter 3, African American men are not only more likely to develop prostate cancer but are also more likely to die from it. In fact, black men from any country are more prone to prostate cancer than any other men. We talked about many reasons why this could be—factors ranging from socioeconomic to genetic. And even though we don't understand exactly why this is, the main thing that we do understand very clearly is that *black men with prostate cancer have a serious condition that needs to be approached with the intent to cure.* If you are a black man diagnosed with prostate cancer, you and your doctor need to go after it *now*, aggressively.

## Stage T1c Cancer

Of all the categories of prostate cancer, this is probably the one that's hardest to make precise predictions about, because it contains a broad spectrum of tumors—from the tiniest, which need no treatment, to some that are quite extensive. We studied nearly 1,200 men with stage T1c disease who underwent a radical prostatectomy at Johns Hopkins between 1988 and 2000. We found two major determining factors in these men: a PSA level greater than 10 ng/ml or a biopsy Gleason score of 7 or higher. In men without either of these risk factors, the odds of having an undetectable PSA level at ten years was 96 percent. For men who had either of these risk factors, ten years after surgery, 73 percent had an undetectable PSA level. In this study, about one-third of the men had high-risk T1c disease. Beyond this, there are two distinct subcategories of stage T1c disease.

*Low-Volume T1c Cancer*

The advantage of any screening program for cancer is that it's designed to detect cancer early. The disadvantage of such programs, including the ones for breast cancer, is that some cancers may be found at such an early stage that they don't need to be treated. This can be the case in men with T1c cancer: a number of these men have low-volume cancers. Do you? And does this mean you're one of those lucky men whose cancer won't ever grow enough to cause trouble? The findings reported by the pathologist on the needle biopsy, your PSA density, and your free PSA percentage can help here. If the pathologic findings suggest that you may have a small tumor, your PSA density should not be more than 10 or 15 percent of the weight of your prostate. If it's higher, this suggests that something more than benign disease is responsible for your elevated PSA level and that the needle biopsy just didn't sample it adequately. Similarly, if the PSA is coming from BPH, your free PSA should be high—above 15 percent. If it's less than 15 percent, then it is likely that cancer, not benign disease, is causing your PSA to rise—in which case, the cancer is probably more significant than it seems.

*If you're a healthy man under the age of sixty with many years still ahead, watchful waiting is not for you. You should strongly consider curative treatment.* The expert pathologist Jonathan Epstein of Johns Hopkins says he does not know which cancer is so small in a young man that it won't grow to the point of threatening his life over time. Also note that even if you meet all of the criteria below, there is still a 25 percent chance that you have more cancer than the evidence suggests and, if you are in this group you have the most to lose.

But if you're over age sixty and you have been diagnosed with a small cancer that may never be life-threatening, you may be a candidate for watchful waiting, or expectant management. Expectant management, which we'll discuss more thoroughly in the next chapter, means monitoring the situation and not making a decision about treatment until it's more clear that your cancer poses a significant threat. Here are some factors that can help predict which cancer is significant and which is not. *Note: These factors apply only if the cancer is not palpable and if the biopsies have included at least six cores.*

## Stage T1c Cancer Is Significant If . . .

It's found in three needle cores, OR
It's present in greater than half of any one needle core, OR
The Gleason score is 7 or higher, OR
The PSA density is greater than 0.1–0.15, OR
The free PSA is less than 15 percent.

## Stage T1c Cancer Is Probably *Not* Significant If . . .

It's found in only one or two needle cores, AND
It makes up less than half of each needle core, AND
The Gleason score is 6 or lower, AND
The PSA density is less than 0.1–0.15, AND
The free PSA is greater than 15 percent.

The key word here is "predictive." (Remember, any clinical stage is a prediction. The only certainty is pathologic stage.) This prediction is the best we have, based on all we know, and it's only about 75 percent accurate. This means that about 75 percent of the men who are predicted to have low-volume cancer actually are found to have it when they undergo radical prostatectomy. There's a caveat here, too: it all depends on your pathology. It is possible that the doctor's needle did not adequately sample the prostate for all the difficulties with needle biopsy that we discussed earlier in this chapter.

What about the remaining 25 percent? The news is good: although there's more cancer, it is almost always confined to the prostate and curable. However, 25 percent is a large number of men with significant prostate cancer. *That's why we feel that if you're a younger man who may have low-volume disease, you should be very cautious about embracing an expectant management philosophy.* Prostate cancer is not always forgiving. There are not many second chances with this disease. You need to understand the seriousness here before you take this step. What if the cancer, which is curable now, spreads from one PSA test to the next?

If your health is otherwise good, you expect to live at least ten years, and you decide to select expectant management, you will need to watch this cancer like the proverbial hawk. For starters, if you did not have twelve samples taken during your biopsy, you should have this done now. This will help you be more certain that there isn't more cancer than the original biopsy suggested. If these samples do not reveal more cancer, you should have a rectal exam and PSA test every six months and have a yearly biopsy to make sure the primary tumor has not changed. Unfortunately, as we discussed above, PSA is not perfect in estimating the growth of a tumor. In one Johns Hopkins study, 25 percent of men with progressively growing cancers showed *no increase* in their PSA. What do we know about expectant management in men who appear to have these small tumors? So far, most studies of this have been short-term, because this condition has been recognized for less than a decade. But several studies suggest that 25 to 50 percent of these men who are followed closely will develop progression of cancer within three to five years. At that point, if they choose to undergo surgery, most—but not all—of them will have curable disease.

### Very High PSA

You have T1c disease, but your PSA level is through the roof. It is still possible that you may have curable disease? There is an unusual form of prostate cancer in which men with curable disease can have very high PSAs—as high as 300 ng/ml, for example. How can this be? The cancer is in the transition zone—the site where BPH develops. This ring of tissue surrounds the urethra, and if cancer is here, it may be trapped in the center of the prostate by a thick band of smooth muscle. In this location, tumors can grow to be quite large without escaping the prostate. This is the site, too, of the low-grade Gleason tumors, as discussed above, that probably wouldn't be diagnosed if it weren't for a TUR procedure. For reasons we don't understand, tumors here are usually well differentiated, and *men with transition zone cancer can usually be cured*. How do you know if you have it? First, cancers in the transition zone are hardly ever felt during a rectal exam, because they're smack in the middle of the prostate. Second, they're hard to diagnose, and a typical patient will have undergone two or three negative biopsies before the cancer is found. And finally, the tumors are usually less than Gleason 7. If these criteria apply to you, you may well have curable cancer.

## Acid Phosphatase

Acid phosphatase is an enzyme that, just like PSA, is secreted by the prostate gland. When a prostate becomes cancerous, the ductal system stops working properly. So, like PSA, acid phosphatase builds up in the prostate, leaks out, and is reabsorbed by the bloodstream. That's why elevated acid phosphatase levels can signal that something's wrong with the prostate. However, unlike PSA, acid phosphatase is made by many organs other than the prostate. For example, after radical prostatectomy, PSA falls to zero, but acid phosphatase still remains in the normal range; thus, acid phosphatase is not as specific as PSA for detecting prostate cancer.

There are two ways of looking at acid phosphatase: radioimmunoassay and enzymatic assay. The radioimmunoassay test is *not* helpful. Acid phosphatase is often elevated in men with BPH, and therefore this test gives little useful information. The enzymatic test, however, can be helpful, because, if it is elevated, it usually signifies advanced disease. But, like PSA, acid phosphatase can be tricky. There are many men with advanced disease in whom acid phosphatase is not elevated.

The PSA test is much more sensitive, and its increasingly widespread use has led some doctors to question the value of acid testing phosphatase. For instance, in one study of 460 men with prostate cancer, twenty-one men had elevated prostatic acid phosphatase (Pap) scores. But for seventeen out of these twenty-one men, advanced cancer had been detected either by an abnormal digital rectal exam or PSA score—so the Pap test provided helpful information for only four men out of the whole group! (This is what scientists call a low yield of unique information.) And sometimes when Pap is elevated, it's wrong—a false positive, creating needless anxiety and confusion. Therefore, acid phosphatase is no longer considered a must-have test before a doctor can determine the best therapy. It is most helpful in determining the extent of an advanced tumor.

## Transrectal Ultrasound and Staging

Most studies have found transrectal ultrasound to be a rather mediocre predictor of the presence of cancer that has penetrated the prostate wall and to be downright poor in finding cancer that has reached the seminal vesicles. Remember, most lesions that show up on ultrasound are not cancer, and most cancers are not seen on ultrasound. In two studies, only 30 percent of tumors that had spread to the seminal vesicles could be found by ultrasound. One investigation of thirty men undergoing radical prostatectomy found ultrasound's sensitivity in spotting cancer that had worked its way beyond the prostate wall was a measly 5 percent. Another study, comparing ultrasound and pathological staging in 121 men, found ultrasound's overall accuracy in staging was only 66 percent—better, but still not reliable enough. And a multicenter study of 230 men found that ultrasound correctly staged 66 percent of locally advanced cancer and only 46 percent of cancers confined to the prostate.

Ultrasound's main difficulty is its inability to "see" microscopic cancer spread. So, to sum up: no definitive decision about a man's course of treatment should be made on the basis of ultrasound alone, and ultrasound readings shouldn't be the cause of a man's exclusion from surgery that potentially could cure his disease.

## Bone Scan (Radionuclide Scintigraphy)

In a bone scan, doctors inject into the bloodstream a radioactive tracer, a chemical that's attracted, like a magnet, specifically to bone. (This substance is harmless and soon passes out of the body.) Then, using a device called a gamma camera, doctors take pictures of the bones. Normal bone absorbs the radioactive tracer at a lower level. But in areas of new growth—of bone regeneration, as in a healing fracture or cancer—the tracer accumulates; more is absorbed, and this surplus shows up as a "hot spot" on the image.

Bone scans are not perfect. Many men feel that if their bone scan is negative, they're home free. Unfortunately, that's not always true. Microscopic prostatic cancer cells, as we've discussed earlier in this chapter, can sneak out of the prostate and move into bone. But these cells are called micrometastases for a reason—they're tiny. It could take five, ten, or even fifteen years for them even to show up on a bone scan. Thus, a negative bone scan doesn't mean you don't have micrometastases, so it's not very sensitive. Worse, it's not terribly specific. Any form of bone disease will show up as a hot spot mimicking cancer: a new or old fracture, infection, arthritis—anything that's got to do with the bone in question. For example, one man went through a terrible scare because a hot spot suggested the prostate cancer had spread to his skull. It turned out to be an old football injury. The man's cancer was removed, and his PSA remains undetectable. But he and his family experienced needless stress at an already stressful time. Thus, routine bone scans are not useful in men with localized prostate cancer. The likelihood of metastases is extremely low, and most of the lesions the scan does pick up aren't cancer anyway.

Today, bone scans are rarely performed on patients with PSA levels less than 10 ng/ml unless they are experiencing bone pain or have signs of more advanced disease (Gleason score greater than 7 or a clinical stage of T3 or greater). Here, a bone scan can be very helpful. If it demonstrates that cancer has spread to bone, then the treatment at this point is clear—immediate hormonal therapy. If the bone scan is inconclusive, more tests will be necessary to find out what form of bone disease is present. Plain X-rays can rule out the presence of benign conditions, such as an old fracture, arthritis, or Paget's disease (in which there is an overgrowth of bone). If these X-rays are clear, it is possible that there is a small bit of underlying cancer—in which case, the next step is usually an MRI scan of bone. If the answer is still not clear, rarely, some men undergo biopsies of bone to exclude metastases.

## Optional Imaging Tests for Staging Prostate Cancer

Thank goodness that we have such powerful tools as the PSA blood test and the Gleason score to help us understand what we're dealing with in each man's particular prostate cancer. The one thing we don't have in our diagnostic workshop is the ability to image the cancer accurately. Such imaging would make life so much more simple! For example, we wouldn't have to guess where to put the needle during the biopsy; we'd already know. And we would have a much better idea whether a man really had a small amount of cancer in his prostate or whether there were a lot of it hiding up on top of the prostate, where our needles can't reach.

But we don't have accurate prostate cancer imaging today. We hope that this will change soon—that with improvements in MRI,

PET scanning, antibody-based probes, and other techniques, we will be able to define the location and extent of cancer not only within the prostate but at distant sites to which it may have spread. Having said that, we're going to cover what we do know about imaging—the advantages as well as the limitations.

### MRI Scan

Magnetic resonance imaging (MRI) is painless and noninvasive; it gives a three-dimensional scan of the body, producing images that are like slices of anatomy. It creates better pictures than CT scans (see below), but it's expensive and time-consuming (an average scan takes about forty-five minutes). Also, being inside an MRI machine, according to one typical patient, is "like being a sardine in a can." Some patients (5 percent or fewer) actually become claustrophobic while they lie in the machine's tubelike embrace. To help prevent this, some hospitals play soothing music while patients are being imaged. (One bit of advice for men about to undergo an MRI scan, although it's easier said than done: it really helps to relax, close your eyes, and, if you can, try to go to sleep.) The newest generations of MRI machines are moving away from the torpedo-tube design and are more open.

The appeal of MRI is that it produces beautiful images of the prostate. The problem is that we can't rely on these gorgeous images to stage a man's prostate cancer accurately. Several years ago, we hoped a new transrectal coil would fine-tune the accuracy. (Like the probe in transrectal ultrasound, this allowed pictures to be taken through the rectum instead of through the abdomen.) Although it helped, it still did not provide the accuracy we had hoped for. Then came another variation of this approach called magnetic resonance spectroscopy imaging (MRSI). Some doctors believe this helps identify whether a suspicious shadow is cancer.

Some institutions place great faith in these techniques and rely on them for determining the location and extent of cancer. In several studies supporting the use of these images, doctors used MRI techniques to estimate the location of cancer before surgery and compared it to that of the actual cancer found in the radical prostatectomy specimen. However—as we talked about earlier—on average, there are seven separate tumors in each radical prostatectomy specimen. And in most men, the tumor is bilateral (on both sides of the prostate)—which makes this a bit like shooting ducks in a barrel. In men already diagnosed with cancer extensive enough to warrant surgery, it doesn't take dazzling, microscopic precision (which MRI techniques are still unable to achieve) to aim an imaging device at the prostate and hit cancer. Two studies have borne this out. One suggested that the ability of MRI and MRSI to estimate tumor volume ranged from 3 percent to 433 percent. That's certainly a wide range! Another tightened the definition for locating the tumor by insisting that the diameter estimated by imaging be within 50 and 150 percent of the true diameter of the tumor, as confirmed by the radical prostatectomy specimen. This reduced the true detection rates to 37 percent. Doctors who report good results say that their ability to use these images improves when the radiologist knows the findings of the rectal examination, where the needle biopsies showed cancer, and the PSA level. Another difficulty is that most of these studies are performed after a man has had at least one biopsy; we know that bleeding from the biopsy can obscure the results. Although there are strong advocates of this technique, I have seen too many patients who have been told that the tumor extended outside the prostate on the left—when, in fact, there turned out to be little tumor on the left or the major tumor extended outside the prostate on the right. An imprecise road map is not terribly useful. For this reason, we limit the use of MRI to men in whom the cancer appears to be more extensive and we are interested in whether it has spread to the pelvic lymph nodes. However, there are newer, faster machines on the horizon that use stronger magnets. When these new machines are combined with the use of intravenous contrast agents (called dynamic contrast-enhanced MRI) the accuracy may be improved.

## LMRI Scan

Nanoparticle-enhanced lymphotropic MRI scanning (LMRI) provides a more accurate way to assess lymph node involvement. It involves injecting tiny iron oxide particles into the bloodstream. These nanoparticles slowly make their way into the lymph nodes, where they are gobbled up by white blood cells—which, in turn, cause changes in magnetic properties that can be detected by MRI. In normal lymph nodes, the iron particles are distributed uniformly. But if there are metastases, small defects can be seen. Although the use of this technique in prostate cancer has been limited, early results appear successful. The availability of LMRI is not widespread, but when a man's lymph node status may affect his therapy, this might be an ideal alternative to surgical lymphadenectomy (see below).

### CT Scan

Getting a computed tomography (CT) scan basically means having a circular series of X-rays taken by a machine that goes around the body. Then, a computer puts the pictures together, generating images that, as in MRI, are like slices of anatomy. The CT tube in which a patient lies is bigger than that of an MRI machine, so claustrophobia is not such a problem, and this technology is faster than MRI. However, the pictures aren't terribly good either. (One way doctors can enhance CT images is to give patients an intravenous dye; however, this can cause an allergic reaction in some people.)

When it comes to imaging the prostate, CT has turned out to be something of a dud. It can't visualize cancer in the prostate, and it's not very good at showing cancer that has spread beyond the prostate. This is mainly because CT looks for sizable masses. It can't spot tiny invasions; and sadly, this is how most prostate cancers spread to new territories. (For example, the overwhelming majority of metastases to the lymph nodes start out on a microscopic level.)

In detecting localized spread of prostate cancer (beyond the prostate wall or into the seminal vesicles), CT has been found to have a sensitivity of 50 percent at best. It also has an unfortunate false-positive rate in diagnosing prostate cancer in the seminal vesicles. We do not recommend routine CT scans for men who appear to have localized disease. In men with advanced disease, where we are concerned that cancer may be in the lymph nodes, MRI is the preferred means of imaging.

### ProstaScint Scan

This test uses an antibody stuck to a radioactive isotope called indium. This antibody, injected in the bloodstream, is designed to zoom in on prostate-specific membrane antigen, or PSMA, a protein that's made on the surface of prostate cells and is highly expressed in advanced cancers. The idea is that this test—a nuclear medicine scan of the abdomen and pelvis—could show the extent of disease, highlighting cancer in the prostate and in the area immediately around it, and could even spot pockets of cancer elsewhere, such as in the lymph nodes. The test has much promise. For now, however, ProstaScint scans are difficult to read, and there seems to be a great deal of subjectivity in interpreting them. Because the results are often inscrutable, many physicians are reluctant to rely on this test—which leads to the question, why perform a test if you're not confident in the result? New approaches using 3-D imaging may make this scan more helpful. Also, the antibody that is currently used is targeted at portions of the protein that are inside the cell, which means that the test can identify only those cells that are already dead. But new antibodies and approaches, aimed at the portion of the protein that is outside the cell, seem to be much better. These antibodies are also being used experimentally in an attempt to direct chemotherapy or radiation therapy toward cancers outside the prostate.

## PET Scan

Positron emission tomography (PET) is a noninvasive technique also called functional imaging. It has the unique ability to show specific biochemical processes, such as tumor glucose metabolism, within the body. PET scans use radioisotopes that release positrons (positively charged electrons) as they decay. The release of these radioactive substances can be measured with a radiation detector and then shown on a computer screen using CT. Tumors, just like normal cells, use glucose, and in some cancers, PET imaging has been helpful in showing this, using a radioactive tracer called FDG. But in prostate cancer, this technique is disappointing—mainly because most prostate cancers have a relatively low rate of glucose breakdown, and the FDG doesn't accumulate in high enough concentrations for us to learn very much. Also, it's hard to see the nuclear forest for the trees; because FDG is also excreted by the kidneys, it appears in the ureter and bladder, so the prostate and pelvic lymph nodes do not show up clearly. Scientists are actively exploring new radioactive tracers, including choline, DHT, acetate, and PSMA. But for now, the use of PET scanning for determining the location and extent of prostate cancer should be considered experimental.

### Chest X-ray

The presence or absence of cancer in a man's lungs can help doctors stage prostate cancer. But metastases to the lungs in men with localized prostate cancer are very rare. A chest X-ray is definitely optional, but not necessary. The greatest value of this test is in detecting heart and lung disease rather than the spread of prostate cancer.

## Lymphadenectomy

Just as the best way to stage cancer is to look at it after the fact (after it's been removed during surgery), the best way to check the lymph nodes in the pelvis for cancer is to go in there and get them—to remove them surgically and let a pathologist examine them. If a large, suspicious-looking lymph node is seen on an imaging study, it is possible to do a needle biopsy (similar to a needle biopsy on the prostate) without surgery. However, when prostate cancer metastasizes to the lymph nodes, the nodes rarely become enlarged. Thus, if it's essential to know the status of the lymph nodes, surgical removal is necessary.

The lymph nodes can be tested during a prostatectomy operation (see chapter 8), but this technique, called frozen section analysis, often misses small amounts of tumor. So again, if it's absolutely essential to know whether cancer is in a man's lymph nodes, the best approach is surgical removal.

The least invasive approach is called a laparoscopic pelvic lymphadenectomy. Picture someone ice fishing—cutting a tiny, inconspicuous hole, dropping a line, and bringing out a big fish. That's the idea here; laparoscopic surgery is much less invasive than traditional surgery that involves an incision, and the benefits to patients include shorter hospitalization, quicker recovery time, less postoperative pain, and a better cosmetic result—a few tiny holes, for example, instead of a scar several inches long. Alternatively, a procedure called a mini-lap (mini-laparotomy staging pelvic lymphadenectomy) can be performed. This requires a slightly longer incision, but the recovery period is about the same. (This is more familiar to most urologists than the laparoscopic technique.)

## Who Should Get It?

The only man who should be subjected to one of these procedures is someone to whom it will make a dramatic difference in the decision-making process. For example, say a man has a large, palpable cancer that invades the muscles in the pelvic side wall (stage T3), a Gleason score of 8, and a PSA level of 30 ng/ml. There is no reason for this man to go ahead with a lymph node dissection. His disease is already extensive, and treatment for him should be aimed at controlling the cancer and relieving symptoms and pain. To put this man through the rigors of a procedure that ultimately won't help him is neither helpful nor kind. Instead, this technique is most helpful in men who appear to have clinically localized prostate cancer (T2a or T2b disease) but a grade of Gleason 8 or greater. If a man with Gleason 8 disease has any cancer in the lymph nodes, he has an 85 percent chance of having metastatic disease within five years. On the other hand, if the lymph nodes are negative, he has a good chance of being cured at five years. Here, the status of the lymph nodes can provide critically important information. But in men with Gleason 7 or less, the information from the lymph nodes is not as important. As we will discuss in chapter 7, men with Gleason 7 disease and positive lymph nodes have only a 15 percent chance of having metastatic disease at five years. And there is some evidence suggesting that even men with lymph nodes may live longer if their prostate is removed. Thus, we only perform staging pelvic lymphadenectomies in men with Gleason 8 disease who are candidates for surgery and who are potentially curable.

## To Sum Up

Take a deep breath. You've had a lot to deal with, and in this chapter alone, a tremendous amount of information to digest. You are not alone. For most men, the diagnosis of prostate cancer is unexpected—like a sudden punch in the stomach. As with any other unexpected calamity in your life, you've got to face it square-on and collect all the facts. At your fingertips are three facts you will probably come to know as well as your Social Security number—your PSA level, Gleason score, and clinical stage. With just these three facts, almost immediately you have a good idea where you stand. The cancer either appears to be clinically localized to the prostate—the most common scenario in the United States today because of improved diagnostic testing—or the cancer has spread locally, but does not appear to be present at distant sites; or rarely, less than 10 percent of the time, the cancer has been caught later, and it has spread either to the lymph nodes or bone. Once you have reached the point of knowing where you stand, your next move is to examine the options for treatment and find the one that you feel is best for you.

Another thing: *all of these statistics are based on men who were diagnosed with cancer a decade ago.* If you have just been diagnosed with prostate cancer, there is no question that you're better off—chances are, you've been diagnosed a lot sooner and at a much more curable stage. What you have just read, then, is the worst-case scenario. These statistics are all we have; the long-term success stories of you and other men newly diagnosed haven't been written yet. With the explosion of new treatment strategies for advanced disease, our ability to control cancer is only getting better and better. There is more hope now than ever. Do not let yourself get discouraged.

Now on to chapter 7 where, based on what you now know, we'll examine your options.

# 7

# WHAT ARE MY OPTIONS?

## ▶▶▶ READ THIS FIRST

What's the best treatment for prostate cancer? This is a trick question. There is no single best treatment, because prostate cancer isn't a "one-size-fits-all" disease. It's different in every man. There are many factors—not only the clinical stage of your cancer but your own age and general health—involved in choosing the treatment that's right for you.

Twenty years ago, most men who had prostate cancer were diagnosed at an older age and with more advanced disease. Most treatment efforts were palliative, aimed at relieving symptoms (as opposed to curative, aimed at eradicating the cancer), and men often died within a few years. Today, thankfully, the tables have been turned. *Now, most American men are diagnosed with localized prostate cancer that is curable.* It is possible today to prevent a man from dying a painful death of prostate cancer fifteen or twenty years in the future. Now, the goal is to achieve this *and* leave the patient with an excellent quality of life—cured of cancer, continent, potent, and as if nothing had ever happened. If you have localized disease (this includes locally advanced disease), you have three main treatment options: expectant management, surgery, or radiation therapy.

The best thing you can do now is educate yourself—not just about prostate cancer but about the doctors who treat it. You're building a bridge here, and you can go only so far by yourself. Ultimately, you are going to have to find a physician you trust to help you find your way through this very complicated disease.

## What Are My Options?

Prostate cancer is a complicated disease—so complicated, in fact, that it's unique in every man. Your brother-in-law had prostate cancer? Your neighbor, too? And now you—three men with three distinct cancers. There is so much variability here. Because the disease is completely different from man to man, you may find the treatment that's best for your neighbor is not the one that's best for you. You can't go by anybody else's experience with prostate cancer, because you've each got your own custom-made case. And yet, you're all part of the same club, a group nobody wants to join—the reluctant brotherhood of men with prostate cancer.

What's the best treatment? This is a trick question. There is no single best treatment, because, again, prostate cancer isn't a "one-size-fits-all" disease. There are many factors—not only the clinical stage of your particular cancer but your own age and general health—involved in choosing the treatment that's right for you. Your personal preferences are paramount here: Some men, for example, would rather take action—even if their cancer is incidental—than drive themselves crazy with worry, living from one PSA test to the next in expectant management. To other men, the idea of surgery is so disturbing that they would rather take their chances with diet, meditation, and other lifestyle changes than go under the knife. For some men—such as an eighty-one-year-old man with diabetes and congestive heart failure—any form of aggressive treatment, with side effects and recovery time, would not only be unhelpful but could produce complications that would make the "golden years" needlessly unpleasant. For others—a seventy-six-year-old man who swims 2 miles a day, who has two teenage children and parents who died in their nineties—not going after this disease aggressively would be uncharacteristic and unthinkable. Only you know how you really feel about this.

Twenty years ago, most men who had prostate cancer were diagnosed at an older age and with more advanced disease. Most treatment efforts were palliative, aimed at relieving symptoms (as opposed to curative, aimed at eradicating the cancer), and men often died within a few years of diagnosis. Today, thankfully, the tables have been turned. Now, most American men are diagnosed with localized prostate cancer that is curable. The use of PSA testing has given us a five-year lead time in diagnosis. It is possible today to prevent a man from dying a painful death of prostate cancer fifteen or twenty years in the future. Now, the goal is to achieve this *and* leave the patient with an excellent quality of life—cured of cancer, continent, potent, as if nothing had ever happened, and as if the diagnosis and treatment of cancer were just a rough patch on the road. If you have localized disease (this includes locally advanced disease), you have three main treatment options: expectant management, surgery, or radiation therapy. As you work through your decision about treatment, ask yourself questions like these: What's more important? Knowing that you're cured of cancer but realizing that there's a trade-off—in other words, you might have some side effects from treatment? Or, would it be better for you to get the treatment with the fewest side effects, hoping that you may die of something else before cancer catches up?

## If You Have Localized or Locally Advanced Disease

As we discussed in chapter 6, prostate cancer grows relatively slowly for many years. When it's localized (confined within the prostate), it can take years for a tumor to double in size. And here is the confounding thing: cancer can stay in the prostate indefinitely. It takes a long time and many steps involving subtle genetic changes before a normal cell, which is designed to live and die, becomes a cancer cell—before some switch is activated that makes the cell think it's immortal—and before such cells start dividing endlessly. (As we've discussed earlier, in high-risk men, some of these steps are shortened.) But, although we're working to improve our means of prediction, as yet, nobody can "mind-read" localized prostate cancer. There is no crystal ball to tell us what it's going to do.

If localized prostate cancer is found in a sixty-five-year-old man, for example, it could stay in the prostate for years and he may die *with* prostate cancer, not *of* it. This is what happens to hundreds of thousands of men, and it's one of the factors that can make treatment decisions so cloudy. But—and this is the crux of the issue—once it escapes the prostate to distant sites, such as the lymph nodes and bones, today there is no way to stop it. It can rarely be cured, although it can often be controlled. (And with an explosion of new treatment strategies for advanced disease, our ability to control cancer will keep getting better.) Just a few years ago, once cancer had spread to bone, the average life expectancy was three years. (Again, as new treatment strategies are tested and made available, this is expected to change—see chapter 12.)

So if you have localized disease, the big, blunt question you need to ask yourself is this: *How long are you probably going to live?* Nobody wants to think about this question, but there it is. In men over sixty-five who don't have heart disease or another form of cancer, life expectancy can vary tremendously, from two years to thirty-seven years. The factors, in order of importance, that can shorten your life expectancy are hypertension, smoking, diabetes, consuming more than four drinks of alcohol a day, and not exercising. In contrast, factors that can help you live longer are getting regular exercise, eating a diet low in fat and high in fruits and vegetables, and having a high HDL (the "good" kind) cholesterol level.

The next question is whether your cancer is curable. What is the chance that the cancer has extended to the seminal vesicles or the lymph nodes? Remember, even if the cancer has penetrated the capsule, it can still be cured in most cases. But it's harder to cure the cancer if it's involved the seminal vesicles, and prostate cancer is rarely curable if it involves the lymph nodes. You probably have a pretty good estimate of this from the Partin and Han tables in the last chapter.

And next, how old are you? This is different from the question about your life expectancy. If you are in your fifties or younger, even if the odds of cure don't appear to be in your favor, you will tolerate surgery better than an older man, and you should probably consider it. If you are older, the situation gets a bit more complicated. Men over seventy who undergo radical prostatectomy are more likely to have problems with impotence and incontinence. (Note: Both of these can be treated, and the rates of complications vary significantly, depending on the expertise of the surgeon who performs the operation.) Men over seventy are also more likely to have more cancer than younger men. For example, in men with stage T2 cancer, the tumor is more often organ-confined in men in their fifties than in men in their seventies. Why? Because the cancer has been there longer and had a chance to grow and possibly become more malignant. The Johns Hopkins urologist H. Ballentine Carter studied five hundred men with T1c disease who underwent radical prostatectomy. He found that older men were more likely to have Gleason 7 tumors (in the midrange, moderately well differentiated) than men in their fifties, and that age was a statistically significant factor in the prediction of curability.

Let's go back to our sixty-five-year-old man. He's in otherwise good health, and he can reasonably expect to live at least fifteen or twenty more years. His cancer is curable now. If he does nothing about it, he may miss his golden opportunity for a cure. Remember, right now we have no way of estimating the biological potential of prostate cancer. We can't determine if it's harmless or deadly; we don't know if or when it will make that leap beyond the prostate. Even in its earliest stages, prostate cancer doesn't always spread considerately, in logical, easy-to-predict steps.

At the other end of the spectrum is the man in his eighties. Even if his cancer is organ-confined and curable, it's not likely that he will live long enough for aggressive treatment to be worthwhile. Older men are less resilient; as we mentioned before, aggressive treatment is much harder on them. What's the point of risking incontinence, a result of surgery, or rectal bleeding, a result of radiation, in an eighty-five-year-old man? If his disease progresses to the point where he has difficulty with urination, there are many ways to treat such symptoms, ranging from a TUR (transurethral resection of the prostate, to relieve urinary obstruction) to hormonal therapy. For most older men, *the number of years of life*—the long-term survival—is not nearly as important as the *life in those years*—the quality of life.

## Why Do I Need to Be Treated? Making Sense of Some Controversial Studies

There are doctors out there who steer their patients with curable disease toward avoiding all treatments. Their main basis for this is studies that suggest the death rate for men who don't get treatment is low, about the same as for men who don't have prostate cancer. For a number of years, doctors who saw no value in treating prostate cancer quoted a study from Sweden, where the traditional mainstay of treatment is watchful waiting. This study suggested that men with localized prostate cancer rarely died from it. It's pretty clear now that this study had many flaws, one of which was in the interpretation. In that study, at ten years, only 13 percent of men had died from prostate cancer. But the disease had progressed in another 50 percent of the men, and most of these men eventually needed castration or hormonal therapy to treat urinary obstruction, bleeding, or pain.

Now that more time has passed, we know even more about how these men fared. That's the thing about this kind of "outcome" study. If you're going to find out whether localized prostate cancer can go on to kill a man, you need to follow him for many years. When these Swedish men were followed for fifteen years or longer, more men went on to die from prostate cancer, and even more men developed local progression and distant metastases. This finding is sobering, because many of the men in this study—like most American men who are candidates for expectant management—had "good," slow-growing, low-grade tumors. Their average age at the time of diagnosis was seventy-two, one-third of them had T1a disease, and half had Grade 1 disease (the Swedish researchers did not use the Gleason scoring system). Of important note: The risk for progression after fifteen years was similar for men who were diagnosed before or after age seventy—which shows that even in older men, relatively indolent cancers can progress and become fatal, if left untreated and if the men live long enough.

In Sweden, watchful waiting means ignoring early prostate cancer and sending the man home, telling him to come back when he has some symptoms—when the cancer has spread—and eventually treating him hormonal therapy. Sweden also has the third-highest death rate from prostate cancer in the world. In Sweden, *50 percent more* men die of prostate cancer than women die of breast cancer. In the United States, where we actually treat and cure prostate cancer, *fewer* men die of prostate cancer than women die of breast cancer.

This is not what watchful waiting, or expectant management, means in the United States (more on this below). But it's the most cost-effective solution in a socialized system of medical care. It doesn't require expensive therapy or skilled therapists. The only drawback is that men die and men suffer—needlessly. These statistics are particularly distressing when we consider this: today, when localized prostate cancer is diagnosed in men who have a life expectancy of longer than fifteen years, the decision not to offer these men potentially curative therapy may be a death sentence. Because in most patients, the disease is going to progress.

### The Scandinavian Study

But out of all this suffering and death from prostate cancer has come one of the most important studies ever to be carried out in evaluating localized disease. The Scandinavian Prostate Cancer Group, made up of physicians from Sweden, Finland, and Iceland, embarked on a courageous trial in 1989. The results of their initial study and their follow-up report, both published in the *New England Journal of Medicine*, have changed the way prostate cancer is perceived in Sweden, Finland, and Iceland. In the first report, nearly seven hundred men with localized prostate cancer were randomly assigned either to watchful waiting or to surgery (radical prostatectomy). What happened to these men provided the first concrete evidence of something American doctors had known anecdotally for years—that *treating localized disease reduces deaths from prostate cancer*. During the average follow-up of six years (the first report), twice as many men in the watchful waiting group died of prostate cancer—which meant, the scientists concluded, that *radical prostatectomy can reduce prostate cancer deaths by about half.*

At ten years after the study began (the results published in the second paper), half of the men in the watchful waiting group who died in the first ten years died from prostate cancer. And, because radical prostatectomy reduced the likelihood of dying of prostate cancer by 40 percent, at ten years there was a statistically significant improvement in death from all causes in the group that underwent surgery. Surgery was of greatest benefit to men who were younger than age sixty-five at the time their cancer was diagnosed. (We will have more to say about the importance of age later in this chapter.) In that age group, after ten years, 19 percent of the watchful waiting patients had died of prostate cancer, but fewer than 9 percent of the men who underwent surgery died from cancer. Also, surgery reduced the risk of local recurrence of cancer by 67 percent and of the cancer's spread to distant sites by 40 percent. The impact on distant metastasis is all the more impressive here because hormonal therapy was given more often to the men in the watchful waiting group than to the men who underwent radical prostatectomy. The study's authors concluded, "We expect the benefits of this surgery will increase during longer periods of follow-up."

One important note about this study: Most—75 percent—of the Scandinavian men were diagnosed with cancer advanced enough to be felt during a physical exam, with an average PSA level of 13 ng/ml. This is in sharp contrast to the United States today, where 75 percent of men are diagnosed, on average, five years earlier and at a much more curable stage—with nonpalpable cancer detected because of a change in PSA level. However, although these men had more advanced disease than we commonly see today in American men, they are very similar to the men who underwent surgery in the early 1990s, before the widespread use of PSA screening.

In 1992, 104,000 men underwent a radical prostatectomy in the United States. If we apply the outcome from the recent Scandinavian trial to these figures, we would expect that there would be at least 5,000 fewer men dying of prostate cancer ten years later, which is close to what we have experienced. In comparing these findings to today's patients, the authors note that it may take much longer to see the difference in survival, "but the removal of small tumors may facilitate surgery and result in fewer side effects." In an article accompanying the 2002 report, the Scandinavian researchers looked at the side effects in all of the men, and by four years they found that the quality of life in both groups was the same—largely because the progression in the watchful waiting patients required them to receive additional treatments and hormones.

## Other Studies

What about studies from the United States? A review article published in the *New England Journal of Medicine* summarized a number of other studies involving expectant management. In these studies, the authors reported, the men treated with expectant management were carefully selected from a large group of patients because they were felt to have slow-growing cancers that were unlikely to spread. These patients were not representative of the usual patient who walks into a doctor's office—in other words, they were almost all "best-case scenarios." Even so, ten years later, 40 percent of the men in these elite groups who had Gleason scores from 5 to 7 had metastases to bone, and by fifteen years, that number had increased to 70 percent. Again, what we see here is that prostate cancer marches on; it continues to progress in most men—even those with the mildest-looking disease. And if a man with localized prostate cancer does not get effective treatment and he lives long enough, he will very likely die of prostate cancer.

One of the most recent investigations of expectant management was a large study conducted by doctors in Connecticut and published in the *Journal of the American Medical Association*. Here, the researchers looked at men who were treated with expectant management and the number of men who died of prostate cancer five, ten, and fifteen years later. It concluded that men with low-grade cancers (Gleason 2–4) faced a minimal risk of dying from prostate cancer. (Remember, those Gleason 2–4 tumors are rarely diagnosed today and make up only about 2 percent of men with localized prostate cancer.) For men with Gleason 5–7 scores, the investigators concluded, the risk of death from prostate cancer is a "modest" one that increases slowly over at least fifteen years of follow-up. "These men face a risk of dying from prostate cancer," the researchers conceded, "but it is unclear from a population perspective what percentage of these men will actually benefit from treatment" and from aggressive screening to detect the progression of their cancer.

There is a huge problem with this study, one that goes to the heart of prostate cancer treatment itself: Why were these men treated with conservative therapy in the first place? Mainly because they were in the group of men we'll talk about later in this chapter, men who were considered too old or too ill to live longer than ten years. Most of these men beat prostate cancer on a technicality—they died of other causes before they lived fifteen years. (Indeed, when this study was finally analyzed, only 6 percent of the patients were still alive.) In other words, they didn't die of prostate cancer because some other disease killed them first. Thus, this study grossly underestimates the risk of dying from prostate cancer in men who actually lived fifteen years. And in doing so, the study fails to tell a young, otherwise healthy man—who could live for twenty or thirty more years—the true probability that his cancer will progress and kill him.

### The PLCO Study

The Prostate, Lung, Colon, and Ovarian (PLCO) cancer screening study is a $100 million attempt by the National Cancer Institute to determine whether early diagnosis will reduce death from prostate, lung, colon, and ovarian cancers. For prostate cancer, men are screened once a year for five years with PSA testing (only every three years by digital rectal examination) and then followed for thirteen years. This is similar to the screening intervals used in a study to determine mammography's effectiveness in spotting breast cancer. However, prostate cancer is much slower growing than breast cancer, and some doctors worry that five years isn't going to be long enough for PSA's yearly rate of change to be as meaningful as it has the potential to be.

Another worry is that the screening isn't being done in the best possible way up front. The study was planned a long time ago, using the then-state-of-the-art PSA cutoff of 4 ng/ml. But we have learned more about PSA testing (as we discussed in chapter 5), and now know that many men with PSA levels lower than 4 ng/ml have prostate cancer. Also, the study does not take into account some of the improvements in PSA testing, such as the use of free PSA and PSA velocity. So a long-term study that does not use the best techniques appears, to some investigators, to be of limited value.

The investigators heading this study have had great concern that their control group might be "contaminated" by PSA screening outside of the study—that a man might have a PSA test on the recommendation of his family physician or because he read about it in the newspapers. This "contamination" could markedly affect the ability of this study in the long run to compare men who have been screened with men who have not. For this reason, these NIH investigators have made a concerted effort to discourage PSA testing through scientific presentations and the use of the media. They are also active in getting this message out to potential patients. These efforts may have helped to protect the integrity of their study, but at what cost? Several of these patients, men who avoided screening based on these doctors' advice, have come to Johns Hopkins and been diagnosed with more advanced disease that was difficult to cure.

Recently, we've learned of another problem with this study. After one year, only about 20 percent of men who had a positive digital rectal examination, and at most 40 percent of men who had a PSA level greater than 4 ng/ml, actually underwent a biopsy. At three years, these numbers had risen slightly, to 28 percent and 55 percent, respectively. What this means, then, is that even if men are found to have an abnormality that could suggest cancer, there is no strong encouragement for them to pursue it.

And finally, in this study, treatment is up in the air—once a diagnosis is made, the choice of treatment (or no treatment) is left up to the patient and his physician, with no mandate to pick the most effective treatment to cure the man's cancer. (This is in contrast to the studies that demonstrated the efficacy of mammography, in which women diagnosed with breast cancer underwent radical mastectomy.) Remember that the end point here is death from prostate cancer. How can we know if PSA testing makes a difference in life expectancy if men pick ineffective therapy? And finally, the age range for the study is not ideal; it includes men up to age seventy-four. The unfortunate fact is that many of these men probably won't be alive to see the end of the twelve-year follow-up period. It is unlikely, then, that they will live long enough to provide any new insights into the long-term effectiveness of treatment.

Many scientists believed that this study would provide meaningful information on the value of screening for a fifty-year-old man who responds promptly to an abnormal finding and then undergoes treatment. Unfortunately, it will not. At best, this study may provide some insight into the value of screening in men who are relatively noncompliant in seeking a biopsy and who may not, then, receive effective treatment. Many of us now believe that our European counterparts (see below) have a better chance of providing meaningful information.

Who would design a study like this? Epidemiologists who are interested in the effects of prostate cancer on a large group of men. The question they are trying to answer is different from the one so many scientists and patients would like to see answered. Their question: If screening in the United States was not carried out perfectly—if all men were not screened, if everyone who had an abnormality did not undergo a biopsy, and if everyone did not seek treatment, what effect would that have on their chances of dying from prostate cancer?

### The ERSPC Study

The European Randomized Study of Screening for Prostate Cancer (ERSPC) is a massive trial involving more than 200,000 men in eight countries: Belgium, Finland, France, Italy, the Netherlands, Spain, Sweden, and Switzerland. Men are screened with PSA tests every four years (every two years in Sweden), and a biopsy is indicated for men with a PSA level higher than 3 ng/ml. So far, between 80 and 90 percent of men with an abnormal PSA test have undergone a biopsy. The study's investigators believe they will have meaningful results by 2010.

### The PIVOT Study

Another attempt to shed light on prostate cancer treatment is the national PIVOT (Prostate Cancer Intervention Versus Observation Trial) study, led by a Minnesota internist and a Seattle urologist and funded by the Department of Veterans Affairs and the National Cancer Institute. Its aim is to find out which works better for clinically localized prostate cancer—radical prostatectomy with early intervention (such as radiation therapy) in case the cancer comes back, or expectant management with treatment for symptoms if the cancer spreads.

"We're not looking at radiation as a primary treatment," comments the internist who's heading the study, "because studies indicate that radiation is at least not better than radical prostatectomy." Instead, the PIVOT study will "compare watchful waiting with the most frequently recommended, and probably the best, of the early intervention approaches—radical prostatectomy."

Like the PLCO study, the PIVOT study is long; 731 men will be followed for up to fifteen years. Only men with prostate cancer who are considered candidates for surgery can take part in the study; they are assigned to one of two groups—either they'll undergo a radical prostatectomy or they will be followed closely with expectant management and treated as needed for specific symptoms or metastases.

## Regional Studies

In chapter 3, we talked about where in the world you live and how that can affect your risk of developing prostate cancer. Where you live also can affect the treatment you may receive. Several studies have pointed out wide geographic variations in how aggressively prostate cancer diagnosis is sought and treatment is given. For example, a recent study from the American Cancer Society compared the death rates from prostate cancer in urban areas, where men have ample access to health care, to those in smaller towns and rural areas. The researchers found that men living in less-populated areas are less likely to have regular PSA tests and are more likely to be diagnosed with late-stage disease. In other words, some American men are living like throwbacks—like men in the 1980s, when there was no way to diagnose prostate cancer early. This study concluded that poorer access to medical care and regular prostate cancer screening, giving men the opportunity to catch and treat the cancer early, leads to higher death rates from prostate cancer in certain regions of the United States. This accounts for 14 percent of the geographic variation in death rates from prostate cancer in white men and 28 percent of the variation in the death rates of black men. Thus, even in the United States, we can see the difference in survival between men who are diagnosed and treated early and men who are not.

Other information comes from an analysis of death rates from prostate cancer in countries around the world. Until recently, the death rate from prostate cancer was falling 1 to 2 percent a year in just a few countries—the United States, Canada, Austria, France, Germany, and Italy. But in many other countries—Portugal, Poland, Hungary, Norway, Sweden, and Finland, for example—the death rate was actually *increasing* by 1 to 2 percent a year. The big difference was the amount of early diagnosis and effective treatment. The good news is that now, across much of Europe, the death rate from prostate cancer is dropping. This is due to improved diagnosis and to advances in treatment, including the widespread use of radical prostatectomy.

## What Do All These Studies Tell Us?

Prostate cancer can be a lethal disease in some men, while in other men, it can move very slowly, with no obvious progression over the course of many years. Population-based studies, such as those described above, may help the U.S. government determine where it should spend its money. But they may not mean much to a man who wants to know whether he will benefit from an early diagnosis and treatment. There is no one-size-fits-all answer here. With that in mind, now it's time to take what we've talked about, look at all the treatment options, and decide which one is best for you.

## Expectant Management

Expectant management is certainly not a new approach. It's long been a mainstay of prostate cancer treatment; in fact, for years, one-third of men with prostate cancer have been treated with watchful waiting. In this chapter, we've talked a lot about watchful waiting, especially in Sweden, where surgery was shown to be a better approach—especially for younger men. However, expectant management in the United States is not the same as watchful waiting in Sweden. In Sweden, doctors sent men home and told them to come back only when they had symptoms of advanced disease—at which point men either began hormonal therapy to treat metastatic disease or underwent palliative treatment to relieve urinary tract obstruction. That's not what watchful waiting means in the United States.

In fact, we're mainly using the term "expectant management" because it means to be followed carefully, to delay definitive treatment only until it becomes clear that the tumor is growing. It's the old "wait until you see the whites of their eyes, then fire" approach. Wait for evidence that cancer is on the move, and then take action.

This has the immediate advantage of allowing men to avoid unpleasant treatment and its side effects. For men with curable disease, though, it has one major disadvantage—the risk of missing the window of curability. When cancer escapes from the prostate, it doesn't send out a press release announcing the event; it just goes, as silently as it appeared in your body in the first place. Then it's too late to close the proverbial barn doors. We can't put cancer back in the prostate. We can do our best to cure it if it's still locally advanced. If it spreads to the lymph nodes or bone, however, the best we can do for now is control it.

## Who Should Opt for It?

### Men Who Probably Don't Need to Be Cured

To put it bluntly, at the top of this list should be men who are too old or too ill either to undergo the rigors of treatment or to live another ten years—long enough for such treatment to be worthwhile. These men are very unlikely to die *of* prostate cancer, and if the cancer progresses, their symptoms can usually be managed well with hormonal therapy. (Frankly, these men should not have had a PSA test and biopsy in the first place.) Also in this group should be men who don't want to experience the side effects associated with surgery or radiation.

Why should older men consider it? In the Scandinavian trial we discussed above, surgical treatment of prostate cancer did not improve the long-term survival of men who were already sixty-five or older when they were diagnosed. Why? Because many men in the watchful waiting group died of other causes before their prostate cancer progressed. However, many older men worry about the progression of cancer—that if it's not treated effectively, it may spread locally, causing symptoms, or that it may spread to bone. They worry that, even if they don't die *of* prostate cancer, they could suffer from its side effects. For these men, just delaying treatment until there is some sign that the cancer is progressing may be enough.

### Tumors That Probably Don't Need to Be Cured

Some men have prostate cancer that is truly incidental and not yet something to worry about. These include some men with stage T1a cancer and older men with stage T1c disease who have favorable pathology, low PSA densities, and high free PSA (see chapter 6).

Remember, in the United States, expectant management doesn't mean "do nothing," and it doesn't mean your doctor has written you off—it means you get treatment for specific symptoms when you need it. It can mean active treatment as soon as there are signs that the tumor is progressing. It can mean hormonal therapy or spot radiation to ease bone pain. It can mean a transurethral resection of the prostate (TUR) or other procedure to bring relief when the prostate cancer becomes large enough to obstruct the urinary tract. It can mean a host of options aimed at tackling specific problems, prolonging life, and easing pain.

Besides its initial freedom from side effects, expectant management has another advantage at first—it's the cheapest option, because there's no expensive treatment to pay for. If you have no symptoms, you simply live your life and return to the doctor every six months or so for a checkup.

---

### EXPECTANT MANAGEMENT WITH CURATIVE INTENT (EMCI)

This is not watchful waiting; it's *proactive monitoring*—watching men with low-volume, low-risk cancer and intervening with curative treatment only if necessary. The Johns Hopkins urologist H. Ballentine Carter is leading the research in this new area, and it's tricky business. The first challenge is to find the right candidates. Next is to figure out how best to follow them. Then, the challenge is determining the triggers for intervention—the subtle signals that tell doctors, "It's time to cure this disease, right now."

"If we're going to be able to intervene and cure men, the men must have curable disease to begin with," says Carter. The best candidates seem to be men older than sixty-five with low-volume T1c disease (see chapter 6 for a discussion of this). These men have a PSA density of less than 0.15, a free PSA greater than 15 percent, and favorable pathology, as determined by at least a twelve-core biopsy. This relatively narrow group may broaden over time to include younger men, Carter notes, "as our experience with EMCI grows, and we are more confidently able to identify those men unlikely to experience progression."

Another challenge is finding the best markers—ways to show that cancer is progressing at a time when the cancer is still curable. Changes in PSA, including measurements of free PSA and PSA density, were somewhat helpful, but because 25 percent of men with cancers that are progressing have no increase in their PSA levels, the best way to check for cancer progression is to look at actual prostate tissue—in other words, biopsies—at least once a year, or sooner, if there are any changes in PSA level.

Carter is leading an important expectant management study at Johns Hopkins, with more than three hundred men currently taking part. First, these men undergo at least a twelve-core biopsy to make sure their disease has not been underestimated. Then, they are followed closely, with a PSA test and rectal examination every six months and a yearly biopsy. Progression is defined by what the pathologist sees in the biopsy—cancer present in more than two cores or in more than half of any one core; or a Gleason score of 7 or greater, or an unusual increase in PSA that prompts another biopsy.

So far, with an average follow-up time of two years, 35 percent of the men developed progression of cancer and 7 percent of the men requested curative treatment, even though they showed no evidence of progression. (Anxiety is another important factor in determining whether EMCI is right for you, Carter says. If you are going to worry and aren't comfortable with this approach, it is better to seek curative treatment.) With this close monitoring, was the chance for a cure lost during expectant management? Carter's evidence suggests that it wasn't. He compared thirty-eight men who were treated with surgery after a period of expectant management with a matched group of patients who underwent surgery at Johns Hopkins as soon as they found out they had prostate cancer. Based on the findings at radical prostatectomy, an equal number of men in both groups turned out to have curable disease.

Carter stresses that this approach is still investigational. However, so far—using this careful plan for enrolling patients and following them—it does not appear that the window of curability is being missed.

## When Expectant Management Is Not a Good Idea

Expectant management should not be an option for a younger man with localized, curable disease, because his window of curability may silently close, and he may live long enough to die from prostate cancer. If you have curable disease and opt for expectant management, you will have to live with uncertainty about the future. At present, we simply cannot guarantee that a man's cancer won't spread. Despite all that we have learned about the use of PSA testing and other tools as prostate barometers, we cannot tell when the disease is just beginning to progress, even if it hasn't yet escaped the prostate. In about 25 percent of men with growing prostate cancer, there is never a significant, telltale rise in PSA level.

So if you're a man under age sixty-five with a life expectancy greater than ten years and localized, curable prostate cancer who decides to watch and wait—with the hope that if the cancer grows, it will be caught in time—think hard about this risk. *You are the man with the most to lose.* You should return to your doctor at regular intervals—every six months—for repeat digital rectal examinations, PSA tests (even though, as discussed above and in chapter 6, PSA doesn't always go up correspondingly when cancer advances), and periodic prostate biopsies to help doctors find out if the cancer that's in your prostate is staying put or if it's on the move. PSA tests alone aren't sufficient to monitor the growth of the cancer because, as Carter reported, in 25 percent of men with cancers that were progressing, PSA levels did not change. You also need to understand the risks you could be facing down the road if cancer spreads—the long-term symptoms and the side effects and costs of treatment for advanced disease.

### When Expectant Management May Be a Safe Gamble

But what if you're in your mid-sixties or older and you have small T1c or T1a cancer? You're young and healthy enough to have surgery, and your disease is certainly considered curable—in fact, it's microscopic, possibly incidental prostate cancer. Why seek treatment now?

### Men With Stage T1c Disease

This is cancer that was found by needle biopsy performed after an elevated PSA score. A significant number—some 10 to 30 percent—of men with a PSA level greater than 4 ng/ml have insignificant cancer; the percentage is even higher for men with a PSA level lower than 4.

Is it truly insignificant? We have to balance what we know. One fact is that, at autopsy, between 30 and 40 percent of men are found to have some evidence of cancer in the prostate. This is cancer that never caused any problems—cancer that, for all practical purposes, didn't exist. It was just there. Another statistic is that, for an American man, the lifetime risk of being diagnosed with prostate cancer is 17 percent. Now, with any good screening program—and with PSA and its kin, we are detecting prostate cancer earlier and earlier—comes the inevitable risk that some cancers may be detected *too early*. This is a well-known phenomenon in breast cancer screening. Perhaps, then, the real question we need to ask for a man with stage T1c disease is, has he had his biopsy before his time? Did we jump the gun? Unfortunately, as we discussed in chapter 6, there is no reliable imaging technique that can show us a man's prostate and tell us how much cancer is actually there. Also, if a man's initial biopsy suggests that only a small amount of cancer is there but only six cores of tissue have been removed, that man needs another biopsy. Needle biopsies sample only about one-thousandth of the prostate. Before you can even think about expectant management, you need to make sure that you're dealing with the right scenario—that your prostate has been biopsied adequately, and that you really do have an insignificant cancer.

## If You Have T1c Disease, Can You Afford to Wait?

There's more about insignificant and significant T1c cancer in chapter 6, but here are some factors that can help predict which cancers are truly incidental and which need to be treated. If your cancer is incidental, your pathology should suggest low-volume disease (cancer in one or two needle cores, involving less than half of any core and a Gleason score of 6 or less), *and* your PSA level should not be more than 10 percent of the weight of your prostate. If it's higher, this suggests that something more than benign disease is responsible for your elevated PSA level. Similarly, if the PSA is coming from benign prostatic enlargement (BPH), your free PSA should be high—above 15 percent. If it's less than 15 percent, then it is likely that cancer, not benign disease, is causing your PSA to rise—in which case, the cancer is probably more significant than it seems. The key words here are "likely" and "probably." Even the expert pathologist Jonathan Epstein of Johns Hopkins says that he does not know which cancer is so small in a young man that it won't grow to the point of threatening his life over time, and that using these estimates, 25 percent of men with T1c cancer still have a significant amount of cancer.

### Men With Stage T1a Disease

If you have not had a transurethral resection of the prostate (TUR), you can skip this section. Stage T1a disease only refers to men whose cancer was found when another prostate problem, BPH, was being treated. There used to be two polarized schools of thought about this: One was that everybody with this small cancer needed treatment as soon as possible. "We can definitely cure it now. Time's wasting—let's get going!" some doctors said. They urged patients to have their cancer "nipped in the bud," treated when the chances of curing it were at their peak. The other group was not nearly so optimistic; these doctors believed that treatment didn't really prolong life by that many years anyway, so what was the point? (Amazingly, a number of doctors still feel this way, as discussed above.)

Beware of extremes. One of the first lessons a doctor learns in medical school is that "There are always two things you never say—always and never." The truth is probably somewhere in the middle.

Before the 1970s at Johns Hopkins, the approach was that if a man had cancer found at a TUR but not a tumor large enough to be felt in a rectal exam (men with stage T2 cancer), then his cancer was the incidental kind, with low malignant potential and not much clinical significance—the kind of cancer men die *with*, not *of*. And so they weren't treated.

In 1976, Johns Hopkins investigators embarked on a pioneering study using tumor volume to predict cancer patients' prognosis. They analyzed the medical histories of more than one hundred of these men who were not treated and followed their progress for an average of seven years. Their findings: One group of these men did reasonably well; their cancer rarely progressed. But another group did not fare so well; their cancer continued to grow.

What was the difference between these two groups? The clue, investigators found, was in the percentage of cancer removed during the TUR. This work provided the now standard classifications for stage T1 disease. (TURs are not performed as commonly as they used to be; there are many other treatments for BPH. And when a TUR is performed, the tissue is often vaporized instead of removed in little chips, so there is nothing to send to a pathologist.)

When 5 percent or less of the tissue was cancerous, only 17 percent of the men went on to develop more advanced cancer within seven years; this is now the classification for stage T1a disease. But when more than 5 percent of the resected tissue was cancerous, 68 percent of these men went on to develop cancer progression within seven years; this now is the classification of stage T1b disease. "It is felt that the amount of cancer in almost all of these patients is significant enough to warrant therapy," says one of the investigators.

Further analysis has shown that when men with stage T1a disease undergo radical prostatectomy, about 25 percent of them turn out to have a significant amount of cancer in the prostate—the kind of cancer that's found in men with palpable tumors. This is because, as we discussed in chapter 6, the biopsy is not perfect. It's a glimpse at what is probably within the prostate, and from that, pathologists make their most educated guess.

So some men with stage T1a cancer require treatment. Some don't. How to tell the difference? Our old friend PSA comes back to help us again. As it turns out, the level of PSA three months after TUR can be helpful in identifying the men at highest risk of cancer progression. If the PSA is less than 1.0 ng/ml, virtually all of the men with stage T1a disease have an insignificant amount of cancer. "And we feel that these men can probably be followed with careful digital rectal examinations and PSA tests every six months or a year," says one of the study's chief investigators. If the PSA level is greater than 10 ng/ml, all of these men are likely to have significant cancer remaining, and all should have definitive therapy before it's too late.

What about the patients in the middle, with PSA levels between 1.0 and 10 ng/ml—the range for about half the men with T1 disease? Currently, there's just no way to predict exactly how much cancer remains in the prostate—and, therefore, who will need treatment and who won't. Some doctors have advised these men to undergo a repeat TUR, but there's no real evidence to suggest that this will provide any helpful information. It's hard on the patient, too. Also, a repeat TUR may make it more difficult for a surgeon to perform a subsequent radical prostatectomy if the man then has to undergo yet another procedure.

Other investigators are enthusiastic about the use of ultrasound and random needle biopsies as follow-up measures for these men, but the long-term success rate for these procedures has yet to be determined; cancer could still slip outside the prostate and not be caught in time. The safest guideline here may be the patient's age: if he's younger than sixty, aggressive, curative therapy should be strongly considered.

## What Happens to Cancer Cells Over Time?

Some men who opt for expectant management take solace in the fact that their cancer cells are well differentiated. But unfortunately, having well-differentiated cancer cells today does not mean they'll stay that way forever. There are two concepts here; one is genetic drift. As a cancer progresses—as its cells double again and again—the DNA becomes less stable. The cancer develops new mutations; it becomes more aggressive. As the tumor progresses, well-differentiated cells deteriorate into poorly differentiated cells. The other concept is heterogeneity, or clonal selection. By the time a prostate cancer is large enough to be diagnosed clinically, its cell population is mixed—a diverse group of cells, all jockeying for position in one location. In this varied group are both well-differentiated and poorly differentiated cells—cells driven by hormones and cells untouched by hormones. And although an initial biopsy may find well-differentiated cancer cells, almost certainly some poorly differentiated ones have mingled in there as well. With time and further growth, these poorly differentiated cells grow at a faster rate than their more sedate, better-differentiated counterparts. Eventually, they will outpace the stately progression of the well-differentiated cells and dominate the tumor. So having a well-differentiated cancer, one that's localized to the prostate, may be only a temporary condition. And unfortunately, we can't tell which well-differentiated cancers are going to stay that way.

## What About Lifestyle Changes?

There is a new subgroup of men who are choosing expectant management with a different strategy in mind: they do not have small tumors or the lowest Gleason scores. Some of them are very young—in their forties and fifties, with tumors that their doctors have described as slow-growing. These men are deciding to avoid treatment now and heal themselves, with lifestyle changes—dietary changes, antioxidants, herbal compounds, meditation, and complementary medicine. (Complementary medicine is discussed in chapter 12.) They have a lot of support—on the Internet, especially, and also from diet specialists who claim to have the answers for beating prostate cancer (as well as heart disease and various other illnesses).

## Why Diet?

The rationale for diet and lifestyle changes goes back to the men we have heard so much about in this book—those remarkable Asian men, whose risk of getting prostate cancer is so much lower than ours, until they move to the United States. Then, their risk starts to climb. This is why so many scientists worldwide believe there is something in the Asian diet that prevents prostate cancer.

The men in this group who are shunning traditional curative treatment are doing it with the belief that if they start eating these same foods and taking high-powered dietary supplements, their cancer will go away. Nobody knows where this approach will lead; it's too new. One day, diet may very well help American men prevent cancer from forming. But the idea that starting a diet after cancer develops can make the disease go away is just not sound. Look at it this way: Smoking causes lung cancer. Men who don't smoke hardly ever get lung cancer (issues of secondary smoke aside), and if you stop smoking now, your risk of developing lung cancer begins to plummet. But what if you stop smoking after you find out you have lung cancer? Does the cancer go away? No, sadly, it doesn't. The reasons for this go back to the complicated chain of reactions we discussed in chapter 3—the domino effect of damaged DNA causing other genes to mutate, eventually resulting in cancer. Mutated genes cause the cancer to grow; these genetic errors are repeated and get worse every time the cells divide. Once the DNA has been damaged, there is no turning back. You can't, as they say, unring the bell. Even if you stop the original inciting agent, the factor that caused cancer in the first place, you will not cure that cancer by this means alone. You may prevent new cancers from forming, and optimistically, you may even slow down the progression of the cancer that's already there. But that first cancer is there to stay, unless it is stamped out by treatment. Those genetic errors are irreversible.

To the best of our knowledge, prostate cancer arises from oxidative damage (discussed in chapter 3). A normal prostate cell is transformed into a cancerous cell because of mutations to DNA caused by oxidative damage. But is it possible that fat itself can make the cancer grow more? We don't know for sure. It is possible that changes in diet and lifestyle could slow down cancer, but again, there's no evidence that they will make the cancer go away. Breast cancer, lung cancer, and colon cancer are caused by similar oxidative damage. But here, too, there is no evidence that dietary therapy can make these cancers disappear.

TABLE 7.1

### TREATMENT PROS AND CONS

| Ideal candidate | Radical Prostatectomy | Radiation Therapy |
| --- | --- | --- |
| **Age** | Under age 70 | Over age 60 |
| **Stage** | T1b, T1c, T2 (and some men with T1a disease) | T1, T2, T3, T4 |
| **Main advantages** | Mental satisfaction of knowing that the prostate has been completely removed | Less invasive |
| **Main disadvantages*** | Side effects:<br>Impotence 10–75%<br>Incontinence 2–20%<br>Death 0.2% | Side effects:<br>Significant rectal injury 1–2%<br>Impotence 20–70%<br>Death 0.2% |

*Note: Side effects vary greatly, depending on the skill of the surgeon or radiation oncologist.

### If I Decide to Get Treatment, What Are My Choices?

For tumors that are confined to the prostate—stages T1 and T2—there are two main choices: surgery (radical prostatectomy) and radiation therapy. Radiation also is used when the cancer has spread just outside the gland to kill cancer cells and shrink the prostate. High-energy X-ray beams are aimed at the prostate and sometimes at nearby lymph nodes; sometimes this is combined with implanted radiation seeds.

---

## WHO SHOULD CONSIDER SURGERY?

**T1a:** Most men with T1a disease have truly incidental cancer that rarely progresses. However, studies of radical prostatectomy patients show that about 25 percent of men with T1a cancer have significant disease. If a man has had a simple prostatectomy for treatment of BPH, and if, three months after that procedure, his PSA is less than 1 ng/ml, he probably has insignificant cancer and is an ideal candidate for expectant management. If he is younger than sixty or has a PSA greater than 1 ng/ml at three months after this procedure, he should consider treatment.

**T1b, T1c, T2:** Decision should be made based on the Partin and Han tables, a man's age, and his overall health. For older men with T1c disease, the presence of low-volume disease should be considered/excluded.

**T3a:** Men with T3a disease are usually not good candidates for a radical prostatectomy. However, some patients with minimal spread of cancer and Gleason scores lower than 8 may benefit from surgery, especially if they are in their fifties or younger. About 25 percent of these men turn out to have organ-confined disease.

---

## Which Treatment Is Better for Localized Disease?

A better question might be, "Which treatment is right for me?" There are several important considerations here: your age, overall health and stage of cancer, the side effects associated with different treatments, and finally—most important—your own wishes.

When prostate cancer is localized in men with a life expectancy of fifteen years or more, the goal for treatment is cure. This sounds obvious, until we remember that when prostate cancer is advanced, the cancer can be controlled, but—for now—not eradicated.

Which treatment is better? We know for certain (see the discussion of the Scandinavian study earlier in this chapter) that radical prostatectomy saves lives. It cures cancer, and for years, the results of radical prostatectomy have been the gold standard against which all other forms of treatment are compared. Having said that, radiation is much better now. Most physicians agree that, for men with prostate cancer in its early stages it would be difficult to show a definite difference in cure rates between radical prostatectomy and external-beam radiation. The results with both treatments are good.

For many men, a big advantage of radical prostatectomy is simply knowing that the prostate—and the cancer inside it—has been completely eliminated. It's out of there. The disadvantages are the side effects, namely the risks of impotence and incontinence. And radical prostatectomy is no walk in the park. It is major surgery, and the body must be strong enough to handle it. (For more on the potential complications with radical prostatectomy, see chapter 8.) In men under sixty-five who undergo treatment by a surgeon who is an expert, the side effects of surgery and radiation therapy are similar, with the exception that rectal problems are rare following surgery. In men over seventy, surgery carries a higher risk of incontinence and impotence. Note: The side effects of surgery are highly variable, depending on the skill and experience of the surgeon.

Radiation therapy's great advantage is that it isn't surgery. For this reason, it has been the preferred option for men who are older or who have other medical problems. In the past, there was also concern that the long-term effectiveness of radiation was unproven, as most men who received it were old enough to die of other causes. More recently, however, there have been short-term studies reporting that radiation can be effective in younger men. Radiation has side effects of its own—impotence and injury to the rectum (see chapter 9). To some degree, the chances of side effects with external-beam radiation are less operator-dependent than with surgery or seed implantation, although your best bet is to receive treatment at a center where experienced radiation oncologists treat many men with prostate cancer.

In choosing the treatment that's best for you, it's important to decide which side effects you are more comfortable with having and which ones you would rather avoid risking. More information on each of these choices follows in this chapter, and the next chapters cover these treatments in significantly greater detail.

### Radical Prostatectomy Is a Better Option for . . .

The ideal candidates for radical prostatectomy are the men most likely to benefit from it: men whose cancer is curable, who are fit to undergo the procedure without an increased risk of complications, and who are going to live long enough to need to be cured. Men who are curable with radical prostatectomy have organ-confined cancer or even cancer that has penetrated the prostate wall *if* the cancer is well to moderately well differentiated and it's possible for doctors to get what's called a clear surgical margin—that is, if they can cut out all the tumor.

The ideal candidates for surgery, then, are men in their forties, fifties, and sixties, in otherwise good health, with curable cancer. (Some otherwise healthy, fit men in their seventies may be individually selected for this treatment as well.) This includes men with stage T1b, T1c, T2a, T2b, and T2c cancer. It also includes some men with stage T1a (discussed above) and T3a disease.

## Radical Prostatectomy Is Not a Good Option for . . .

Radical prostatectomy is not helpful for men with disease that has spread widely beyond the prostate. It also is not ideal for older patients.

Once prostate cancer escapes the wall of the prostate to the point where it widely invades the seminal vesicles, pelvic lymph nodes, or bone, it can rarely be cured. The principal treatment goal in this case is to control the tumor locally; this can be done with radiation, hormonal therapy, or a combination of both. With late-stage cancer, the goal is simply to do everything possible to fight the cancer and buy more time, with the hope that one of the very exciting new treatment strategies currently being tested will be shown to work and will be available in the near future. The main line of treatment for late-stage prostate cancer has traditionally been hormonal therapy, chemotherapy, and spot radiation to treat painful metastases. But this is changing, and many promising new therapies are being tested (see chapter 12).

### Why Is Age a Factor?

Several reasons. One is that men over age seventy, as we discussed above, often have more advanced cancer than the clinical findings might lead a doctor to suspect and are therefore less likely to be cured because the cancer has been there longer. As men age, the prostate enlarges from BPH, so by the time a doctor can feel a cancerous lump in these men with larger prostates, it's probably bigger than the cancer that can be felt in a younger man with a smaller prostate. Studies have shown that for men with T2a disease, the likelihood that the cancer is confined to the prostate is less for men over seventy than for men in their fifties. Similar findings have been shown for men with nonpalpable T1c cancer.

Also, older men are more likely to suffer side effects from surgery than are younger men; they're more likely to have incontinence because, as men get older, their muscles get weaker—all the muscles, including the ones responsible for urinary control. The problem is that the sphincter muscles involved are the ones men don't normally need to use (because the prostate and bladder neck bear the main burden of holding back urine and keeping urination a voluntary experience). Also, because most older men have BPH, their bladder has thickened from the extra work needed to overcome the obstruction caused by the enlarged tissue. For these men, instead of three gatekeepers, the lone stalwart holding back an overmuscled bladder is a weaker, untested sphincter that's never been asked to work this hard before and may have some trouble adjusting to the job.

Sexual dysfunction is also more common for a couple of reasons: First, as men age, in addition to losing muscle strength, they lose nerves, too. By age sixty, men have lost about 40 percent of all the nerves in their bodies. And during radical prostatectomy, nerves are often injured—some permanently, some temporarily. So if a man has fewer nerves to begin with and some of these are damaged, the critical number of nerves necessary for erection may be lost. Yet another aspect of aging is that the nerves don't heal as well—again, making recovery of sexual function less likely. And finally, because men over age seventy aren't likely to live as long as men twenty years younger, it's difficult to show that radical prostatectomy actually does more than radiation therapy to lengthen life expectancy in these men.

### Radiation Is a Better Option for . . .

In the past, men who underwent radiation treatment were said to be negatively selected—they got radiation therapy because radical prostatectomy had been ruled out as the best option for them. They were generally older men, men in poor health who weren't considered strong enough for surgery, or men who had disease that extended beyond the prostate to the point where it could't be removed surgically (stage T3 or T4).

However, because evidence now shows that radiation (discussed in chapter 9) works well in younger, healthier men with longer life expectancies, radiation therapy is a valid option for men of any age or stage.

## Why Not Have Both Treatments? A Word on Combined Approaches

Although some men appear to have clinically localized cancer, there's a good chance that their cancer has spread beyond the prostate. For these men, the combination of radiation and surgery might sound like a promising option. However, if your cancer extended beyond the confines of the prostate and is not curable with surgery, it is unlikely that having your prostate removed will solve the problem. The only guarantee there is that you will have side effects from two treatments.

Some surgeons recommend hormonal treatment to shrink the prostate (and, they hope, the tumor) before radical prostatectomy, believing that this will make the cancer more curable. But hormonal therapy is not a vacuum cleaner—it can't whisk the cancer cells back into the prostate once they've escaped. There are now a number of very good studies that have followed men who were given hormonal therapy before radical prostatectomy with the hope of rounding up stray cancer cells. These studies have shown that the men who received hormonal therapy were just as likely to have their PSA levels rise. For this reason, there is no reason to give hormonal therapy before radical prostatectomy. Also, this approach may mislead a surgeon into thinking the cancer picture is rosier than it actually is and thereby encourage a less-aggressive cancer operation.

The findings in surgery determine the course of the operation—more or less tissue is removed, depending on what the surgeon sees and feels when the body is opened up. If, for example, there is any hint that the cancer has escaped the prostate along the nerve bundles that lie on either side of it, these nerves should be widely excised—

cut out, along with as much nearby tissue as possible. But if a man has received hormonal treatment, the surgeon may be reassured—falsely—about the extent of disease. "Nah," a surgeon may think, "there's no way the cancer could ever reach out this far, not after that hormonal treatment I started. I'll leave these nerve bundles in and give this guy a break—now he can keep his sexual potency." As a result of such well-meaning thinking, the surgeon may leave malignant cells behind instead of doing what any good surgeon normally does in a cancer operation—cutting out as much tissue as possible in an aggressive, no-holds-barred attempt to cure the disease.

There's another extremely important fact you should know about hormonal therapy: It's effective *only while a patient is on it.* The day you stop taking it is the day it stops working. Inevitably and almost immediately, the cancer cells begin growing again. If a surgeon has been timid or overconfident during surgery and not removed all the tissue that needed to be removed, the cancer is going to come back—hormones didn't kill it.

However, hormonal therapy before radiation is another story. It has been shown to improve the results for men with high-risk (of having spread outside the prostate) localized cancer. Several studies have found that if a man receives hormonal therapy before beginning radiation therapy and stays on hormones for several years afterward, not only is his chance of beating prostate cancer better than that of a man who receives radiation therapy alone, but he is more likely to be alive several years later.

### So What Do I Do?

First, educate yourself. Learn everything important there is to know about your own cancer—your clinical stage, PSA level, and Gleason score. Consult the Partin and Han tables in chapter 6. Explore all your options. We've done our best to cover them all in this chapter, and specific forms of treatment are covered in greater detail in the next chapters. Get a second opinion, and a third if you need it, and talk to other patients. If you can't get some names from your doctor, call a prostate cancer support group (see Where to Get Help at the back of this book) or another organization that specializes in prostate

## WHAT IF YOU'RE IN THE "GRAY ZONE"?

W hat if you're in your sixties, in reasonably good health, and a good candidate for either treatment? You're certainly in good company; thousands of men fit this description. How do they—and how should you—determine the better of these two good options? Here, after weighing all the facts, is where your own judgment matters most.

It may help to think of the worst-case scenario for each option. Picture yourself five years from now. What if you opted for surgery and you're still experiencing complications? Your cancer was cured, but you've had significant long-term problems with urinary control, or maybe your sexual function has never come back. How would you feel?

Or what if you selected radiation therapy—external-beam or brachytherapy (radiation seeds)—and have problems with erectile dysfunction, rectal irritation or bleeding, or difficulty with urinary flow?

Which of these situations would bother you the most? You may find—by imagining the worst in addition to the best possible outcome—that you'll learn the most about yourself and how you should be treated.

cancer. Be your own advocate and take heart: there is much you can do to make sure you get the best treatment possible.

The Partin and Han tables can be extremely helpful to you and your doctor in making the decision about treatment. In the best cases, they can identify men who are likely to be cured. But what if the probabilities in the tables suggest that cure is unlikely? Say a man has a PSA level between 10 and 20 ng/ml, a palpable tumor involving one entire lobe of the prostate (stage T2b disease), and a Gleason score of 7. What should this man do? Here, age plays a major role. Say this man is in his early fifties. Even though cure is not certain, it's possible, and it's clear that if he does nothing, he will probably die of his disease. Because the side effects of surgery are much milder in men this age, surgery or radiation are certainly both reasonable options and offer the possibility of cure.

On the other hand, say he's in his seventies. The question here is whether a man who may not live long enough to die of prostate cancer should be put through an operation with an uncertain likelihood of cure. Surgery has more side effects in people in their seventies. So, for this man, radiation therapy is a better, more reasonable option.

TABLE 7.2

## OPTIONS IN THE TREATMENT OF PROSTATE CANCER

| Clinical Extent of Disease | Stage | Options |
| --- | --- | --- |
| Localized | T1, T2 | Radical prostatectomy |
| | | Radiation therapy |
| | | Expectant management |
| Locally extended beyond the prostate | T3, T4 | Radiation therapy plus Hormonal therapy |
| Metastasized to lymph nodes and bone | N+, M+ | Hormonal therapy |
| | | New medical approaches and Chemotherapy |
| | | Spot radiation for pain |

## Final Thoughts on Treatment

What if you don't like any of the options? Maybe you're worried about the complications of surgery and the efficacy of radiation therapy. Maybe you're also questioning whether your cancer really needs to be treated, because right now you feel terrific. And what about all the health stories in the newspaper and on TV? Every day, there's another new breakthrough in cancer treatment. Look at the Human Genome Project—maybe those scientists will discover the "prostate cancer genes" next week. Maybe some new form of treatment will come along—maybe gene therapy. After all, it's working in other diseases—it's just a matter of time before it works in prostate cancer, too. What if you bite the bullet, and undergo one of the "mainstream" treatments for prostate cancer and open up the newspaper the next morning and see the headline "Cure for Prostate Cancer Discovered—No Side Effects!"

Or maybe, like some men, you think you can achieve a time-out by putting your prostate on a "block of ice" for a while by taking hormones. The problem there is, as we'll discuss later in this book, some prostate cancer cells respond to hormonal therapy. But others don't—and unfortunately, it is the cells that don't that eventually could kill you. So if you take hormones, your PSA will plummet—even though, as we'll discuss later on, this is not the same as making the cancer go away completely—and the tumor may shrink clinically. But the cells that can eventually prove fatal *aren't affected at all.* So taking hormones does not cure you, and it doesn't really put the problem on hold. It doesn't stop the clock in the cells that are immune to it.

But what about the miracle cure that could come along any day now? Again, there's the "test of time" issue. Even if a new form of treatment were developed today, it would take fifteen years before we knew whether it really worked. That's the problem with prostate cancer. Localized disease progresses very slowly; this is why we can't tell if a treatment is working right away. And this is why you won't hear anything in the near future about a new form of treatment that is *proven* to work. This problem also comes up any time a treatment is changed. In order to reduce side effects, treatments are sometimes modified, but this can potentially reduce their effectiveness.

So, as nice as it would be for a new form of treatment that cures cancer without side effects to come along tomorrow, the truth is that this can't happen, because there is no way to know whether that treatment will actually cure prostate cancer. The answer to that question, every time it's asked, takes many years to determine.

How can you think calmly when you're riding a roller coaster? Most men who find out they have prostate cancer feel physically great. They have no symptoms. They're taking some doctor's word for it— not only that there's a cancer growing inside them but that the cancer could kill them if they do nothing. Or, unfortunately, as is the case with some doctors (discussed earlier in this chapter), men are being told the opposite. They're given false assurances that the cancer will grow slowly and it's okay if they don't do anything but watch its progress.

Throughout this book, we've emphasized that your best hope of surviving prostate cancer is to educate yourself in order to learn all you can about a disease that's deceptively simple—but which is actually so complicated that many doctors don't understand it.

Now we're at the crossroads. *Educating yourself is just half the battle—the half you can control. The other half involves a leap of faith: You must find a doctor you can believe in, and then you must be able to accept that doctor's advice.* We talk about finding a good surgeon in chapter 8, but this is more than that—your doctor must be adept and knowledgeable but must also inspire your trust. Ultimately, in matters of illness, this is something everybody must do. Even we doctors (keeping in mind the old adage "The doctor who treats himself has a fool for a patient") must put our trust in the hands of another physician when we get sick. This is because—as educated as you may be, or as much as you've learned about this disease, or as accustomed as you are to taking charge of your life—you can't be objective, and somebody needs to be. Make sure this somebody is the best you can find, and then be prepared to follow the plan this doctor believes is best.

Getting through any course of treatment is a hard job. Every form of treatment takes its toll. It's a lot harder if you're spending precious energy and strength fighting—disagreeing with your doctor, or nitpicking and double-checking even the simplest morsel of advice. The time for questioning is now. Get it all out there—every question, every complication you can think of. Write it all down, meet with your doctor, and don't start anything until you're satisfied that you're doing the right thing. And then, once you've done this, release the burden from your shoulders. Let go and allow the doctor to take over. Spend your energy and strength following that advice, recovering from treatment, and beating this disease.

# 8

# RADICAL PROSTATECTOMY

## ▶▶▶ READ THIS FIRST

Never underestimate prostate cancer. It is a formidable adversary that springs up in several places at once inside the prostate. A cancerous prostate has, on average, seven separate tumors growing inside it. Thus, to cure the disease, we can't just take out a few of these spots of cancer; we must eliminate the entire prostate. *If cancer is confined to the prostate, there is no better way to cure it than radical prostatectomy.* The goal of all other forms of treatment for prostate cancer is to be as good as the gold standard, radical prostatectomy. Today, radical prostatectomy cures the vast majority of men with cancer confined to the prostate, even if it has penetrated the wall, or capsule, of the prostate. And if the operation is performed by an experienced surgeon, preserving potency is common, and few suffer from serious incontinence.

And yet *radical prostatectomy is not for everybody*. It is intended for the younger man with curable disease, the otherwise healthy man who can reasonably expect to live for at least another fifteen years. In other words, it is for the man who is not only curable, but who's going to live long enough to need to be cured. It is not something that an older man or one burdened by other health problems should have to put himself through.

The radical prostatectomy operation that's performed today has evolved over the last twenty-five years. My role in this operation began in the early 1970s. I wondered why so many side effects were occurring and whether it was possible to avoid them. To solve this problem, I took an anatomical approach and learned how to create a bloodless field to save the anatomical structures that previously had been unrecognized and damaged during surgery. Later, noticing that there was a cluster of arteries and veins consistently located in the same region in adult men as the microscopic nerves we first discovered in stillborn infants, I speculated that these blood vessels might be the key to preserving potency during surgery. On April 26, 1982, I performed the first purposeful nerve-sparing radical prostatectomy on a fifty-two-year-old professor of psychology. This man regained his sexual function within a year and has remained complication-free and cancer-free ever since. Today, the neurovascular bundle of Walsh is widely recognized as the landmark used in nerve-sparing surgery. Over the last twenty-five years, I have continued to refine the procedure, making certain that it is an excellent cancer operation and attempting to speed up the recovery of urinary control and sexual function.

## THE LAPAROSCOPIC/ROBOTIC PROCEDURE

Laparoscopy is the use of a lighted tube that enters the body through a tiny hole, through which a surgeon can thread a scalpel. The idea here is that "less is more"—the tiny hole means a smaller incision. More recently, a robot connected to special instruments has taken laparoscopic surgery to another level, providing new refinements to the procedure.

In this chapter, we cover the advantages and disadvantages of all three procedures: open surgery, laparoscopic, and robotic radical prostatectomy. The most important point you should know is that the outcomes from all three procedures are definitely operator-dependent—

*which is why, whichever procedure you select, it is essential that you have an experienced surgeon.* This is just as important, maybe even more so, with the laparoscopic/robotic techniques. Remember, the operation is not performed by the machine but by the surgeon who tells the machine what to do.

We also discuss in detail the complications that can occur in the months after the operation. For a detailed discussion of the results of all forms of treatment for localized disease—surgery, radiation, and cryo/thermal ablation—see chapter 10.

## Radical Prostatectomy—The Gold Standard

Never underestimate prostate cancer; it is a formidable adversary. In its own way, prostate cancer is much like the Hydra, the many-headed, hard-to-kill monster of Greek myth. It's what scientists call multifocal, which means it springs up in several places at once inside the prostate. A cancerous prostate has, on average, seven separate tumors growing inside it. Thus, to cure the disease, we can't just take out a few of these spots of cancer; we must eliminate the entire prostate. *If cancer is confined to the prostate, there is no better way to cure it than with radical prostatectomy.* The goal of all other forms of treatment for prostate cancer is to be as good as the gold standard, radical prostatectomy. (Note that when we talk about radical prostatectomy in this book, unless otherwise stated, we are referring to the anatomic radical retropubic procedure.)

Having said that, we must add right away that radical prostatectomy is not for everybody. It is intended for the *younger man with curable disease,* the otherwise healthy man who can reasonably expect to live for at least another fifteen years. In other words, it is for the man who is not only curable, but who's going to live long enough to need to be cured. It is not something that an older man or one burdened by other health problems should have to put himself through. What if you're somewhere in the middle of these two ends of the spectrum? What if you're a young, active man, and the Partin Tables say there's a fifty-fifty chance your cancer can be cured? If surgery is the best way to cure you, then you should do it. What if you're a man in his early seventies, in excellent health, with curable disease and a family history of longevity? There is no question that older men are more prone to side effects after surgery than younger men, and you must consider the quality of the years ahead. How would you feel if you never regained full control over urination? Also, what if you had complications and were not cured—remember from chapter 7 that older men often have more advanced disease, because it has been there longer. On the other hand, if you select a less effective form of treatment, have a long life, and your cancer comes back, you may end up asking yourself "what if"—what if you had gone for surgery the first time around? For older men, this can be a tough decision.

Many men of any age hate what this decision entails—that forced look in the mirror, the necessary assessment of their own health aside from prostate cancer. You may find it helpful to look back at the section in chapter 7 on the Scandinavian study. Although this study clearly demonstrated that surgery increased survival, the main beneficiaries of this were men who were younger than sixty-five at the time of surgery. For men over age sixty-five, there was no improvement in cancer-specific survival—mainly because many men died of other causes before they died of prostate cancer.

Today, radical prostatectomy cures the vast majority of men with cancer confined to the prostate, even if it has penetrated the wall, or capsule, of the prostate. And preserving potency—by not removing one or both of the nerve bundles adjacent to the prostate, which are responsible for erection (surgeons didn't even realize these bundles existed twenty-five years ago)—does not compromise cancer cure; a recent study found that the odds of cure are just as high. Serious bleeding is very rare, and if the operation is performed by an experienced surgeon, the preservation of potency is common, and few suffer from serious incontinence.

## Evolution of an Operation

Surgery to remove the prostate as a treatment for cancer was first performed in 1904 at Johns Hopkins by Hugh Hampton Young, the pioneering first director of the Brady Urological Institute. Young's procedure, called the radical perineal prostatectomy, was a success. Six and a half years later, when the patient died of other causes, an autopsy showed that his prostate cancer had been cured.

In the late 1940s, another approach called the radical retropubic prostatectomy was developed, and like Young's operation (which still is used today, although not as often as the retropubic approach), it proved extremely effective in stopping prostate cancer in its tracks—if, that is, the cancer was confined to the prostate.

Both the radical perineal and retropubic operations had a definite downside—two devastating side effects, incontinence and impotence. Every man who had a radical prostatectomy was impotent, and as many as 25 percent had severe problems with urinary control. Worse was the extreme, often life-threatening bleeding that went along with the retropubic approach. It's no exaggeration to say that the operation used to be performed in a sea of blood. In that era, many men believed that the side effects from surgery were almost worse than having the disease. So understandably, when radiation treatment for prostate cancer was introduced in the 1960s and popularized (see chapter 9), doctors as well as patients welcomed this alternative therapy. Although doctors realized that it probably did not cure prostate cancer as well as surgery, it certainly had fewer side effects.

The harshness of the procedure and its aftereffects were the catalysts for change, inspiring the anatomical discoveries that have drastically reduced these side effects. As a result of these discoveries, when radical prostatectomy is performed by an experienced surgeon, most younger men should remain potent, and few men should have serious problems with urinary control. Today, radical prostatectomy is the most certain way to cure men with cancer that's confined to the prostate.

### Crafting a Kinder, Gentler, Better Operation

How did radical prostatectomy change? My role in this operation began in the early 1970s. Like many urologic surgeons, I was appalled by the blood loss in these men. With the goal of finding surgical methods to lessen the bleeding—so we could actually see what we were doing instead of blindly feeling our way—I studied the anatomy of the venous drainage surrounding the prostate and developed some new techniques, which did two things. First, with less bleeding, the operation became safer. And with what we call a bloodless field, critical structures—which previously had been unrecognized and damaged simply because there was too much blood in the way to see them—could be looked for and saved. More precise dissection and reconstruction reduced the likelihood of significant urinary incontinence to 2 percent, and even those 2 percent are not incontinent all the time. (We're still working to improve this—more below.)

## Breakthrough in Understanding Potency

But what about impotence? It had been widely assumed that penile nerves inevitably were damaged by the radical prostatectomy. Previously, many doctors thought the nerves that controlled erection ran through the prostate and would be destroyed as a necessity if you removed the prostate—the idea of "to make an omelet, you have to break a few eggs." These nerves were the "broken eggs"—severing them was the price of curing cancer.

It didn't make sense to me that the nerves from one organ would run through another organ. But this had always been the assumption, even in medical textbooks. One highly respected anatomy textbook, for example, stated merely that the nerves that enable erection were "extremely small, difficult to follow in the adult cadaver," and that their location was known "merely through experimental studies."

Around this time, something unbelievable happened. In 1977, one of my patients returned for a follow-up visit three months after surgery and reported that he was totally potent. To me, this news was staggering—how could this man be potent if the nerves that control potency were inside the prostate that I had removed? Furthermore, if this could happen to one man, then why *only* this one? Why weren't *all* men potent after radical prostatectomy? The key was finding these elusive nerves. If we could just figure out where they were—and then find a way to save them but still cure prostate cancer—then men would no longer be faced with an either-or situation. They could be cured of cancer and remain potent.

If this were a detective novel, then here's where we would say something like: "The place: Leiden, the Netherlands. The year: 1981. Here's where the whole case blew wide open." And really, it did—thanks to a urologist named Pieter Donker. I was in Leiden for a conference; Donker, who had recently retired as professor of urology there, was studying anatomy and tackling unanswered questions.

No one had successfully dissected the nerves to the bladder because they were difficult to identify in adults. However, these nerves are not nearly so obscured in infants. I asked to see the laboratory where he was working to trace these nerves, in a cadaver of a still-born male infant. I asked Donker if he knew what happened to the other end of this plexus of nerves—the ones that controlled penile erection. "I've never looked," he said. We got to work. Four hours later, we were jubilant. We could see clearly that the nerves were outside the capsule of the prostate—and that, indeed, it was possible to completely remove the prostate and preserve sexual function!

Over the next year, we worked together on this project long-distance, and then we met again. In the infant cadaver, the location of these nerves had become clear. But how could we apply our findings in stillborn infants and find these tiny, microscopic structures in the deep, complicated recesses of the pelvis in adult men? (An infant's nerves are easier to see for many reasons, including the fact that infants have less fatty fibrous tissue than adults.) It was like having a schematic drawing and trying to identify a burned-out transistor in your television set. During this year, I had noticed something important: there was a cluster of arteries and veins that traveled along the edge of the prostate in the exact location where these nerves were found in the infant cadaver. Perhaps these blood vessels acted as they do elsewhere in the body—maybe they provided a scaffolding for these microscopic nerves. And maybe we could use these bundles as landmarks. Donker agreed. I returned to Baltimore and tested this theory while performing an operation called a radical cystectomy, removal of the prostate and bladder, in a sixty-seven-year-old man. I had never seen or heard of a patient who had been potent after this operation. But ten days after surgery, this man stated that he awoke in the morning with a normal erection.

A month later, on April 26, 1982, I performed the first purposeful nerve-sparing radical prostatectomy on a fifty-two-year-old professor of psychology. This man regained his sexual function within a year, and has remained complication-free—and cancer-free—ever since.

Better understanding of the anatomical terrain also led to several important observations. Now that we've learned exactly where the scalpel can and cannot go, depending on the extent of a man's cancer, it has become possible either to save these nerves deliberately or to remove more tissue by cutting these bundles away—in surgical terms, to create wider margins of excision—than we previously had believed possible. It used to be that surgeons never excised these nerves because they were adherent to the rectum; instead, surgeons just cut the nerves and unknowingly left them in place. However, with these anatomical techniques, we now have a better chance of removing all the cancer. Many people call this a nerve-sparing operation, but a more accurate description is that it's an anatomic radical prostatectomy, because there are actually two things going on here: one is preserving the nerves; the other is creating wider margins— by excising them when necessary, removing as much tissue as possible around the cancer—making this a better cancer operation.

At the same time these discoveries were taking place, an anatomist provided an entirely new insight into the location of the sphincter responsible for urinary control. Previously, we believed that the pelvic floor muscles opened and closed like sliding doors. But this was not the case; it turns out that the sphincter is a tubular structure embedded in the veins that had once bled so much during surgery. This observation explained why the anatomic approach improved the results of urinary continence: In controlling the venous bleeders and making the bloodless field, we did a better job of preserving this sphincter.

Before every radical prostatectomy, I tell my patients that we have three goals: removing all of the tumor, preserving urinary control, and preserving sexual function. Sexual function is number three, because if it is lost, there are many ways to restore it.

Men who are impotent following radical prostatectomy have normal sensation, normal sex drive, and can achieve a normal orgasm. The one element they may be lacking is the ability to have an erection sufficient for intercourse, and that can be restored by drugs such as Viagra or by other means. (For more on erectile dysfunction, see chapter 11.)

## Perfecting the Radical Prostatectomy

Baseball pitchers use videotape to perfect their fastball; tennis players use it to get a better spin on their serve. The video camera is a staple for most athletes, in fact: no respectable football coach would dare contemplate next week's game without spending hours seeking wisdom

## WILL I BE FERTILE AFTER SURGERY?

For most couples, there is good news after a radical prostatectomy: They can safely discontinue birth control measures. That's because the vas deferens (see chapter 1), which carries sperm, is completely divided, and there is no way that a woman can become pregnant during intercourse. But what happens to the sperm that continue to be produced by the testes? They are absorbed by the epididymis (this is what happens after a standard vasectomy as well). However, many men who undergo radical prostatectomy today are younger and may not have completed family planning. If you're not ready to close this door forever, the safest thing to do is store sperm before surgery (a process called cryopreservation). This is the most cost-effective way to ensure that you can have a baby someday, if you choose. There is also a plan B available for men who have already undergone radical prostatectomy and then decided that they want to have children. This is a process called intracytoplasmic sperm injection (ICSI). It's somewhat complicated and expensive. Basically, it involves using a tiny needle to harvest sperm from the testis or epididymis. These sperm are then injected directly into eggs that have been harvested from the patient's wife. After a period of incubation, they are then implanted. But the best bet, if there's even a remote chance that you may want more children after surgery, is to plan ahead and store your sperm.

from hindsight, going over this week's effort on the gridiron, play by play.

So why don't surgeons do the same thing? How are we ever going to improve our technique if we don't analyze our own work this way?

Over the years, I have come to believe that very small differences in surgical technique can have a major impact on outcome. Recently, I put this theory to the test, watching my own operations. Using a high-quality, three-chip video camera, I videotaped the operations on the men discussed below (see Continence and Potency: Quality of Life After Radical Prostatectomy). Then, eighteen months after that study began, I reviewed these tapes. My goal was to make a good operation even better by minimizing the operation's two major side effects—incontinence and impotence. This is what I wanted to find out: When a patient is continent and potent immediately after surgery, what made the difference in this man? I spent my summer vacation examining these videotapes, sometimes stopping them frame by frame, looking for insight. (Another bonus of the video camera is that it allows surgeons a view of the entire operative field, not just the small area where we focus as we operate.) It took many hours of intense scrutiny to watch sixty of these two-hour operations, but gradually I was able to identify four slight variations in my technique—in controlling bleeding from the dorsal vein and dividing the sphincter—that appeared to make the difference in the men who recovered sexual potency the soonest.

Perhaps most exciting was that a new finding came out of this research: it turns out that some men have a significant anatomical variation. Previously, everyone believed that the neurovascular bundle took a fairly straight pathway from its origin in the sacrum along the lateral surface of the prostate to the urethra. But I learned that in many patients, the bundle curves around the apex of the prostate and is tucked just beneath the sphincter and held there by a small group of vessels. And that, if one attempts in good faith to preserve as much of the sphincter as possible, the neurovascular bundle can be damaged and recovery of sexual function delayed. Indeed, the eight men who at eighteen months had not yet recovered full sexual function all seemed to have this variant curve.

Part two of this project was to make the study "blind." I went back over the operations again—this time without identifying the patient or the outcome—to see if the steps I had identified checked out. Fortunately, they did.

Incontinence is a long-term, significant problem for only about 2 percent of our patients at Johns Hopkins, and I was unable to find evidence that anything I did or did not do during surgery would make a difference there. Clearly, it had nothing to do with preservation of the sphincter. There was one man with perfect preservation of the sphincter who was still wearing a pad one year after the surgery. For this reason, I am now taking a different approach.

To the best of my knowledge, this is the first time any surgeon in any field used retrospective reviews of video footage of an open surgical procedure to improve a surgical technique. I believe many surgeons could benefit from regularly reviewing their operations in this way. Because many surgeons use different techniques, it's likely that each surgeon may be able to identify other important, arbitrary

## FOR BEST RESULTS, FIND A HOSPITAL WHERE THEY DO A LOT OF RADICAL PROSTATECTOMIES

When it comes to finding a hospital for radical prostatectomy, a Johns Hopkins study has found a simple rule for potential patients to keep in mind: experience counts, especially if you want the best chance of being cured.

"Radical prostatectomy is a complex, notoriously difficult surgical procedure," says the epidemiologist Bruce J. Trock. The study confirms what many in the medical community have known for years: the best re-sults—fewest side effects and greatest control of cancer—are found at academic medical centers where the urologists specialize in this com-plicated operation.

The study, headed by the Robert Wood Johnson scholar and Hop-kins urology fellow Lars Ellison, compares the recurrence of prostate cancer at a hospital to the number, or volume, of prostatectomies per-formed at that hospital. What does hospital volume have to do with the results of surgery? A lot, explains Trock, who also took part in the study—particularly when the procedure is a hard one for surgeons to master. For radical prostatectomy, he says, several studies have examined the link between hospital volume and short-term problems, such as surgi-cal complications and death up to one year after surgery. But this study, published in the *Journal of Urology*, is the first to examine whether hos-pital volume is related to cancer control—the likelihood that cancer will come back—after prostatectomy.

Ellison and colleagues evaluated more than twelve thousand men aged sixty-five or older—patients from hospitals in Arizona, California, Connecticut, Iowa, Utah, and Washington State—who underwent radi-cal prostatectomy between 1990 and 1994 and who were followed through 1999. The researchers determined hospital volume based on the number of prostatectomies performed in men aged sixty-five or older during 1990–1994—low (1–33), medium (34–61), high (62–107), or very high (108 or more). Then they looked for evidence of prostate can-cer recurrence in these men—the start of hormonal therapy or radiation therapy more than six months after radical prostatectomy.

They found that the low-volume hospitals had more patients with low-grade disease and local tumor stage, both of which indicate a better prognosis. This suggests that hospitals with less experience prefer to operate on the men most likely to do better, explains Trock. Even so, low-and medium-volume institutions had significantly higher rates of treat-ment for cancer recurrence—25 percent and 11 percent higher, re-spectively—than did very high volume institutions. However, hospital volume did not seem to affect the number of deaths from prostate can-cer or otherwise. Trock believes this is due to the study's relatively short follow-up time of five to nine years and the low rate in general of death from prostate cancer after radical prostatectomy.

The higher recurrence rates at lower-volume institutions could be because the surgeons' experience—and also their techniques—vary widely. Ellison and colleagues found as much as a 25 percent difference in cancer control between low- and very high-volume hospitals. "The anatomy of the prostate and biology of a tumor can vary tremendously among patients," concludes Trock. "Surgeons at high-volume institutions encounter the full range of this diversity and are prepared to deal with it."

In another study not yet published involving surgeons at a number of large institutions, investigators found that the *total* number of radical prostatectomies a surgeon performed—not in a week or year, but over a cumulative period—made a difference in cancer control. Patients who underwent surgery by a urologist who had performed more than 250 radical prostatectomies had the best chance of being cured.

variations that may help patients. Also, for surgeons whose patients seem prone to more side effects than usual, the review of early successful cases may help them identify ways to modify their technique, and improve the outcome in future patients. If I had videotaped that first successful operation in 1977—after which the man was potent immediately—I would have discovered the location of the nerves four years sooner.

### Are You in Good Hands? What to Look for in a Surgeon

Doctor A is a nice, personable young doctor whose empathy for your condition appealed to you immediately. That's great. Now what else do you know about him? He's got a terrific bedside manner, but is he a board-certified urologist? What training has he had? Does he know—and use—the nerve-sparing techniques, the anatomical approach to radical prostatectomy? How many of these operations does he do a year? What success has he had in preserving potency and continence? (If he can't or won't give you his rate of success as compared to reports from other surgeons or to results published in medical journals, this may be a red flag, and perhaps you should look elsewhere.) You should be able to get a good idea of his success rate in numbers or percentages. And if he hasn't done very many of these operations—ideally, hundreds—you might want to find a more experienced surgeon. Look at it this way: Do you want to be one of the patients he's learning on? Do you want to be part of someone's learning curve?

When you're looking for a surgeon, you don't necessarily want some brand-name academician or a specialist in other areas of urologic surgery. You want to find a doctor who performs *this particular operation*. Often. Preferably, a doctor who does this operation several days a week. Even better, a surgeon who has dedicated his or her life to doing this one operation.

Doctor B is another nice doctor, a respected, fatherly man who's been operating in your town for as long as anybody can remember. Just looking at him inspires confidence. Swell. But does he also keep up with the latest research? Does he continue his education regularly, brushing up on old surgical skills as well as mastering new techniques? Does he operate on nearly every man who has prostate cancer? (This is not a desirable quality in a surgeon.) Or does he screen his patients carefully, making every attempt to spare any man with cancer that can't be cured by surgery the unnecessary ordeal and side effects of an operation?

Dr. C is Mr. Technology. His hospital is widely advertising the new million-dollar robot it just acquired (and now must pay for). This robot, Dr. C promises, will do everything: reduce blood loss, get you back to work earlier, and give you a much better likelihood of retaining continence and potency than the old-fashioned, "traditional" prostatectomy. When you meet with him, Dr. C says that he's only taken the robot out for a few test spins; he's done only a few of these procedures so far, but already, the results seem to be better than for his patients who underwent the old procedure. Here's the problem: new or old procedure, *it's still the same guy!* The robot, however sophisticated, is not performing the surgery; it's just a tool in the hands of Dr. C. More than this, there is no instrument—laparoscope, laser, or robot—that can do the thinking as well. No tool can make some of the difficult decisions—which are unique for every operation, because every man is different—that must be made during a radical prostatectomy. A million-dollar scalpel doesn't know when, where and how to separate the urinary sphincter and nerves responsible for erection from the prostate without leaving cancer behind. It's the surgeon behind the machine, not the machine behind the surgeon, that ultimately makes the difference—no matter what the ads say.

There's no getting around it: radical prostatectomy is a tricky operation, one of the most difficult in medicine. There can be tremendous, at times life-threatening, blood loss. Does your surgeon have the proverbial nerves of steel? A good surgeon can handle unexpected or excessive bleeding without panicking, but also—thinking of your long-term quality of life—won't damage the microscopic nerves necessary for erection. An experienced surgeon knows how to preserve these nerves *and when it's safe to do so.* You don't want someone whose knee-jerk reaction to the biopsy is to cut, cut, cut. For example, if the biopsy is positive on the right side and your surgeon says, "We'll take out the nerves on the right side and on the left, too, for good measure—I'm interested in getting out all the cancer," you should find another surgeon. For one thing, the biopsy being positive on the right side doesn't mean the nerves on the right side are involved in the cancer. For another, it's unlikely that such a surgeon will actually remove the nerves on either side. A more probable scenario is that he'll cut the nerves and leave most of them in place. Excising these nerves widely is as difficult as preserving them, because they're adherent to the rectum, and it takes great skill to cut them out completely. Or there's also the surgeon who says, "We don't care about side effects; I'm just there to get out all the cancer. We can always put in an artificial sphincter [for control of incontinence] and give you shots or a penile prosthesis [for impotence]." Again, probably not the right surgeon for you. Your ideal surgeon should get out all the cancer *and* make every effort to minimize side effects.

Remember, you don't want a surgeon who's "pretty good" at removing the prostate. And you can't assume that every urologist does this well. There are no second chances here; this is a one-shot operation. *You are looking for the one surgeon who will perform the one radical prostatectomy you will ever receive in your life, the one operation that will cure your cancer.* You want a surgeon who isn't going to leave some cancer behind and who knows how to minimize trauma to your body during surgery so you don't wind up incontinent, impotent, or both. (Note: Unexpected trouble can crop up in any operation; nobody can help that. But the unexpected is less likely to happen with an experienced surgeon.) So ask questions, such as:

- How many of these operations are performed at his hospital per year (you want the answer to be sixty-two or more) and how many have you personally performed in your professional career (more than three hundred is a good answer)?
- What percentage of your patients have positive margins?
- In patients like me whom you have operated on, at one to two years, what percentage have to wear a pad, and how many have recovered erections sufficient for intercourse? How do you collect data on your patients? Do you know their long-term outcome? (If the answer is something like, "Only if they let me know," find someone who keeps better tabs on his or her patients. Urologists who don't know their own results may not realize that their technique should be better. And if the urologist can produce statistics but you don't like those results, get another opinion.)
- How often do your patients require radiation therapy after surgery or treatment with hormones? (If the number is greater than 15 percent, this suggests that the doctor either doesn't do a very good job selecting surgical candidates or is not completely removing all the cancer during surgery. It also suggests that you need to get a second opinion. But you should get a second opinion anyway. *Always get a second opinion.*)

Finally, ask to talk to the urologist's patients. Find out how they're treated—how hard is it to get the doctor when you have a question or need help? If they've had postsurgical complications, how did the doctor treat them?

Finding the right physician may mean that you must travel to a major medical center in another city. This may mean that you'll be away from home for four days. But after that, even though you will be wearing a catheter for a week or two (see below), the recovery from this operation is usually speedy, and follow-up communications can usually be carried out over the telephone (for example, if you have your follow-up PSA tests done in your hometown, you can have the results sent to your surgeon and discuss them—or any complications or troubling issues, such as incontinence or impotence—over the phone).

## HOW COULD THE STANDARD OF CARE
## BE IMPROVED NATIONALLY?

Why are the results of radical prostatectomy so uneven across the country? In the hands of an expert, the complication rate from this operation is low. But many of the patients with bad results—lifetime incontinence, for example, or worst of all, an immediate return of cancer—are men who should never have undergone the operation in the first place, because they were not good surgical candidates and/or because their cancer was not curable when it was diagnosed. It's unfortunate that so many men with prostate cancer must heed the advice *caveat emptor*—Buyer, beware.

The burden of making sure the doctor is competent shouldn't have to weigh so heavily on the patient's shoulders. For example, it seems absurd that a would-be buyer at an Internet auction house can instantly learn the track record and customer rating of a seller before committing to doing business, but a man who is looking to place his life in the hands of a surgeon must do his own research—and even then, hope he's asked all the right questions and left no important stone unturned. There should be a similar system for monitoring the performance of urologists and all physicians.

The information is already out there. Insurance companies know how long a surgeon's patients are in the hospital, how many must be readmitted for complications, how many eventually need placement of an artificial sphincter to control incontinence, and how many need postoperative radiation or immediate treatment with hormonal therapy. If the insurance companies and managed care organizations were really interested in seeing that their patients received the best care, they could identify surgeons who have the highest volume of patients and lowest rate of complications. This might stimulate the physicians whose patient outcomes were not as good to improve their skills—or to decide that performing one operation a month was not the best thing for them or their patients.

The next step would be for an organization to collect patient-reported outcomes. Again, this is something insurance companies could do—find out exactly how patients are doing and then put together a roster of surgeons who provide the best service. To some, this might seem like unnecessary interference; after all, the idea of "letting the market decide" is a cornerstone of private enterprise, capitalism, and the American way. But this is different from buying a car that turns out to be a lemon. If you have winced at the results of a botched operation, feeling at once sorry for the patient who came to you, hoping you could repair the damage, and outraged that medical care in this country is so variable, you might agree that the system ought to be improved. What about the surgeons whose work is not up to the national standard? One obvious solution is that they could work to improve their technique. It's never too late to learn. (See Perfecting the Radical Prostatectomy.)

In an attempt to help others learn, I produced a detailed one-hour-and-forty-five-minute DVD, and through the generosity of the Mr. and Mrs. Robert C. Baker Foundation, distributed fifty thousand of them free to every urologist in the world who wanted one. On a recent visit to India, I had the rewarding experience of speaking to a urologist who had never done a radical prostatectomy before—but who, after studying the DVD, successfully performed the operation, losing less than 1 unit of blood. Although the full DVD is intended only for urologists, you can view the illustrations and see selected video clips by going to http://urology.jhu.edu and clicking on "Anatomic Radical Retropubic Prostatectomy—Detailed Description of the Surgical Technique."

Undeniably, the results of surgery are best when patients are in the hands of experts. For the sake of men with prostate cancer and their families, it's time for this information to be made available to everyone.

## The Anatomic Retropubic Prostatectomy

### Questions You May Have Before Surgery

*Why Do I Have to Wait Several Weeks for the Operation?*

There should always be a delay of about six to eight weeks between the time a man's prostate cancer is diagnosed and the time he can undergo surgery. Many men are frustrated by this. They think, "I've got cancer, it's curable, and I want it out of there right now!" They see the delay as the operating-room equivalent of an overbooked airport, with planes stacked up waiting to land and interminable layovers. But this is not the case. The main reason for the six- to eight-week lag time between diagnosis and surgery is not to accommodate a busy hospital's schedule; it's so you can have a better cancer operation.

Immediately after the needle biopsy, which often involves a dozen punctures of the rectum, your body reacts—as it does to any injury—with inflammation and bleeding. Now is not the ideal time for surgery. A biopsy is what doctors call an insult to the body, in this case, to the wall of the rectum, which is riddled with tiny holes and weakened. Think of how much easier it is to tear perforated paper than regular, intact paper. The body needs time to recover from this relatively minor insult so it will be ready for the really big one—major surgery. Even after two weeks, the punctures may have healed, but the prostate is now adherent to the rectum; it remains stuck to the rectum until the inflammation resolves. If surgery were attempted at this point, it would not be easy to release the rectum from the prostate—and the last thing the surgeon wants to do is make a hole in the rectum. In an attempt to protect the rectum, the surgeon may cut too close to the prostate, possibly leaving cancer cells behind. But after giving it a few more weeks, the inflammation heals, and the prostate is no longer sticky. The normal anatomy is restored, and it's easier for the surgeon to see the terrain.

At Johns Hopkins, we studied more than nine hundred of my patients who underwent surgery between 1989 and 1994, evaluating the delay between diagnosis and cure. Some of these men were treated early, within two months. Others had surgery three, six, and nine months, or even more than a year after diagnosis. We found no significant difference in the long-term cancer control rates of these men. Let these results reassure you that *there is no immediate urgency to perform surgery after you are diagnosed with prostate cancer*, especially if you have stage T1c disease and a biopsy Gleason score lower than 7. Take your time, and find the right doctor and hospital (see above).

### Should I Stop Taking Aspirin, Herbal Remedies, and Vitamins?

Before surgery, when you give the doctor your medical history, be sure to say so if you've had any unusual problems with bleeding in the past (from dental work, for example). Aspirin and drugs such as ibuprofen (Advil, Motrin) can cause excessive bleeding; if you are taking aspirin or a similar drug regularly, make sure you stop *at least ten days before the operation*. Also be sure to tell your doctor if you are taking vitamins—particularly high doses of vitamin E—herbal compounds, or other dietary supplements. These supplements still count as medications, even if they "just came from the health-food store," and they can affect blood-clotting mechanisms. Thus, you should stop taking them as well.

## What About Donating My Own Blood?

This is another point to discuss with your doctor. Many men who undergo radical prostatectomy need a blood transfusion during the procedure. The best blood for you to get, obviously, is your own; if your hospital allows this, it's a good idea to donate 1 or 2 units of your blood ahead of time. (This is another good reason for the six- to eight-week delay; it gives you plenty of time to make up your own blood bank.) However, there is some difference of surgical opinion here. Some surgeons say that their patients never lose any blood and therefore don't need any blood transfusions. For these physicians, the most important thing during the operation is to clamp, ligate, and clip every little bleeder—every blood vessel that bleeds. My philosophy is somewhat different. The nerves that control erection are surrounded by blood vessels; in fact, that's what the neurovascular bundle is, a knot of blood vessels. When exposing these vessels, there is often bleeding, and if a surgeon aggressively clamps every bleeder, it is unlikely that the nerves will survive. So, with the patient's long-term outlook—controlling cancer plus maintaining quality of life— as my main goal, I must sometimes "spend" a little bit of blood. If I see something bleeding, I may wait until I've completely released the tissue surrounding that bleeder to see what's beneath it—and then control just that bleeding vessel, leaving the nerves beneath it intact. If a patient gives his own blood and receives a unit or two of it during surgery, there is no harm; in fact, it may improve his quality of life immediately after surgery. Many argue that banked blood today is very safe, and that the main risks of a transfusion (getting the wrong blood or infected blood) are not avoided by donating your own blood. Advocates of giving your own blood disagree. So you need to ask yourself—if you will need a transfusion, whose blood do you want, your own, or someone else's?

You can give 1 unit of blood a week beginning two or three weeks before surgery. The day you start giving blood, take one iron tablet three times a day and continue until the day of your last blood donation. And while you're giving blood, don't take aspirin, ibuprofen, vitamin E, or any similar medication; if this blood will be going back into your body during surgery (presumably because you've lost enough to need it), the level of these drugs may be high enough to interfere with the clotting of your blood during surgery.

### Does It Matter If I've Had Previous Prostate Surgery for BPH?

This is how some men find out they have prostate cancer—when the prostate tissue removed in a TUR procedure or open prostatectomy (another procedure for BPH) is evaluated by a pathologist. It's more difficult for surgeons to perform a radical prostatectomy after an open prostatectomy, but that doesn't mean it can't be done. It often is, and with great success. You may need to wait about twelve weeks after a TUR, until the inflammation from this operation has gone down, before having a prostatectomy.

## Countdown to Surgery

One of the most important steps in recovering from a radical prostatectomy is the recovery of the gastrointestinal tract—mainly, this means the return of normal bowel movements. This return to normal happens much faster and with fewer complications if the bowels are empty when you undergo surgery. Thus, to help speed things along after surgery, you can work on improving your digestive tract before surgery. Be sure that your bowels are moving well for about two weeks before the operation; increase your daily intake of fiber, fruit, and liquids. Note: Iron supplements (which you should be taking if you are giving your own blood—see above) can sometimes cause constipation. If necessary, take a stool softener, or talk to your doctor about using a bulking laxative (such as Citrucel). Stick to clear liquids during the day before surgery. Then, on the night before surgery, take a laxative, and don't eat anything after midnight. On the morning before surgery, give yourself an enema.

### Anesthesia

Your two best options are spinal or epidural anesthesia. The great advantage to both of these approaches, as opposed to general anesthesia, is that there is less bleeding during surgery. Also, both reduce the likelihood of blood clots forming in the legs after surgery (perhaps be-

## ARE YOU IN SHAPE FOR SURGERY?

In any man, the prostate is not terribly accessible. It's way down there, deep in the pelvis, and in the retropubic procedure (as opposed to the perineal approach, discussed later in the chapter), the surgeon must go through the lower abdomen to find it. This is not only much more difficult in a man who is overweight; the extra fat can also interfere with performing a good cancer operation, preserving urinary control, and preserving potency.

If you are overweight, your surgeon may operate only on the condition that you lose weight beforehand. It is in your best interest to meet this challenge—it may be that your life will be saved twice, because men who are overweight are medical time bombs. Heart disease, stroke, diabetes—you're at high risk for all of these, and if you smoke or have high cholesterol, the risk skyrockets. In blunt terms, what's the point of curing your cancer if you're not going to live long enough to benefit from it?

Here, as an example of what can be done in just two months, is a diet plan developed by one of my patients, who was diagnosed with prostate cancer at age fifty-three. I agreed to operate on him under the condition that he lose at least 30 pounds.

Here's how he explains it: "I needed to lose the weight for my own health benefit, and a leaner patient would simplify the surgical procedure, improving prognosis for success. I dropped from 224 pounds to 189 pounds between November 8 and January 8. I had surgery on January 15, stronger and leaner. Here's how I did it:

- "Goal-setting and plotting expectations kept me motivated to lose weight continually.
- "Actual weighing-in only took place twice a week, Monday and Thursday. There is too much weight shift due to water retention to recommend weighing in every day. I wanted to avoid setbacks. Every weigh-in should result in a legitimate loss.
- "I didn't starve! It took only four days to get used to a daily diet, which roughly followed this pattern: Breakfast—Ultra Slim-Fast; tea or coffee. Lunch—salad (I was creative, using a variety of vegetables), cup of soup; Dinner—tossed salad, Stouffer's Lean Cuisine. These are delicious, come in many varieties, and provide a 'unit dose' of calories, about 230 to 290. I favor the spicier ones.
- "I wrote down everything that I ate or drank, meal by meal, in a daily journal. Having to confront my sins in black and white kept me from committing them.
- "Exercise played a key role. I worked out daily, varying the thirty- to forty-five-minute exercise between NordicTrack, treadmill, jogging, and briskly walking my dog. This burned off one of the meals, so I netted out at two meals per day."

cause there is increased blood circulation in the legs during surgery). With both forms, you can be sedated to the point where you are asleep and don't remember anything about the operation. Rarely, some men like to remain conscious and hear what's going on, but they can't feel it. For many patients, however, this is just one more thing to worry about. They say, "I don't *want* to know what's going on." Don't worry, you can be sedated (with a mild drug such as Valium (diazepam), which will make you sleep) as well as anesthetized. Most men don't remember anything about the operation. In spinal anesthesia, a tiny needle is used to inject a local anesthetic into the small of your back through the dura, the membrane lining the spinal cord, and into the spinal fluid. In epidural anesthesia, a local anesthetic enters the body through a tiny plastic tube inserted between the vertebrae of your spine, near the small of your back. This bathes the area outside the membrane lining the spinal cord, temporarily numbing the nerves in your lower body. Within minutes, you'll feel numb, relaxed, and heavy from the waist down.

### During Surgery: What Happens

How much information do you want? In this next section, we're going to take you through the radical prostatectomy, step by step. But if you want to know even more or actually see these steps, you can find them on the Johns Hopkins Urology Web site: *http://urology.jhu.edu*. (Under "Video Resources," click on "Anatomic Radical Retropubic Prostatectomy—Detailed Description of the Surgical Technique.")

Let's begin with a quick review of the territory. (It might help if, as you read this, you refer to figures 8.1–8.8.) For a surgeon, this is precarious terrain indeed. The prostate (fig. 8.1) is located deep in the pelvis, surrounded by structures that are fragile and vulnerable to injury—the rectum, the bladder, the sphincter responsible for urinary control, some large blood vessels, and the bundles of nerves that are responsible for erection.

The operation begins with a 3-inch incision through the skin that extends from the pubic area halfway to the navel (a longer incision is not necessary and may delay your recovery). Next, the muscles in the abdomen are separated in the midline and spread apart. *They are not cut*, which is one of the reasons men recover from this operation

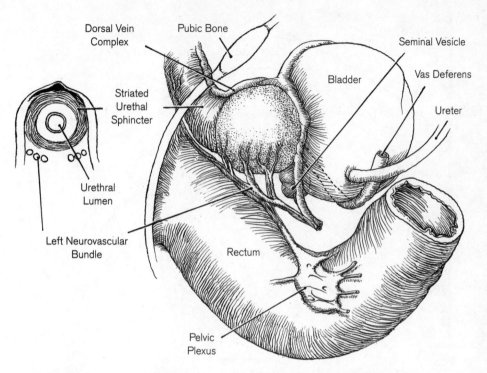

**FIGURE 8.1   The Radical Retropubic Prostatectomy, Step by Step**

You're looking at the prostate and surrounding terrain—the rectum and bladder; key nerves; veins; and the urethral sphincter, a tube-shaped structure that helps control urine. You can also see one of the two neurovascular bundles, the package of nerves critical for erection, which sit on either side of the prostate. [Figures 8.1–8.8 by Leon Schlossburg, reprinted from Patrick C. Walsh, *Radical Prostatectomy: A Procedure in Evolution*, Seminars in Oncology 21 (1994): 662–71. Used by permission, W. B. Saunders Company.]

quickly, with little pain and with no long-term injury to their abdominal muscles.

The next step is the staging pelvic lymphadenectomy—dissection of the pelvic lymph nodes to make sure they're free of cancer (fig. 8.2). To do this, we remove a triangle of tissue on each side of the bladder; these triangles contain important lymph nodes. In the past, these lymph nodes were then rushed to a pathologist for what's called frozen section analysis (the tissue is frozen, then sliced into very thin sections and examined under the microscope). We don't do that very often. In most men, these lymph nodes are usually removed as part of the operation and sent along with the

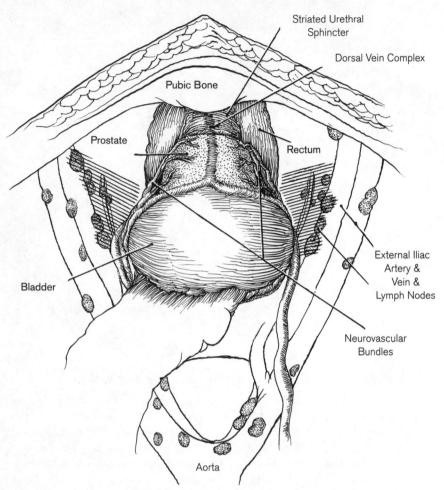

**FIGURE 8.2   The Radical Retropubic Prostatectomy (Continued)**

This is a schematic look at the prostate, bladder, and lymph nodes. It's the view the surgeon has after the abdominal incision has been made. Inside the shaded area are the lymph nodes removed during a staging lymphadenectomy.

prostate to the pathologist, who then examines this entire "specimen," or bunch of removed tissue.

Today, staging pelvic lymphadenectomy (as a separate procedure, done several days ahead of time) is usually performed only in men with palpable disease and a Gleason score of 8 or higher. This is because for lower-grade, well- to moderately well differentiated tumors—Gleason 7 or less—the long-term prognosis is different than it is for men with high-grade, poorly differentiated tumors. With

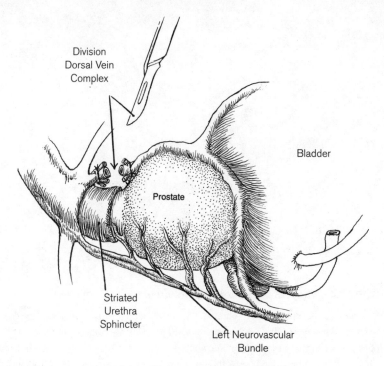

Division
Dorsal Vein
Complex

Bladder

Prostate

Striated
Urethra
Sphincter

Left Neurovascular
Bundle

**FIGURE 8.3** **The Radical Retropubic Prostatectomy (Continued)**

This is how the surgeon helps create the critical bloodless field—carefully cutting the dorsal vein complex, which travels over the urethra and prostate and carries a great deal of blood.

Gleason scores of 7 or lower—even when there is a tiny bit of cancer in a lymph node—without further treatment (such as hormonal therapy), up to 35 percent of men will have an undetectable PSA level, and 60 percent will have no sign of metastases on bone scans ten years later. Although some of these men may be cured, this does not mean the cancer won't eventually come back in other men. However, it can take years longer to return when the tumor is of a lower, better-differentiated grade (less than Gleason 8). So, because these men can live for many years, they often benefit from having their prostate removed. Removing it now will help them avoid problems with urinary tract obstruction and bleeding later, if the cancer does return. Furthermore, we have some evidence that men in this situation who have their prostate removed live longer (see chapter 7).

For men with Gleason scores of 8 or higher, it is very important to know the status of the lymph nodes before going ahead with a

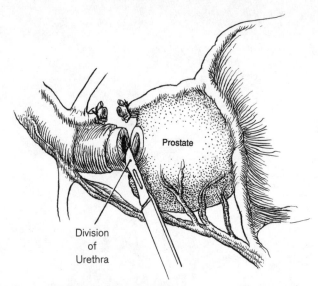

Prostate

Division
of
Urethra

**FIGURE 8.4   The Radical Retropubic Prostatectomy (Continued)**

The surgeon is now cutting the urethra, which runs through the prostate. This is another delicate procedure—cutting the urethra too close to the prostate might mean some cancer is left behind, but cutting it too far from the prostate might mean damaging the urethral sphincter, which helps control urine flow. With great care, the prostate is separated from all the tissue and blood vessels that are connected to it.

radical prostatectomy. Because frozen section analysis may miss small but important deposits of tumor in the lymph nodes, we prefer to carry out this procedure at least several days ahead of time. (As discussed in chapter 6, this can be performed either laparoscopically or with a modified procedure called a mini-lap.)

Some surgeons do not perform lymph node dissection at all, because finding positive lymph nodes is—fortunately—so rare these days. That's understandable. However, one out of one hundred times, lymph nodes turn out to be positive in a patient in whom you would least expect it. Because we have found that these are also the exact patients who would benefit most from having these lymph nodes removed, we continue to do lymph node dissections in all patients. We are emboldened to do this because of the extremely low risk of complications associated with this, the ease with which a complete lymph node dissection can be performed in a short time, and the fact that more good can come from doing it than not.

Next (fig. 8.3), the major vein system that overlies the prostate and

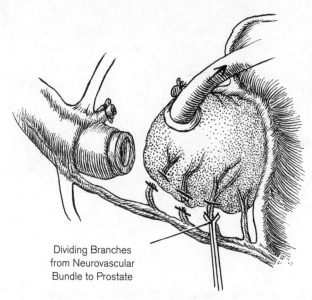

Dividing Branches
from Neurovascular
Bundle to Prostate

**FIGURE 8.5  The Radical Retropubic Prostatectomy (Continued)**

If it's possible—and for most men today, diagnosed with curable cancer, it usually is—the surgeon can preserve the neurovascular bundles on either side of the prostate. To do this, the surgeon gently separates each branch of these nerves and vessels from the prostate.

urethra (this is called the dorsal vein complex) is divided and tied. This is a crucial step; control of these veins makes a huge difference in the surgeon's ability to see what's happening, and it's particularly significant for what happens next—cutting through the urethra (fig. 8.4). If the urethra is cut too close to the prostate, some cancer might be left behind. This is the most common location for a positive surgical margin—for the presence of cancer cells at the cut edge of the removed prostate specimen. Positive surgical margins are discussed later, but briefly, a positive margin can mean one of two things: It can mean that the tumor extends outside the prostate, to a point where the surgeon can't remove it all. But it often means simply that the boundaries of the prostate are indistinct, and the surgeon cut extremely closely along the edges of the prostate. This is the part of the operation where it's most difficult to see exactly where the prostate ends and the tissue outside it begins. If we err on the other side—if we cut too far away from the prostate—the urethral sphincter might be damaged, and such an injury can make a man incontinent. The surgical line here is

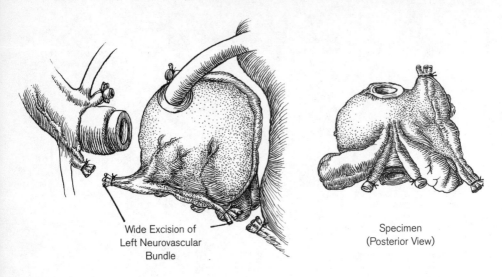

Wide Excision of
Left Neurovascular
Bundle

Specimen
(Posterior View)

**FIGURE 8.6  The Radical Retropublic Prostatectomy (Continued)**

If it is not possible to preserve these nerve bundles—if they have been reached by cancer—
then the surgeon removes them along with the prostate. This is called wide excision. The
surgeon cuts out as much tissue as possible surrounding the prostate in an aggressive
attempt to get every last bit of cancer.

literally not much more than a hairbreadth, and that's why, in this operation, the surgeon's experience counts.

Next, depending on the degree of cancer, the surgeon must make
a decision that will affect the patient's potency—to leave intact the
neurovascular bundles, the wafer-thin packets of nerves that sit on either side of the prostate, or to remove one or both along with the
prostate (fig. 8.5). These are the nerve bundles responsible for erection.

Remember the three goals of radical prostatectomy: removing
the cancer, preserving urinary continence, and preserving sexual
function, in that order. The primary goal here is not to preserve potency; it's to get rid of the cancer in a careful but thorough way. Fortunately, because prostate cancer is now detected early in most men,
it is usually possible to preserve the neurovascular bundles on both
sides. These bundles are outside the capsule of the prostate; even
when cancer penetrates the capsule, it travels only 1 or 2 millimeters—not much more than the width of a pencil point—away from
it before turning northward, toward the seminal vesicles. Because the
neurovascular bundles are, on average, about 5 millimeters from the

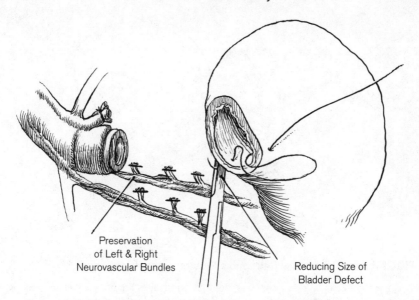

Preservation
of Left & Right
Neurovascular Bundles

Reducing Size of
Bladder Defect

**FIGURE 8.7  The Radical Retropubic Prostatectomy (Continued)**

This shows the situation after the prostate has beem removed. Note how big the opening in the bladder is in comparison to the urethra. This must now be narrowed in size, so the two can be connected.

prostate and because cancer—even when it penetrates the capsule—travels only 1 or 2 millimeters away from the prostate, we can usually preserve both neurovascular bundles without creating a positive surgical margin. Recently, we evaluated one hundred of my patients who had cancer extending through the capsule of the prostate into the area of the neurovascular bundle and compared them with one hundred similar patients operated on by another experienced surgeon. I widely excised the neurovascular bundle in 16 percent of my patients, as did the other surgeon in 63 percent of his. However, the frequency of positive surgical margins was the same—just slightly less than 6 percent. One year later, 84 percent of my patients, compared with 64 percent of the other patients, were potent. This study shows that an experienced surgeon, during open radical retropubic prostatectomy, can maintain that delicate balance—knowing when these bundles should stay and when they must go; how to remove enough tissue to obtain a clear surgical margin, yet preserve the patient's sexual function.

It also helps to have good tools. I use a fiber-optic headlight, which

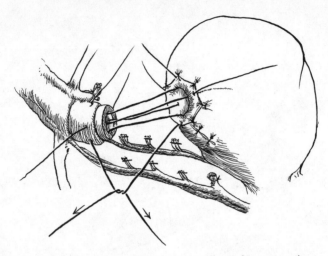

**FIGURE 8.8   The Radical Retropubic Prostatectomy (Continued)**

The operation's almost over now. Here the surgeon rebuilds the urinary tract, pulling the bladder down to bridge the space, connecting the urethra and urethral sphincter.

shines a powerful light directly into the surgical field, and magnifying glasses called loupes, like a jeweler uses. Using 4.5-power loupes provides excellent, three-dimensional magnification, much like the visualization associated with use of the laparoscope, or the robot (see below). What about using nerve stimulation during surgery? Some surgeons believe that this can help them find the nerves. We have studied this extensively, and unfortunately, we have found that the current technology often identifies nerves that aren't there and fails to pinpoint them where they are actually hiding. At this point, nerve stimulation is more of a gimmick, and it can't compare with the accuracy of an experienced surgeon.

In another review, of five hundred consecutive men who underwent radical prostatectomy at Johns Hopkins between 1997 and 2000, 87 percent of men had both bundles preserved, and 13 percent of men had one bundle preserved. Pathological study confirmed that the cancer was completely removed, with no evidence of cancer at the edge of the removed tissue (margins were negative) in 95 percent of these men. Only 5 percent had a positive surgical margin, and only 2 percent had cancer cells at the neurovascular bundle. In half of these positive margins, the cancer was on the *opposite side* of where the biopsy had suggested (again, more evidence for caution before a surgeon should reflexively decide to remove the bundle on the side of the positive biopsy). As we discuss in chapter 10, the vast majority of these men were eventually proven to be cured of their cancer.

However, if it's necessary to remove one neurovascular bundle, it should go (fig. 8.6). Remember, *men can remain potent even if one bundle is removed and can still have normal sensation, sex drive, and orgasm even if both bundles are removed.* And frankly, there are plenty of older men out there who *haven't* had prostate surgery who still have problems with erection. This is an inevitable problem for many men, one of those things that come with the territory of aging. In other words, it may be a bullet you couldn't have dodged anyway. However, it's also important to repeat that there is plenty of help available, and you can still have a normal sex life (see chapter 11).

There is no way for the surgeon to know for certain before the actual operation whether the bundles can be spared. Some surgeons believe that imaging studies, such as MRI and ultrasound, can be helpful, but my experience has been different; in fact, I have often found them to be misleading. Only during surgery is it truly possible to tell where the cancer is. Some urologists believe that the neurovascular bundle must always be excised on the side of a positive biopsy—in other words, if your biopsy showed cancer cells on the left side, then that bundle's got to go. This is not the case, and although well intentioned, it's a bit of a knee-jerk reaction. Actually, the most common site of positive surgical margins is the apex of the prostate (where the sphincter meets the urethra), followed by the posterior (next to the rectum), and last, the posterolateral area (near the neurovascular bundle).

Experienced surgeons don't make any decisions beforehand. We wait and assess the extent of a tumor during surgery. We can see it, and more importantly, we can feel it. During surgery, if we feel cancer on the edge of the prostate—this can only be done during open surgery—the neurovascular bundle should be removed. It should also be removed if, at any point during its release (when we slowly peel it away from the rectum), it seems adherent or sticky. Red flag—this is often a sign that the cancer is beginning to escape the prostate. However, if no firmness is felt and the neurovascular bundle falls away from the prostate, it's safe to preserve it. As a final precaution, we double-check the bundles later in the operation. Once the prostate has been removed, the surgeon carefully examines the specimen, feeling every inch of it for hardness. If there is any suggestion that we need to go back and remove a bit more tissue, we can remove the bundle at that time. Unfortunately, with current laparoscopic and robotic techniques, the prostate cannot be examined until the operation is completely finished.

If the surgeon decides to preserve the nerve bundles, the tiny branches that connect the nerves to the prostate are divided carefully. If, however, one or both bundles must be widely excised, the nerve bundles are cut near the urethra and beside the rectum.

Next, the surgeon goes to work on the prostate, making a cut to separate it at the bladder neck, which links the bladder to the prostate (fig. 8.7). The seminal vesicles are removed, along with the vas deferens on each side (for more on the anatomy, see chapter 1). The goal here is to remove as much surrounding tissue as possible along with the prostate. Finally, the surgeon must carefully rebuild the urinary tract, hooking up the bladder once again to the urethra and urethral sphincter, which is responsible for urinary control. Note that the gap between the bladder and urethra—where the prostate used to be—is now filled by the bladder. Some men worry that the penis will be shortened—that the surgeon will pull it up to meet the bladder. This doesn't happen; instead, the bladder is mobile, and can easily be pulled down to meet the urethra. The surgeon uses sutures, or stitches, to narrow the bladder neck so it matches the size of the urethra (fig. 8.8). The Foley catheter is left in place after the operation to drain urine until the connection has healed and is watertight.

## After Surgery

A drain will be left in the abdomen until nothing flows through it (this usually takes a day or two), and a Foley catheter, inserted in the penis and anchored by a tiny balloon in the bladder during surgery, will remain in place for one to two weeks. Note: To minimize your risk of getting a urinary tract infection, which often happens in men who have a catheter, you should begin taking an antibiotic such as Cipro (ciprofloxacin) or Levaquin (levofloxacin) the day before the catheter is scheduled to come out, and keep taking it for five days. On the day the catheter is due to come out, be sure to drink extra fluids. Your doctor will want to make sure that you are urinating with

## THE NERVE GRAFT BANDWAGON

Some urologists believe they'll have a better chance of curing cancer if—just to be on the safe side—they cut out both neurovascular bundles and put in nerve grafts to restore the potential for erection they just cut out. Hey, there's a great idea! Except that in the PSA era, where most cancer is diagnosed at a curable stage, it is hardly ever necessary to cut out both neurovascular bundles.

If a man has bilateral capsular penetration (cancer on both sides of the prostate) to the point where it's necessary to remove both neurovascular bundles, then this man is probably not curable with surgery, because cancer has already spread to distant sites. Out of 2,700 radical prostatectomies I performed over a fifteen-year period, only seven potent men had both neurovascular bundles removed. Four of these men were not cured, because they had positive lymph nodes, positive seminal vesicles, or a positive margin elsewhere; in the other three, it was not necessary, because there turned out to be no capsular penetration on that side. Because of this, I have come to believe *it is almost never necessary to remove both neurovascular bundles.* A man who needs both bundles removed probably shouldn't be undergoing the surgery anyway, and a man who doesn't need them removed is going to be a lot better off with nerve-sparing—preserving what he's already got—than with a nerve graft—trying to replicate what should have been left alone to begin with. Also, in many patients, it is possible to remove part of a bundle and still preserve potency.

Now, having said all that, I should add that the idea of nerve grafts in radical prostatectomy patients—although recently revived—is not that new. In fact, the first experimental work on nerve grafts to restore sexual function was reported from the Brady Urological Institute at Johns Hopkins in 1989. We found an ideal animal model. In the rat, the nerves responsible for erection are relatively large, distinct structures, compared to what men have—tiny clusters of nerves and blood vessels that fan out broadly at both ends, making it impossible to perform a precise nerve graft. The experimental studies in rats were encouraging, and in the early 1990s, collaborating with a neurosurgeon, I carried out a study of nerve grafts in patients who underwent wide excision of one neurovascular bundle. We followed the patients for more than five years, and unfortunately, there was no difference in the recovery of sexual function in men who received a nerve graft and those who did not. At the same time, another trend was emerging; with the widespread use of PSA testing, more men were being diagnosed with localized cancer, and as a result, fewer men needed to have a neurovascular bundle removed.

Recently, surgeons have been taking another look at nerve grafts. Some urologists have reported that in men who had both neurovascular bundles removed and received nerve grafts (using small nerves taken from the side of the foot), 30 percent had recovery of sexual function. However, in reviewing these surgeons' results, I found that 58 percent of the patients who underwent nerve grafts had no evidence of capsular penetration on either side—and thus, they didn't need to have either nerve bundle removed in the first place. Also, it is not clear whether the men who recovered sexual function were the ones who actually needed the nerve bundle removal—the men with cancer that needed to be cut out—or the men with organ-confined cancer—who had less disease, and whose nerve bundles should have been spared anyway.

What about nerve grafts in men who have one bundle removed? This same group of surgeons states that when they remove one neurovascular bundle, only 25 percent of their patients are potent. However, at Johns Hopkins, without a nerve graft, 64 percent of the patients who have one neurovascular bundle removed are potent. Would a nerve graft improve these results even further? The argument is not terribly convincing. In a study done at Hopkins several years ago, we analyzed the factors that influenced a man's recovery of potency after surgery. It turned out that men who had more extensive disease—capsular penetration or cancer involving the seminal vesicles—were less likely to have recovery of sexual function, even if both neurovascular bundles were preserved.

Also, nerve grafts are not without their own risks. Potential side effects include the development of numbness or nerve damage on the side of the foot (at the site where the to-be-grafted nerve is removed) and the possibility of a delay in walking after surgery. Also, removing a nerve, closing that site, and then grafting the nerve in the pelvis prolongs the surgery and may cause men to lose more blood. Before nerve grafts become an added component to many radical prostatectomies, they need to be studied in many men in a randomized, controlled study.

*The Bottom Line:* Men with more extensive localized disease—cancer that spreads slightly outside the prostate—are less likely to recover sexual function regardless of the status of their nerves and are unlikely to be helped by placement of a nerve graft. If it is likely that a man will need to have one neurovascular bundle removed, the best thing he can do to ensure his recovery of sexual function is to find a urologist who can do a good job of preserving the nerve bundle on the other side. (Again, this does not mean that a man can't still have a normal sex life; see chapter 11.)

a strong stream. (Note: The time it takes to recover urinary control varies, and it is not likely that your urinary control will be perfect immediately. Your doctor just wants to make sure there is no urinary obstruction.)

The main reason for using the catheter is that it allows the newly connected bladder and urethra (this is called the anastomosis, if you hear your surgeon using this term) a chance to heal. The drain is there to evacuate any urine that might leak from this connection as it's healing; it must stay in place until nothing more flows through it. *It is critical that the Foley catheter stay in place.* If it is inadvertently pulled out or removed too soon after surgery, this can be disastrous and may lead to permanent incontinence. Your catheter should be securely taped to your thigh, and you should examine its mooring often. The catheter may take some getting used to, but remember— it's only temporary, and its presence is helping the body heal. While you're at home, keep the catheter connected to a large drainage bag most of the time, and avoid using a leg bag. The leg bag doesn't hold as much urine, and if the bag becomes full and you don't realize what's happening, the urine can back up into you because it has nowhere else to go. Depending on your surgeon's preference, the catheter will be left in place for one to two weeks.

### Bleeding Around the Catheter

This looks scary, but it's pretty common, especially if you strain to have a bowel movement. Don't worry; it will stop. Also, don't worry if you see some blood in the urine. This usually has no significance and almost always resolves on its own—usually by the time the catheter is removed. Sometimes this bleeding happens spontaneously, and sometimes it's due to overexertion (walking too briskly, for example) or is a result of taking aspirin or ibuprofen. If you see blood, flush it out by drinking a lot of fluids. This will dilute the blood so that it won't clog the catheter, and it will also help stop the bleeding.

### Leakage Around the Catheter

Another scary phenomenon, this, too, is usually nothing to worry about. Leakage can occur when you're up walking around or when you're having a bowel movement. It can usually be managed with the use of diapers or other absorbent materials. Important: If your catheter stops draining completely, lie down flat and drink a lot of water. If after one hour there is no urine coming through the catheter, it is possible that your catheter has become clogged or dislodged. Call your doctor right away.

### Urinary Sediment

Another common, disconcerting problem, this can manifest itself in several ways. You may see some old clots, which appear as dark particles, after you have had bloody urine. These usually go away on their own. Also, the pH balance of the urine (its acidity) changes throughout the day. After a meal, for example, urine often becomes alkaline. There are normal substances in the urine called phosphates. These can precipitate if the urine has too little acid and can cause cloudy masses to appear in the urine. (The urine also may appear cloudy if you have a urinary tract infection—see below.)

### Bladder Spasms

These can be extremely painful. Fortunately, bladder spasms are not very common. The men most likely to have them are those who have been troubled by urinary symptoms before surgery (usually, men who have had BPH), who have developed a thickened bladder wall and a hair-trigger bladder that is easily irritated. In this case, the irritant is huge—the catheter—and the bladder is trying its best to push it out by contracting. The spasms may happen at random, or they may be provoked by an activity, such as having a bowel movement or going for a walk. If you have a bladder spasm, lie down until the contractions improve. If you have frequent spasms, you may be helped by medication. Nonsteroidal analgesics (such as ibuprofen) work quite well because they relax smooth muscle. For persistent spasms, tranquilizers such as Valium (diazepam) are usually able to control the problem.

### Pain

You'll be dealing with the catheter mostly at home; the economic trend these days is for patients to leave the hospital as soon as possible after any procedure, and prostate surgery is no exception. Fortunately, radical prostatectomy patients are actually *able* to go home and generally be more active sooner than ever. It used to be that men would have to stay in the hospital for a week after radical prostatectomy because they were unable to eat. We always blamed this on the operation, assuming that, somehow, the surgery caused the intestines to hibernate. It took between two and four days for men to resume normal bowel activity. As it turned out, this slowdown was caused by the pain medications—the narcotics we routinely gave after surgery. Today, we administer pain medication more judiciously.

At Johns Hopkins, immediately after surgery, men receive painkillers through an automated delivery system. This intravenous drip provides a baseline of pain relief, and if a patient needs more, he can press a button and increase the dosage. The next day, all radical prostatectomy patients—those who have open surgery as well as those who undergo the laparoscopic or robotic procedures—stop taking narcotics and switch to a nonsteroidal anti-inflammatory drug (NSAID) called Toradol (ketorolac). They are able to eat a clear liquid dinner on the night of surgery and start back on solid foods the next day, when they're up and walking around. One or two days after surgery, they are able to leave the hospital. Regardless of the surgical approach, most patients report little pain, and the pain they do have isn't where they most expect it—right along the incision. Instead, it's usually on one side or the other; it rarely hurts equally on both sides. The pain comes from irritation of the abdominal muscles; sometimes it occurs where the drainage tubes stick out of the body. It always goes away on its own.

When you leave the hospital, as soon as your doctor says it's okay, you can eat and drink whatever you wish—even alcohol, in moderation. The main thing is that you *avoid becoming constipated*. Remember, the prostate sits on top of the rectum; when it's removed, this part of the rectum is thin, fragile, and particularly vulnerable to injury for the first three months after surgery. Therefore, it is critical that you do not have an enema or your temperature taken rectally anytime soon. And it's absolutely essential that you have a bowel movement every day. For many men, this is easier said than done; pain medications, inactivity, and slight dehydration (from not getting enough fluids before or after surgery) all can add up to constipation. To help keep things moving, you'll probably be given stool softeners or laxatives for several days. If you do become constipated, take mineral oil and milk of magnesia (but again, do not use an enema—you could perforate your rectum).

### Caring for the Incision

You can take a shower as soon as you are discharged from the hospital. Your surgeon will probably remove the skin clips (the surgical equivalent of staples) before you leave the hospital and put Steri-Strips in their place. These are surgical tapes that hold the edges of the incision together nicely. They'll probably be kept on for about a week—until the body's own healing process gradually takes over. (Their presence seems to encourage a thinner scar to form.) To protect these strips, tape some plastic wrap over the incision before you shower. Some men develop an infection in the incision several days after they get home from the hospital. This usually manifests as some drainage—either a clear fluid or an unsightly mixture of blood and pus. Don't worry; this can be treated simply with some hydrogen peroxide and a cotton swab. Soak the cotton swab in hydrogen peroxide, and stick it through the opening in the incision.

### Urinary Tract Infection

Having a catheter often means getting a urinary tract infection; the two seem to go together. If you develop an infection while the catheter is still in, you may notice that your urine becomes cloudy, or you may see some pus in the drainage around the catheter. Talk to your doctor, who will probably prescribe an antibiotic such as Levaquin (levofloxacin) or Cipro (ciprofloxacin).

### When Can I Resume Normal Activities?

Until the catheter is removed, take it easy. You can eat and drink whatever you want, take long (but not strenuous) walks, and make as many trips as you'd like up and down stairs. Also, you can drive a car and go back to work two to three weeks after the surgery. Exactly how soon you should resume all activities will depend on how quickly you seem to be recovering, but once the catheter has been removed, most men feel well enough to return to their normal routines (including golf) by four weeks after surgery.

Expect to have some incontinence. This is normal, and it, too, is not permanent. It will go away eventually—don't be discouraged. Also, expect to have some trouble with erections (see chapter 11).

Finally, you'll be encouraged to sit in certain positions, to do leg exercises to boost your circulation, and to walk around almost immediately. This also is crucial—among other things, it can help reduce your risk of developing blood clots.

## Other Procedures

### The Radical Perineal Approach

In the radical perineal prostatectomy, the prostate is removed through a small incision in the perineum, the space between the scrotum and rectum. (This is the original operation devised by Hugh Hampton Young, the Johns Hopkins surgeon who pioneered radical prostatectomy in 1904.) Similar to the retropubic procedure (in which surgeons reach the prostate through the abdomen) in terms of before-surgery preparation and recovery, the radical perineal approach offers some advantages over that technique: there's less bleeding, because the major vein system that overlies the prostate (the dorsal vein complex) is not removed. However, this also means that surgeons aren't able to cut out as much tissue as in the retropubic approach—so if the cancer has penetrated the prostate wall, positive surgical margins may be more likely than with the retropubic approach. If the likelihood of cancer appearing in the pelvic lymph nodes is low (see the Partin Tables in chapter 6), there's no need for an abdominal incision. Many men, however, do have a laparoscopic lymph node dissection before getting a perineal prostatectomy just to be sure cancer hasn't reached the lymph nodes. There are also reports that the return of PSA after surgery may be higher with the perineal procedure than with the retropubic approach. Thus, if you are at high risk of having capsular penetration, or cancer reaching the wall of the prostate, you should have the retropubic procedure.

Some studies suggest that the odds of incontinence with the perineal approach are lower than with the retropubic technique, although there is a higher risk of another complication, fecal incontinence, because the anal sphincter is stretched. One study suggested that as many as 9 percent of patients had fecal incontinence during an average week after the procedure.

Another drawback with this approach is that the operating quarters are cramped, making it more difficult for surgeons to see, and thus protect, the neurovascular bundles, the thin packets of nerves that sit on either side of the prostate and are essential for erections. Therefore, preserving potency is not as certain. The operation is not ideal for overweight men, particularly men with a large "barrel" abdomen. Also, for the surgeon to get at the perineum, it's necessary for the patient to be folded up, almost like a pretzel, with his legs held up in stirrups. This can lead to the compression of nerves, a condition called neurapraxia (the same problem that can affect the nerves that control erection if they are injured during surgery) and can sometimes cause sensory or motor problems in the leg and foot. A study by researchers at Duke University Medical Center found that neurapraxia developed in 21 percent of 111 men who underwent radical perineal prostatectomy. In almost all of these men, the symptoms were temporary. The researchers concluded that this problem could be prevented if the time the patient spends in the position (called the exaggerated lithotomy position) is limited.

### During Surgery: What Happens

You will be given general anesthesia, which means you'll be unconscious during the procedure. To reach the prostate, surgeons make an incision just above the rectum. The prostate is gradually separated from the rectum, bladder, urethra, and vas deferens. The seminal vesicles are removed along with the prostate, and then the bladder is linked once again with the urethra.

### The Laparoscopic/Robotic Radical Prostatectomy

Someday, all operations will be performed less invasively, and big abdominal incisions will be a thing of the past. Laparoscopy is the use of a lighted tube that enters the body through a tiny hole through which a surgeon can thread a scalpel. The idea here is that "less is more"—the tiny hole means a smaller incision and possibly a shorter recovery time. Laparoscopic versions of other operations, such as removal of the gallbladder, have turned out quite well, and the promise of a faster recovery has proven true. More recently, a robot connected to special instruments has taken laparoscopic surgery to another level, providing new refinements to these procedures. With all of these advances, is it time for these techniques to be applied to radical prostatectomy?

Radical prostatectomy is one of the most complicated procedures in all of surgery. The tissues surrounding the prostate are delicate, and the surgeon must walk a fine line, excising enough tissue to make certain that all cancer has been removed without adversely affecting urinary control and sexual function.

What about laparoscopic removal of the prostate? Just a few years ago, laparoscopic radical prostatectomy offered no clear benefits; fledgling attempts at this operation were disastrous because of excessive bleeding and difficulty connecting the bladder and urethra, resulting in marathon operations that lasted as long as twelve hours. However, new suturing techniques, popularized by surgeons in Europe, have led to a revived interest in the laparoscopic procedure. Now, surgeons have reduced the operating time to less than three hours and say that the procedure offers several advantages—less bleeding and the ability to make a watertight connection.

*Advantages*

The surgeons promoting this procedure are enthusiastic. They emphasize the definite advantages: First, there is less blood loss. In order to get to the prostate, the surgeon distends the abdomen—inflating it like a balloon—using high-pressure carbon dioxide. This process compresses many bleeding veins. This has definitely resulted in less blood loss and a higher blood count after surgery. (However, this has had only a marginal effect on the need for the transfusion of patients' own banked blood. At Johns Hopkins, where patients donate 1 or 2 units of blood before surgery, only about 1 or 2 percent of patients undergoing either the open or laparoscopic/robotic procedure need a further transfusion of banked blood.) Another advantage is excellent magnification, especially using the robot, which provides three-dimensional magnification. Again, for perspective, open surgeons, by using 4.5-power loupes, can also gain three-dimensional magnification. Finally, one disadvantage of the procedure may well turn out to be an advantage as well: Laparoscopic/robotic surgery, by its very nature, means working in tight quarters. But this means less stretching of, and stress to, the delicate nerves involved in erection and may help with the restoration of potency.

*Disadvantages*

The major downside to laparoscopic/robotic procedures is the surgeon's lack of ability to feel things. Tactile sensation is extremely important during the nerve-sparing procedure. It is vitally important for the surgeon to be able to feel the tissue to make certain that it is safe to preserve the nerves. For example, before we release the nerves in open surgery, we feel the surrounding tissue. If we detect any trace of firmness, we remove those nerves. We check again as the nerves are being released from the prostate. Any sensation of resistance or adhesion—stickiness—is a strong indicator that cancer is there and that these nerves should go. Finally, immediately after we remove the prostate, we give it a thorough going-over as in the physical examination, but this time, without having to feel for hard spots through the rectum. If we find any areas of suspicious firmness, we can take extra tissue from these sites. In laparoscopic procedures, this tactile sensation is muted; it's like using chopsticks to read braille. And with the robot, the surgeon's ability to feel is nonexistent. Also, in laparoscopic/robotic operations, because the prostate specimen is not removed until the end, it is not possible to go back and remove additional tissue if there seems to be a need. There is no question that with advancements in technology, once it is possible for the surgeon to feel tissue, both the laparoscopic and robotic techniques will be improved. But for now, the surgeon using the laparoscope is somewhat handicapped in performing fine maneuvers, because the instruments are located a great distance from the tips of the fingers. With the robot, however, fine maneuvers are made easier by the design of the instrument.

Because of the difficulty in deciding whether the nerves can safely be preserved or because of adhesions, bilateral nerve-sparing (preserving the nerve bundles on both sides) does not happen as frequently as it does in open surgery. Thus, if you are interested in the laparoscopic or robotic procedure and your surgeon says, "If I preserve both nerves, your likelihood of potency is X percent," be sure to ask the follow-up question: How often do you preserve both nerves in patients like me?

It is not clear whether the long-term cancer control rates will be as good as the gold standard—the anatomic radical retropubic procedure. Here's why: During open surgery, surgeons can find out much by feel. Tactile sensation—feeling subtle differences in tissue with our gloved fingers—shows us exactly where to cut; it tells us whether the neurovascular bundle should be preserved or widely excised and whether the structures next to the prostate are suspiciously adherent to it. Here, the laparoscopic surgeon is operating at a distinct disadvantage; one important avenue of information and feedback just isn't available.

During any nerve-sparing procedure, there are often multiple small arteries and veins that must be controlled as the neurovascular bundle is released from the prostate. This is more time-consuming and difficult to perform during laparoscopic/robotic procedures, and to shorten the operation, surgeons have used thermal (heat) energy—electrocautery. Most nerves in the body have a blanket of insulation around them, a sheath called myelin. Unfortunately, the nerves in the neurovascular bundles don't have this protection. This makes them exquisitely sensitive to any form of heat. We have shown experimentally that even the slightest bit of heat produces irreversible damage to the nerves involved in erection. For this reason, the skilled laparoscopic surgeons at Johns Hopkins, Li-Ming Su and Christian Pavlovich, have developed techniques that replicate the open surgical technique, with meticulous tissue handling and avoidance of electrocautery. With this technique, their potency rates mirror the results of open radical prostatectomy at Hopkins.

One other disadvantage for the laparoscopic/robotic procedures can be the cost. These operations sometimes take much longer than the open operation and can turn out to be very expensive. Also, they involve costly tools that can be used only once.

*Outcomes*

We are fortunate at Johns Hopkins to have experts in all three surgical procedures: Open, laparoscopic, and robotic. This has also given us an opportunity to look at the short-term outcomes. Our findings confirm the findings of studies from Vanderbilt University, which did not demonstrate any short-term advantages to the laparoscopic/robotic procedures over open surgery. Patients undergoing all three procedures routinely have a liquid supper on the night of surgery, discontinue narcotic painkillers the next morning, leave the hospital one or two days after surgery, and have their Foley catheters removed nine to fourteen days after surgery. Their recovery times are similar.

This basic sameness in recovery time is an important point—one that might be missed in an era when Web sites promoting laparoscopy feature such statements as "Do you want six weeks of pain and suffering after an open prostatectomy?" This plays on the wide assumption that radical prostatectomy is a painful procedure. But this is not the case. Our patients don't have six weeks of pain and suffering; they recover quickly. In most open surgical procedures, large incisions must be made through muscle, and these incisions truly are painful. But in radical prostatectomy, the muscles in the lower abdomen are separated in the midline; *they are not cut.* Also, because our incisions are now around 3 inches, the muscles aren't even spread very far apart. For this reason, there is no difference in the short-term outcome for patients undergoing open and laparoscopic/robotic radical prostatectomy.

The outcomes from all three procedures are definitely operator-dependent—*which is why, whichever procedure you select, it is essential that you have an experienced surgeon.* This is just as important—maybe even more so—with the laparoscopic/robotic techniques. Remember, *the operation is not performed by the machine but by the surgeon who tells the machine what to do.*

In terms of continence and potency, because there is so much variation in the outcomes of open surgery (again, the best results are at academic medical centers, where experienced surgeons perform many radical prostatectomies each year; see above), it is difficult to have a baseline for comparison. However, at this point, it's safe to say that there have been no dramatic improvements noted with laparoscopic or robotic techniques, with one exception. An experienced robotic surgeon in Michigan has reported 97 percent potency at one year. These patients all had normal sexual function before surgery and appeared to be highly selected, because 98 percent had organ-confined disease. This is very important to emphasize because, as we will discuss below, there can be a major trade-off between cancer control and preservation of potency.

The major goal of radical prostatectomy is to eliminate all prostate cancer. This, then, should be the major endpoint. But because the laparoscopic/robotic procedures are still relatively new, we don't know their long-term results. Until we do have information on how often PSA levels go up (the most critical way to analyze cancer control) in the years after surgery, the second-best thing we can look at is a short-term measure—pathological results showing how often cancer was left behind after surgery. The most critical way to evaluate this is to see how frequently there are positive surgical margins in men when the cancer was completely confined to the prostate. In other words, how often was the entire prostate removed? (This is important because, if the surgery didn't get all of the prostate, it is possible that some cancer cells could remain behind and that they will continue to grow.)

Initially, laparoscopic surgeons were comfortable reporting positive surgical margins of 15 to 25 percent in men with organ-confined disease. In contrast, in more than ten thousand operations performed by all surgeons at Johns Hopkins, the frequency of having a positive surgical margin in a patient with organ-confined disease is only 1.3 percent. Recently, some centers have reported that the frequency of positive surgical margins is the same in open and in laparoscopic surgery. However, they are quoting positive margin rates of 7 percent in organ-confined disease; this rate is still too high. Similarly, on the Internet you may see a report citing positive margins in 23 percent of patients with open surgery but in only 5 percent of patients with robotic surgery. If you go back and read the original paper, you will see that 93 percent of the men who underwent open surgery had organ-confined disease. Clearly, these operations were not done very well if 23 percent of these men with organ-confined disease had cancer left behind! Further, if you look at the 5 percent figure for robotic surgery, you'll see that the definition of positive margins is somewhat unorthodox. The margin was positive on the surgical specimen, but when the surgeon went back and took a tiny piece of tissue further out, no cancer was found.

Surgeons who perform the laparoscopic procedure are acutely aware of this problem of cancer remaining at the margins and have been working diligently to modify their surgical technique to prevent it—recently, by reviewing videotapes of their own operations. The most common site for some prostate tissue to be left behind is at the apex of the prostate. If you are interested in undergoing a laparoscopic or robotic radical prostatectomy, you should be very concerned about this potential problem and should ask your surgeon about the frequency of positive margins in organ-confined disease.

### In Summary

I view the introduction of this new technology as a good thing. It has raised the bar for surgery in general—forcing surgeons to modify their operations, for example, by decreasing the size of their incisions and coming up with new ways to reduce side effects. Who benefits most? Patients. It has made surgeons performing all three procedures aware of the importance of adequate cancer control and understanding the anatomy in an effort to make radical prostatectomy a better operation for everyone. The results across the board have shown, once again, that the most important factor affecting outcome is the expertise of the surgeon.

## Complications

### Early Complications

Like all surgery involving anesthesia, radical prostatectomy carries the risk of death, but *this is extremely rare*. In a Johns Hopkins study of nearly four thousand patients, there were three deaths—one man had a heart attack before surgery as the anesthesia was beginning, and two men died after surgery (one at ten days, one three weeks afterward) from a blood clot to the lung. (For important tips on how to recognize symptoms of this, see below.)

The most common complication during surgery is excess bleeding, usually a result of a blood vessel being injured during the operation. That's why it is absolutely critical that your surgeon has mastered the techniques for ensuring a bloodless field (described above; see also Are You in Good Hands? What to Look For in a Surgeon, also above). Less-common complications during surgery include injuring the rectum or ureters; such injuries can be repaired during surgery, and extra surgical precautions can be taken to avoid permanent damage.

Complications shortly after surgery include:

## Blood Clots

These are among the most common—and potentially most serious—complications of radical prostatectomy. One of the body's most effective defense mechanisms after any trauma is something called the clotting cascade—a chain of events that causes the blood to coagulate. This can help stop bleeding if you skin your knee or even help save your life if you're in a car wreck, but this helpful system can also be activated when it's least welcome—after surgery—and can do more harm than good. Blood clots that form in the legs' deep veins (this is called deep venous thrombosis) can be, at best, painful. At worst, they can be fatal. The leg veins are, basically, a straight shot to the lungs; the nightmare scenario here is for part of a blood clot in the leg to break free and shoot up to the lungs.

Blood clots in the legs and pulmonary embolism, or blood clots in the lungs, occur in an estimated 2 percent of men. At Johns Hopkins, 2 men out of the first 1,300 patients who had the anatomic radical retropubic prostatectomy died of a blood clot. In the 2,800 operations since that time, none of our patients has died of a blood clot. (Note: Both of these men had major underlying heart disease, which underlines what we have discussed earlier—that this operation is not always the best choice for men with significant health problems. If you have serious heart disease—even if your cardiologist gives you the green light for surgery—you may be more likely to experience complications and may not tolerate them as well as other men.)

Clearly, the best way to deal with this problem is to *prevent it from ever happening*. Some doctors do this by administering blood-thinning medications such as mini-dose heparin. Some doctors also give their patients compression devices—various forms of heavy-duty support hose—for the legs. One of these looks like a pair of long johns and is designed to force all blood into the deep veins and keep the flow powerful and continuous. (Sluggish blood flow leads to clot formation.) Other hose have special compression chambers that control blood flow and are designed to "milk" blood up the leg.

*Important: If you have ever had a blood clot, make sure your doctor knows about it.* This could influence the way your anesthesia is administered. Also, men considered at higher risk of developing a blood clot may have a stronger blood-thinning medication administered throughout their stay in the hospital.

These preventive steps are very important, but they're only part of it. The rest falls squarely on your shoulders. Make sure you and your family members know the warning signs of a blood clot, and *if you think you have any of them, seek treatment immediately.* A blood clot is a problem that can be treated easily with anticoagulants (blood thinners and clot-dissolving medications), if it's caught early. But if diagnosis—and therefore treatment—is delayed, a blood clot can be fatal.

### You may have a clot if you have:

* Swelling or pain in the leg, especially in the calf.
* Sudden chest pain—especially if it gets worse when you take a deep breath—or coughing up blood, shortness of breath, the sudden onset of weakness, or fainting. *If you have any of these signs— even if you don't feel anything unusual in your legs—you could have a blood clot in your lungs. Call your doctor immediately!* Don't wait for your doctor's office hours if this happens in the middle of the night! If you can't get to your doctor, go to an emergency room and tell the doctor there that you need to be evaluated for deep venous thrombosis or pulmonary embolism with ultrasound of the leg veins or a spiral CT of the lungs.

Exercise is another crucial factor in helping to avert blood clots. Walking is good; it pumps blood back to the heart. Walk as soon as you're allowed to after surgery. If you stand up, don't stand still for longer than a few minutes at a time—move around. The only way the blood that's in the veins in your legs gets back up to the heart is by the pumping action of the muscles. Your doctor will probably encourage you to do dorsiflexion exercises—pumping your feet up and

## CALL YOUR DOCTOR!

Contact your doctor if you have any of the warning signs of a blood clot. This is part of being your own advocate. It doesn't mean that you have to be militant or obnoxious or that you should call your doctor in the middle of the night just to chat (please don't!).

What it *does* mean, however, is that you have certain rights. If you have a question or problem during office hours, by all means, go ahead and call; you may not always get the doctor, but you'll get somebody who can help.

And if you have a problem that you don't think can wait until morning, call at night. Most doctors have twenty-four-hour answering services; many doctors have partners who share "on-call" time—they split it up, each taking a certain number of nights, weekends, and holidays a year. They do this because they expect to get some calls at night, because they know from years of training and experience that medical emergencies don't always happen during office hours.

This won't be the first phone call your doctor gets in the middle of the night, and it certainly won't be the last. What would you rather do—wind up in the hospital as a result of a serious complication that should have been treated hours ago or "bother your doctor"?

down to exercise the calf muscles. Do these often, about one hundred times an hour in between naps. Also, it is essential that you *do not sit upright in a chair (with your legs hanging down)* for more than an hour at a time during the first four weeks. Try to sit with your legs elevated on a sofa, reclining chair, or comfortable chair with a footstool as much as possible. This accomplishes two goals: One, because it raises your feet, it improves the blood flow from the veins in your legs. Also, it protects the area of surgery from bearing your full weight.

Note: Because patients are in and out of the hospital so fast these days, it's likely that any postsurgical trouble you experience will be when you're at home. That's why it's essential that you and your family be aware of the warning signs of a clot in the leg or a clot that has gone to the lung.

### Bladder Neck Contracture, or Constriction of the Bladder Neck

This is scar tissue that forms where the bladder neck is sewn to the urethra, and it has been reported in between 1 and 12 percent of men after surgery. Its symptoms are usually manifested by a very slow or dribbling urinary stream when—this is the tip-off—the bladder is full. Also, it can sometimes appear as a delay in recovery of urinary control, like a sticky faucet that won't open or close completely. Remember, incontinence immediately after surgery is a very common problem. In the early days after surgery, many men who are experiencing incontinence also worry about having a slow urinary stream. But it's hard to achieve a good stream if there's not much in the bladder, and it's impossible to store up urine in the bladder if it keeps leaking out. Bladder neck contracture is different; the bladder is full, but the best you can manage is a dribble, because the scar tissue is blocking the flow, like a stuck washer in a faucet.

If you have a very slow urinary stream or prolonged incontinence, you should be evaluated with a urinary flow rate and a measurement of residual urine following completion of urination through ultrasound measurement. If your urinary stream is slow and you have residual urine, you have some form of obstruction. This can be confirmed by cystoscopy, and if scar tissue is found, the bladder neck can be reopened in a simple outpatient procedure as a urologist, using a cystoscope (a tiny tube inserted through the tip of the anesthetized penis, through the urethra, and into the bladder), makes a few tiny cuts to relax the tight scar tissue.

To keep the area open, your urologist may recommend that you pass a small catheter through the urethra every day for a month or so after the procedure. This way, the scar tissue won't re-form, and the normal lining of the bladder and urethra will cover the opening as it's supposed to. If the scar tissue is particularly stubborn, your doctor may inject a powerful steroid called triamcinolone into the area of the contracture; this can be effective in preventing the scar tissue from returning.

### Inguinal Hernias

We know—although we're not sure why—that within two years of radical prostatectomy, about 15 percent of men develop an inguinal hernia. It may be that some of these men already had a hernia, but didn't know it. For example, in a recent study of 430 patients, we identified hernia defects (more obvious, or frank hernias, and hidden hernias) in about a third of the men. It is very easy to fix a hernia during a radical prostatectomy. If you have a hernia, tell your surgeon you'd like to have it repaired, and if you think you might have one, ask your surgeon to look for it during the radical prostatectomy.

## Long-Term Issues

### Urinary Continence

Before surgery, many men focus on impotence as the major complication of radical prostatectomy. They're wrong. Recovery of urinary control is far more important and—if it happens slowly or doesn't happen at all—casts a far greater shadow on your life. If something's wrong with your ability to urinate, you'll be reminded of it several times a day—or worse, several times an hour—not just a few times a week or month. And frankly, having to change your adult diaper because you just involuntarily urinated in it can dampen—literally—any romantic thoughts that you do have. Thus, before you go under the knife, you and your urologist need to talk about the risk of incontinence. (See Are You in Good Hands? What to Look for in a Surgeon, above.)

Why does incontinence happen after radical prostatectomy? Let's take a moment to review the male plumbing. Men are equipped with three separate anatomical structures that control urine—a sphincter at the bladder neck, the prostate itself, and the external sphincter (also called the striated sphincter). Radical prostatectomy knocks out two of these—the sphincter at the bladder neck and, of course, the prostate—leaving only the external sphincter to do the work of three. Because of the powerful structures upstream, this external sphincter is never tested or even used much in most men. Thus, we have no way of knowing before radical prostatectomy how strong this sphincter really is. In some men, it's extremely well developed; in others, it's not. Like the rest of the muscles in the body, this sphincter loses its tone with age, and here's where older men have the disadvantage. Men over age seventy have more problems recovering perfect urinary control after surgery than do younger men. Here, too, is where men differ from women: Women have only this one sphincter. In consequence, they have very thin bladders. Men, in contrast, normally have thicker, more muscular bladders to begin with (see fig. 2.1 in chapter 2). Add any element of BPH (benign enlargement of the prostate, which often makes the bladder work harder and become muscle-bound), and a man's bladder can become quite thick. Thus, some men are left with a situation where a burly, thickened bladder is connected to a sphincter that may not have been that effective to begin with.

To make matters worse, at the time of surgery, the sphincter can be damaged, because the major blood vessels that can cause excessive bleeding are intertwined within it. This is why the skill of the surgeon is so important. One of the first steps in a radical prostatectomy is to divide this complex structure. If too much sphincter is taken out or if the sphincter is injured during the surgeon's attempts to stop bleeding, urinary incontinence can result. Thus, it's vital that your surgeon understand the complicated anatomy and know how to preserve the urinary sphincter and carefully rebuild the urinary tract. Urinary incontinence is a huge quality-of-life issue. You must think about it now, before surgery, and do your best—by choosing an experienced surgeon, and afterward, by following the exercises described below—to minimize trouble later.

### The Return of Urinary Control

Some men are lucky. They are dry from the moment the catheter is removed. They can stop their stream on a dime and start it whenever they want to. The great physician Sir William Osler once made a perceptive comment that applies here: "The man who is well," he said, "wears a crown that only the sick can see." Men who are continent immediately after radical prostatectomy are blessed. Most men, however, have variable amounts of urinary leakage. You may be one of the lucky ones; then again, you may not. Most likely, it will take some time for your control of urine to come back completely. For most men, this process happens in three distinct stages: Phase one is when a man can remain dry when he's lying down. In phase two, you're dry when you're walking around. If you can walk to the bathroom and not urinate until you get there, that's a great sign—it means that the sphincter is intact. And in phase three, you are dry when you stand up (using muscles that put pressure on the sphincter) after sitting.

At Johns Hopkins, 79 percent of men are wearing no pads at three months after radical prostatectomy; 88 percent are wearing no pads at six months, and 98 percent are dry at twelve months. (Note: At Hopkins, we consider any man continent if he wears no pad or if he wears a pad that is dry. Many men continue to wear a small pad just to be safe. Your doctor may have a different definition of continence, which you should find out before surgery.) However, most men (even at three months) are not very wet, and when asked in a confidential questionnaire, 96 percent stated that leakage caused little to no bother. It's hard to believe, but urinary control does continue to improve over two years and, in an occasional patient, for even longer than that.

Can you do anything to speed things along and improve your urinary control? First, whatever you do, *do not wear an incontinence device with an attached bag, a condom catheter, or clamp*! If you use any artificial device, you will hurt yourself in the long run. You won't be able to recover your urinary control, because you won't develop the muscle control you need. Until your urinary control returns completely, wear a pad such as a Serenity pad, or disposable diaper such as Depends. You can get these at a pharmacy or grocery store. Some men prefer using a special kind of padded underwear called Sir Dignity briefs; your doctor should have good suggestions and perhaps even some samples for you to try.

Also, until your urinary control has returned to an acceptable level, don't force fluids. When the catheter is in, you're asked to drink a lot of fluids to flush out the system. However, once the catheter is out, you've got to slow the pace considerably. Avoid drinking excessive amounts of fluids, and stay away from caffeine in all forms—coffee, tea, and even soft drinks. Caffeine is a powerful pharmacologic agent that increases the frequency and urgency with which you need to urinate. (Note: If you are being treated for high blood pressure with an alpha-adrenergic antagonist such as Cardura (doxazosin) ask your doctor to put you on a different kind of drug. Also, if you were taking Flomax (tamsulosin) for BPH, you should discontinue it. Cardura and Flomax make the sphincter relax and can make incontinence worse.)

### Exercises You Can Do
Next, every time you urinate, do it standing up. You can't practice the following exercises, which strengthen the external sphincter and speed up your recovery of urinary control, while you're sitting down.

Start your stream, and once it's in full force, stop the stream by contracting the muscles in your buttocks—not your abdominal muscles, not the muscle up in front around the penis. Tighten your buttocks; imagine you're trying to hold a quarter between your cheeks. Hold the urine back for five or ten seconds, and repeat as many times as you can. Note: Perform these exercises *only* when you're urinating; if you keep contracting these muscles throughout the day, you'll overdo it—the sphincter tires easily—and you'll end up wetter than you would be otherwise.

Remember, for many men, the recovery of urinary control is a slow process. The most important thing you can do during this time is not get discouraged. If your doctor told you there was only a 2 percent chance that you would have a long-term, serious problem with urinary control, believe it. This means there's a 98 percent chance that you'll be back to normal someday, even if no crystal ball can say exactly when. It will help for you to discuss your progress at regular intervals with your urologist—even a phone call every so often can make a world of difference in how you see your progress. It may also help for you to take part in a support group so you can talk about the issues that are bothering you with other men who are in the same boat, going through the same process of recovery. You can do this online, from the privacy of your own home (this may be better if you are uncomfortable talking about personal matters in front of others), or you can find a local prostate cancer support group. Ask your doctor.

If you are experiencing no progress, it's reasonable to consider whether something else—other than the natural, gradual return of urinary control—could be causing the delay. One possibility is a *bladder neck contracture*, the formation of scar tissue around the reconnected bladder and urethra.

Incontinence after surgery falls into two basic categories: stress incontinence and urgency incontinence. Stress incontinence is caused by a weak sphincter; urine leaks out when you cough, sneeze, laugh, or run. Urgency incontinence (also called urge incontinence) is when you know you have to go to the bathroom but can't get there in time, and some urine leaks out. Men with urgency incontinence leak right away, when they have the sudden urge to urinate and can't hold it back.

If you have stress incontinence, there are several medications that may help. For example, decongestants, used to treat a stuffy nose and cold symptoms, work by contracting smooth muscle in the nose. The urethra is surrounded by this same smooth muscle. Thus, if you do not have high blood pressure, you may benefit from taking a short-acting decongestant, such as pseudoephedrine (Sudafed), or a long-acting agent combined with an antihistamine, such as loratadine and pseudoephedrine (Claritin-D). However, some of these drugs can cause drowsiness and a dry mouth, and some men find those side effects worse than the urinary leakage itself. Another drug, called imipramine (Tofranil), works through a two-pronged approach. It relaxes the muscle in the bladder and also tightens the muscle tone of the external sphincter. This drug, too, can cause drowsiness and a dry mouth; however, some men find that if they take just one tablet at night, it lasts well into the next day. (Otherwise, the usual dose is 25 mg up to three times a day.)

If you had an enlarged prostate before surgery and experienced a lot of urinary frequency and urgency, you may have urgency incontinence resulting from a hyperactive bladder. Your doctor can check for involuntary bladder contractions with cystometry, a test that measures bladder progress and function by passing a small catheter through the urethra into the bladder. Changes in pressure are monitored as the bladder fills with water.

If you have urgency incontinence, you may benefit from treatment with an anticholinergic medication. A simple, over-the-counter one is diphenhydramine (Benadryl); other choices, available by prescription, are the long-acting drugs tolterodine (Detrol), oxybutynin (Ditropan XL), tropsium (Sanctura), and solifenacin (Vesicare), which target mainly the bladder and have fewer side effects (including dryness of the mouth and eyes, headache, constipation, and rapid heart rate) than other drugs of their kind. Anticholinergic drugs have an antispasmodic effect—they can prevent involuntary bladder contractions and help prevent urine leakage. Other drugs, classed as antispasmodics (which means they fight muscle spasms), can help relax an overenthusiastic bladder muscle that contracts too frequently. These include flavoxate (Urispas) and dicyclomine (Bentyl). Antidepressants also may help by strengthening the internal sphincter and relaxing the bladder.

Many doctors advise their patients to undergo something called pelvic floor biofeedback. This includes a forty-five-minute biofeedback behavioral therapy session—a tutorial on how to use your pelvic floor muscles. Patches are placed on the perineal and abdominal muscles to be sure that you're performing these exercises correctly. Some men find this helpful. However, this is an expensive way for a man to learn how to start and stop his stream, and indeed, critical studies have demonstrated no great benefit to this elaborate and expensive procedure.

### If It Still Doesn't Get Better

The gains made in recovering urinary control can be incremental, often frustratingly so. But there's a point at which it probably isn't going to get any better on its own. If incontinence persists beyond two years (or if your doctor thinks you need extra help sooner), there are several options for treatment.

### Collagen

The sphincter can be bulked up by the injection of collagen—a procedure similar to the one used by plastic surgeons to take away wrinkles in a patient's face. Before you consider collagen injections, you should have cystometry to rule out the possibility of involuntary bladder contractions. You should also be checked with a cystoscope (a lighted tube, inserted into the anesthetized penis and threaded through the urethra into the bladder) to make sure you don't have a bladder neck contracture and to evaluate the anatomy to see whether it's amenable to injection. Collagen injection is performed as an outpatient procedure. It may take three or four injections for you to receive maximal benefit. Some men feel an immediate improvement, which may ebb over the next few days, then return. It usually takes about a month before the collagen settles.

Before you consider it, you should know that collagen is not for everybody. For one thing, some people are allergic to it, so you should have a skin test to see whether you react to this substance. For another, it is not helpful for men who have had treatment for a bladder neck contracture or for men who have undergone radiation therapy. And it simply is not helpful for men who have severe incontinence. A few bits of collagen are like sealing wax; their effectiveness is limited. At best, only about 60 percent of men who receive collagen injections have what they consider to be a good result. Also, because collagen is eventually reabsorbed by the body, even if the treatment is successful, it probably won't last forever; you may need repeat treatments every six to eighteen months.

Before you decide on collagen injections, you need to ask yourself some serious questions: Do I really need it? Am I that uncomfortable? The reason we're saying this is that some men have almost perfect control—almost. They wear a small liner in their pants, and they have to change it only once a day. But in an attempt to become perfect, they undergo collagen injections—and wind up wearing adult diapers that they must change two or three times a day. There's an old saying in medicine that "perfection may be the enemy of good."

### Artificial Sphincter

Men who have severe, prolonged incontinence should undergo placement of an artificial sphincter. This is the gold standard. In this procedure, a soft, sylastic (a material that's flexible and stretchy, like elastic) cuff is positioned around the urethra and connected by tubing to a reservoir for fluid that's installed in the abdomen. The placement of this reservoir is important. It's designed so that when a man coughs or sneezes, or does anything else to increase the pressure within the abdomen—activities that would otherwise result in stress incontinence—that pressure is instantly transferred to the cuff. This temporarily increases the pressure around the urethra and blocks urine from leaking out. The artificial sphincter features a valve, placed in the scrotum, that is used to deflate the cuff and allow urine to pass. The device is somewhat elaborate, but it works very well for men with severe incontinence. The idea is that "the buck stops here"—urine comes out only when you decide it's time. In the past, artificial sphincters had two main complications—the risks of infection and malfunction. Infection can cause erosion of the tissue that holds the device in place (in the urethra and bladder neck), may make incontinence worse, and may even mean that the device must be removed. If the infection is severe, this tissue damage may limit the success of any replacement sphincter. The device may need to be replaced if, for some reason, the original one is a dud. The good news here is that, as technology evolves, these devices keep getting better, and the odds of malfunction are going down all the time.

Another option is what's called the male sling. This procedure, developed by urologist Anthony Schaeffer at Northwestern University, uses Teflon bolsters to compress the urethra at the perineum. The operation is less complicated than the placement of an artificial sphincter, but it has one major disadvantage: to urinate, a man must increase his bladder pressure to overcome the obstruction. As opposed to the artificial sphincter, in which the sphincter is relaxed, this creates more work for the bladder, and over time, this can become a problem. Schaeffer reported in his long-term results that 72 percent of men who had not undergone radiation were using two or fewer pads a day, at an average of four years of follow-up. Nine out of sixty-two patients required the sling to be re-tightened once, and three needed to have it retightened twice. At an average of four years, 12 percent of the patients complained of moderate to severe perineal pain, and seven had undergone removal of the bolster. Long-term follow-up will show us if the sling is durable or whether these men may someday develop problems with erosion or infection. Ideally, natural tissues would be available to reconstruct the sphincter, and new experimental work suggests that using smooth muscle stem cells may help surgeons accomplish this goal.

### Sexual Potency

Chapter 11 is devoted to erectile dysfunction, so you should consider this just an introduction to this difficult subject. The first thing we need to do is make sure we're all talking about the same thing. What do we mean by potency? The medical definition is simple—"an erection sufficient for vaginal penetration and orgasm." Having said that, it's worth repeating that men who are impotent after radical prostatectomy have normal sensation and normal sex drive, and can achieve a normal orgasm. Their only problem may be in achieving or maintaining an erection.

Potency after radical prostatectomy can be affected by many things: a man's sexual function before surgery, his age, the stage of his cancer, the surgeon's skill, and the extent of tissue removed—in other words, whether one or both neurovascular bundles were removed during the operation.

## FIGHTING INFLAMMATION DURING SURGERY MAY HELP MEN RECOVER POTENCY

A s we mentioned above, the nerves involved in erection are gossamer-thin, exceedingly fragile, and tiny—so small, in fact, that until twenty-five years ago, surgeons performing the radical prostatectomy routinely cut them and left them in place, never realizing they existed. Then came the nerve-sparing radical prostatectomy. Now, impotence is no longer considered an inevitable consequence of the operation: surgeons know that if even one of the two bundles of nerves that are responsible for erection can be preserved during the surgery, it is still possible for a man to recover potency.

The problem is, even if both nerve bundles are preserved, potency—the ability to have and maintain an erection—is still not a certainty; also, the recovery of potency may take months. Two men of the same age with the same degree of prostate cancer can have exactly the same operation, performed with the same skill by the same surgeon. Afterward, one or both of them may be potent. There is no guarantee and no sure-fire means of predicting.

In any part of the body, whenever there is injury, there is an immune response. In an attempt to protect themselves, the tissues around the nerves fight back with inflammation—heat, redness, and swelling, sometimes on a microscopic level. But sometimes this reaction proves more damaging than the injury itself. The Johns Hopkins urologist Arthur Burnett believes the key to preserving potency after surgery may be to protect the nerves *during* it—to quell this inflammation almost as soon as it starts.

"We have excellent rates of potency here at Hopkins," he says. "But it's not 100 percent, and it can take months to recover. What accounts for that discrepancy? It may be that the nerves are inadvertently injured with traction, or even that the dissection adjacent to them somehow exposes them to injury—something causes the nerves to sustain an inflammatory setback." Indeed, some nerves are sluggish after surgery because they've been traumatized, a condition known as neurapraxia. It takes time for them to recover. If this is the case, Burnett adds, then what's needed is a way to "preserve, recover, regenerate, or otherwise just regain nerve function that is critical for erection."

These nerves need extra protection; they need the time and necessary ingredients to heal. They also need to be shielded from their own immune response, says Burnett, a surgeon who has also spent the last decade doing research in collaboration with the Johns Hopkins neuroscientist Sol Snyder. For the last few years, Burnett has been working with special proteins called neuroimmunophilins, which are being studied in a host of ailments—stroke, Huntington's disease, and even in organ transplants—for

310 DR. WALSH'S GUIDE TO SURVIVING PROSTATE CANCER

their ability to reduce inflammation and shield nerves from injury. He has found that in rats with nerve injury and erectile dysfunction similar to that found in men after radical prostatectomy, using neuroimmunophilin solutions to bathe the nerves provides "greater preservation of erectile function, despite the injury." It is likely that, someday, using such approaches will allow us to shorten the time it takes for men to recover erectile function.

Another exciting approach to preserving the nerves is called EPO (short for erythropoeitin), a drug commonly used to stimulate the production of red blood cells in people with kidney failure or in cancer patients undergoing chemotherapy. Recently, scientists have shown that a receptor for EPO is abundantly expressed in the nervous system; in laboratory experiments, animals with spinal cord and sciatic nerve injuries have recovered faster when given EPO. With this in mind, Burnett and colleague Mohamed Allaf have found, using their rat model, that EPO also promotes more rapid recovery of erectile function. Because EPO is easy to administer and one of its side effects—increasing patients' hemoglobin levels after surgery—could also prove a helpful bonus, this drug, which has not yet been tested clinically in radical prostatectomy patients, appears to hold great promise.

What about ED drugs? Should men take them nightly in an attempt to speed up their recovery? No one knows for sure, and the only study that tested this idea did not provide convincing results. Among my own patients, I have not been impressed with the results, and consequently I encourage my patients to use them only when attempting sexual activity. (For more on ED drugs, see chapter 11.)

For men in their forties, potency is similar (about 90 percent) in men who keep both neurovascular bundles intact and in men who have one nerve bundle removed. This suggests that all that's needed for men to achieve erection is one of these nerve bundles, and that nature has provided a "spare." Over age fifty, however, sexual potency is better in men who have both neurovascular bundles preserved than in men who lose one bundle. When the relative likelihood of impotence after surgery is adjusted for age, the risk is higher if the cancer has penetrated the prostate wall, if it has invaded the seminal vesicles, or if one neurovascular bundle has been removed. Thus, the men most likely to remain potent are younger, with disease confined to the prostate. These also are the men who will benefit most from surgery. Again, for more on erectile dysfunction, see chapter 11.

## Continence and Potency:
## Quality of Life After Radical Prostatectomy

It used to be, as we discussed early in this chapter, that the long-term quality of life for men undergoing radical prostatectomy was pretty dismal. Every man was impotent, and as many as 25 percent had severe incontinence. The results were so bad that many men felt they'd be better off taking their chances with prostate cancer than submitting themselves to this operation. Now, of course, the picture has changed. Skilled surgeons at three high-volume hospitals (where hundreds of radical prostatectomies are performed each year) reported almost identical results—at one year, 92 percent of their patients wore no pads and 70 percent were potent.

And yet, as surgical procedures go, radical prostatectomy remains one of the most delicate, intricate, and flat-out difficult to perform correctly. Proof of this can be found in the widely varying rates of success of surgeons at hospitals throughout the world—not simply in controlling cancer, but in preserving a man's quality of life in two major areas: urinary continence and sexual potency. The unfortunate fact is that when less experienced or less skillful surgeons attempt this procedure, the results can be disastrous. It has taken more than a decade for the results—the good, the bad, and the ugly, if you will—to surface.

Part of the issue is that it's hard to know exactly what happens after a man leaves the hospital, particularly in areas where men feel so vulnerable. Nobody wants to talk about it. It's different when we look at something as black and white as, say, a man's cancer status. All we have to do is follow his PSA tests, and bingo—we have all the information we need, a definitive means of knowing whether all of the tumor has been removed. But there aren't such objective ways to tell how a man's doing in the other important areas.

In an effort to be as objective as possible, and out of concern that patients may try to minimize their problems when talking about them directly with their physicians, scientists have determined that the best way to collect information is for patients to fill out a questionnaire and mail it to an independent third party. This type of research, in all disciplines of medicine, has launched a cottage industry known as outcomes research. Scientists create validated questionnaires, score the questions, and assign an arbitrary number to patients' quality of life. On validated questionnaires, the questions have been tested and retested to avoid ambiguity. However, I am not always impressed with these scores, because these numbers have little meaning to patients. I also worry that these results don't always reflect the reality of many men's lives. For example, if a man undergoes a hip replacement and is able to enjoy life without pain, dance with his wife, and walk the dog, he may not be back to the 100 percent level he was at age sixteen, but he has a happy life. However, he certainly wouldn't score 100 on a validated questionnaire. Similarly, after a radical prostatectomy, if a man confidentially reports that he is not wearing a pad and that he and his wife are able to have intercourse more than 50 percent of the time with or without drugs such as Viagra (sildenafil), and he says that he is happy with the result, I believe that this type of information is valuable.

With this in mind, we have carried out studies to evaluate men who underwent radical prostatectomy at Johns Hopkins. At many centers, it's up to the patient to report his success in continence and potency. But very often these are the last things men want to discuss, even with their doctors. So the men's information was sent to an independent third party, a data analyst who had no access to their patient records. (All of the men reported that they were potent and that they had a sexual partner before the surgery.) Because we believe that radical prostatectomy is an ideal form of treatment for younger men with curable disease, the men we studied fell into this category. Their average age was fifty-seven; because 59 percent of them had nonpalpable cancer, it was possible to preserve both nerve bundles in 89 percent of these patients. At three months, 38 percent of these men were potent. At six months, 54 percent were potent; at twelve months, the number increased to 73 percent, and at eighteen months, 86 percent were potent (see table 8.1, below). We later carried out another study, after we had developed a surgical refinement involving the bladder neck. In this study, at three months, 79 percent of the patients were wearing no pads; at six months, the number was 88 percent, and at twelve months, it was 98 percent.

TABLE 8.1

## URINARY CONTINENCE AND SEXUAL FUNCTION AFTER
## RADICAL PROSTATECTOMY AT JOHNS HOPKINS

|  | 3 months | 6 months | 12 months | 18 months |
| --- | --- | --- | --- | --- |
| **Sexual Function** | | | | |
| Potent | 38 percent | 54 percent | 73 percent | 86 percent |
| No/small bother | 49 percent | 64 percent | 76 percent | 84 percent |
| **Continence** | | | | |
| No pads | 79 percent | 88 percent | 98 percent | |

The good news is that there are many excellent surgeons at large referral hospitals and academic medical centers who have obtained similar results. Unfortunately, however, the success of radical prostatectomy is not uniform; patients at some centers report much greater trouble with side effects. For example, researchers at the Fred Hutchinson Cancer Research Center in Seattle looked at changes in urinary and sexual function in men from six different communities in the United States. Although there were some flaws in their study design— at six months after treatment, they were asking men to recall how potent they were before surgery (the authors admitted that their data indicated that the men had overestimated the frequency of intercourse and quality of erections before surgery)—the message they got loud and clear was that most men who undergo radical prostatectomy are impotent. Worse, they may even have underestimated the true extent of incontinence in these men. The authors said that at twenty-four months after surgery, 8.4 percent of the men were incontinent—and by this they meant men who had "frequent leakage" (6.8 percent) or "no control" (1.6 percent). If they had used the definition we use at Johns Hopkins—needing a pad at all—then 42 percent of these patients would have been considered incontinent. It's not as easy to ascertain the results of their impotence study, because the authors did not specify whether impotence meant unassisted erections firm enough for intercourse or whether they included patients who were using injection therapy or who had penile prostheses. The authors did not hint at the possibility that these results could be much better—and, in fact, are remarkably better at many major medical centers—if the surgical technique were improved. Most troubling here is that until urologists believe these results can be better—until they're not willing to accept these devastating side effects as routine—they may not understand the need to improve.

One of the worst series of results is reminiscent of the awful situation in the "before" category—before the operation was improved. A 1997 study from Boston reported in the *Journal of the National Cancer Institute* that only 50 percent of their patients were continent and that fewer than 20 percent were potent after radical prostatectomy. We mention this older study here because its authors continue to stand by these results, even today. They suggested with some bravado that the poor results were not because the surgery was faulty, but because their outcome studies were—as opposed to those of other centers—"truly objective." They concluded that nerve-sparing surgery doesn't work, dismissing the far better results achieved at Hopkins and at other centers as unreliable, suggesting that because patients were reluctant to disappoint their surgeons, they were not truthful in discussing their side effects.

Now, there is always a concern that patients may try to minimize their problems to their physicians or—something we must always look out for—alternatively, that there may be an unconscious bias on the part of the surgeon toward minimizing adverse outcomes. But it's difficult to swallow the idea that patients would rather spare their surgeons' feelings than regain urinary continence and sexual potency. I believe that most men who are incontinent or impotent following surgery want help. If the urologist poses these questions with the intention of helping the men overcome these problems and get their lives back to normal, I believe men will tell the truth.

The Hopkins study shows that when radical prostatectomies are performed by experienced surgeons, major side effects are infrequent. We hope these findings will encourage urologists to work on improving their technique. The study from Boston led many urologists who had poor outcomes to believe that no one had good results. But the study at Johns Hopkins, along with the good results at other medical centers, show that the results of surgery can be excellent with proper surgical technique.

The take-home message here is this: any man who wants a radical prostatectomy, and believes it's the best form of treatment for him should seek out centers where experienced surgeons perform many of these procedures, and where the results can be documented through validated, independent outcome studies.

Finally, the Johns Hopkins study revealed some interesting things about men in general. It turns out that some men exaggerated their sexual activity before surgery, and on careful questioning, acknowledged that they really weren't potent or had difficulty with erections before they had the operation. But after surgery, men did just the opposite. Many of them said they were not potent, but their wives disagreed. In separate questionnaires of the patients' wives, 78 percent reported that their husbands were potent at the same time the husbands said they were. But 20 percent of the wives said potency occurred earlier than their husbands thought it did, and 2 percent thought it occurred later. What accounts for this discrepancy? Often, the women sense that their husbands are doing better than the men think they are. This is because the men feel that their erection may not be as strong as it was before surgery—and until they have a very strong erection, many men feel any intercourse that occurs "doesn't count."

At many top medical centers, the rates of potency after radical prostatectomy are quite good. But there are still men at those centers, and many men elsewhere, who experience problems. The important thing to remember is that sexual function—potency—can be restored to all men after radical prostatectomy. The main problem for these men is the ability to obtain an erection. But sensation and the ability to achieve orgasm are intact. Many men don't understand this. They think that they can't have an orgasm if they can't have an erection. They forget that half the people in the world have orgasms without erections—women. This is because orgasms occur in the brain. There are many ways to restore sexual function, and these are discussed in detail in chapter 11.

In this chapter, we've covered everything about radical prostatectomy and the complications that can occur in the months after the operation. But what about the long-term outlook and the biggest question of all—has your cancer been controlled? For a detailed discussion of the results of all forms of treatment for localized disease—surgery, radiation, and cryo/thermal ablation—see chapter 10.

# 9

# RADIATION AND CRYO/ THERMAL ABLATION

## ▶▶▶ READ THIS FIRST

Radiation therapy is an excellent treatment option for many men with prostate cancer. First and foremost, it requires no surgery. This means there's no risk from anesthesia, no recovery time from a major operation—this is a great advantage for older men as well as for men with other health problems that might preclude surgery—and it can be performed on an outpatient basis. Most men who receive external-beam radiation can continue to work during their course of treatment. Men who undergo brachytherapy (implantation of radioactive seeds) usually require just a few days off from work for the procedure and recovery and can return to most normal activities within a week. Traditionally, radical prostatectomy has been considered the gold standard of treatment for prostate cancer. But we now have excellent long-term outcomes with external-beam radiation therapy as well. For men with tumors that have advanced beyond the wall of the prostate, radiation therapy is the standard treatment approach.

The two major approaches are: sending radiation into the tumor from the outside with external-beam radiation therapy and brachytherapy—implanting radioactive seeds directly into the tumor (doctors also describe this as interstitial radiotherapy).

Cryoablation and thermal ablation—killing prostate cells by freezing or heating them—have also been put forth as less invasive forms of treatment for localized prostate cancer. However, there is one crucial problem with both of these forms of treatment—the urethra. With cryoablation (also called cryotherapy, cryosurgery, or cryosurgical ablation) or thermal ablation, the prostate is physically heated or cooled to extreme temperatures, causing all of its cells to die. If this truly happened, the urethra would be killed along with the prostate, there would be no connection between the bladder and the distal urethra (the part of the urethra on the other side of the prostate), and you could not urinate. Instead, the urethra is protected, kept at a normal temperature while the surrounding prostate is either frozen or cooked. With cryoablation, the urethra and surrounding tissue (called the periurethral tissue) are heated, and with thermal therapy, these tissues are cooled.

But this is where the multifocal nature of prostate cancer, which we've talked about earlier, presents a problem. A study from the Mayo Clinic found that 66 percent of prostate cancers were located within 5 millimeters of the urethra; 45 percent were within 1 millimeter; and 17 percent actually touched the urethra. *This means, theoretically, that as many as 83 percent of men could have their cancer spared right along with the urethra.* Any man with localized prostate cancer who is otherwise healthy and can expect to live for many more years should consider this fact very carefully before choosing cryoablation or thermal ablation.

In this chapter, we cover everything about radiation and cryo/thermal ablation and the complications that can occur in the months after the procedure. But what about the long-term outlook and the biggest question of all—has your cancer been controlled? For a detailed discussion of the results of all forms of treatment for localized disease—surgery, radiation, and cryo/thermal ablation—see chapter 10.

Before we begin this chapter, I want to express my thanks to two of my Johns Hopkins colleagues, Danny Y. Song and Theodore L. De-Weese. I have learned over the years that when you want the best answers, you've got to consult the best people. This is why I have asked for their expert advice. They are not just using this technology, they are improving it, redesigning it, and changing the future of radiation therapy for prostate cancer. In the next pages, you will see them quoted directly at times, but their opinions have shaped the entire radiation therapy section of this chapter and the radiation section in chapter 10, on long-term results. These chapters truly give you a second opinion from expert radiation oncologists.

## Radiation Therapy for Prostate Cancer

Like radical prostatectomy, radiation treatment for prostate cancer is not a new idea. In fact, it wasn't too long after the urologist Hugh Hampton Young did that first radical prostatectomy (see chapter 8) that he and another colleague at Johns Hopkins were among the first to pioneer radiation therapy in this country (it had been developed a few years earlier in Europe). The treatment was primitive by today's standards, involving special radium applicators placed in tissue surrounding the prostate—the urethra, bladder, and rectum.

But the next few decades laid the groundwork for some of today's radiation therapies. X-ray treatments were introduced, followed by radium "seeds" that could be inserted into the prostate tumor. These fledging attempts at curing prostate cancer, however, were not distinguished by astounding success. Compared with today's high-powered technology, the low-energy X-ray beams produced throughout the 1930s were imprecise and lackluster, and their ability to penetrate the prostate was mediocre. Radiation treatment, therefore, was not much more than palliative; it could shrink the prostate and relieve pain and symptoms, but it often could not completely eradicate the cancer.

In the 1940s, the impact of hormones on the prostate was discovered (see chapter 12), and radiation was all but abandoned in favor of castration and hormonal drugs. But radiation's exile was not long, thanks largely to scientists who revolutionized the field using an exciting new machine called a linear accelerator. They produced penetrating, high-powered beams that could target radiation doses to a specific site with much less harm to surrounding tissue than previously had been possible. And suddenly, radiation was off the bench and back in the game as a major player—a treatment that actually could cure localized cancer, not just relieve the symptoms of advanced disease.

In the decades since then, radiation therapy has been refined and made even more powerful. There are two standard approaches—sending radiation into the tumor from the outside with external-beam therapy and implanting radioactive "seeds" directly into the tumor (this is called interstitial radiotherapy, brachytherapy, or simply seed implantation). The 1990s saw a minirevolution in external-beam therapy, thanks to the development of a new technique called three-dimensional conformal therapy followed by intensity-modulated radiation therapy. Most recently, image-guided radiation therapy is bringing about yet another revolution in radiation treatment.

## Conformal Radiation Therapy

How does an X-ray machine work? The simplest way to think of it is to imagine yourself getting a suntan. The difference here is that you can't feel or see the X-ray energy hitting your body, and the "sunburn" occurs internally. Actually, what happens is the radiation particles destroy DNA, causing targeted cells to die. Scientists have long known that not all cells respond to radiation in exactly the same way. The effects of DNA damage on a cell are complex, but the cells most susceptible to radiation are the ones that are constantly undergoing division—cancer cells, for example.

Early in the twentieth century, when scientists were first exploring this form of treatment for cancer, they learned that single, whopping doses of radiation did more harm than good; they were more toxic to normal tissues than to cancer. But, they discovered, incremental radiation—smaller daily doses spread out over a period of weeks—worked much better on cancer (although this conclusion is now being re-evaluated; see the section on hypofractionated radiation therapy below). They also found that this was the most effective way to minimize long-term damage to normal cells. That's why today, radiation doses are spread out over several weeks—usually delivered

Monday through Friday, leaving weekends free, for about eight weeks. Each treatment lasts just a few minutes at a time—a total of about twenty minutes spent on the treatment table. That's it. Then you go home and come back the next day.

In the era before prostate-specific antigen (PSA) testing and before today's improved radiation technology, the only way to determine the response to treatment was by evaluating whether men developed local recurrence (as felt on digital rectal examination or by progression of local symptoms) and whether men developed distant metastases. Under these circumstances, early radiation methods appeared to be quite effective. However, once PSA testing became available and began to be used as a way to track the success of cancer treatment, scientists realized that only 20 percent of men with T1 and T2 disease who had been treated with external-beam radiation had low PSA levels after ten years. A study from Toronto, using multiple biopsies, found that even at four years after conventional radiation treatment, 38 percent of men who were believed to be cured turned out to have active prostate cancer. It became all too clear to the radiation oncology field that conventional external-beam radiation therapy wasn't doing the job. In a substantial number of men, it failed to eradicate all of the tumor.

What was happening—or not happening—in the traditional radiation approach was that men weren't receiving enough radiation. The problem in some men, we know now, was similar to what happens when a speaker with an inadequate sound system tries to make himself understood to an audience of 100,000 in a vast amphitheater. Some, maybe even most, of the crowd can hear him, but that still leaves hundreds or even thousands who aren't getting his message. In traditional radiation treatment for prostate cancer, scientists discovered, this inadequate coverage meant that many men who suffered local relapses of prostate cancer did so because they were underdosed.

This made it imperative for radiation oncologists to achieve better local control of prostate cancer. Research in recent years has found that the dose of radiation received has a lot to do with who gets cured and who doesn't. In other words, men who receive higher doses of radiation have lower relapse rates than men who receive less radiation. However, in traditional radiation treatment, delivering a higher dosage almost always meant more, and worse, side effects, particularly to the bladder and rectum.

## 3-DCRT

Enter the high-tech advances. (Note: As you will notice, some of them go by abbreviations, and these all end in "RT," which can be confusing.) The first of these was conformal or three-dimensional radiation therapy, which involved having the patient undergo computed tomography (CT) scanning to determine the radiation treatment design. Before this breakthrough, radiation oncologists planned a man's radiation treatment field based on X-rays of the prostate and surrounding area—usually two images taken at 90-degree angles to each other. "With this method," explains the Johns Hopkins radiation oncologist Danny Song, "the position and shape of the prostate could only be estimated by having contrast material placed in the bladder and urethra, since the prostate cannot be directly visualized on an X-ray." Also, he continues, radiation oncologists relying on these estimates had to incorporate enough of a safety margin of normal tissue around the prostate to make sure that they did not inadvertently miss the target. "Logically, the by-product of this was that there was a substantial amount of surrounding tissue receiving the same amount of radiation as the prostate, leading to side effects such as bladder irritation, diarrhea (from treatment of the rectum), and even skin reaction."

The use of CT scanning made a huge difference in treatment planning. It provided a more precise view of the location and shape of the prostate and surrounding terrain—which, in turn, allowed for a much more accurate treatment design. At the same time, the development of faster computers, with intricate software and imaging systems, provided new help with treatment planning and complex dose calculations. Elaborate computer programs could now zip through sophisticated mathematical calculations of prostate volume and radiation dose per millimeter (or even smaller) of tissue. Amazing technological advances made it possible for doctors to custom design a three-dimensional model and treatment plan so each patient's prostate tumor could get the most precise and thorough radiation coverage possible. This new treatment was called three-dimensional conformal radiation therapy (3-DCRT).

## IMRT

And that was just phase one in the evolving world of radiation therapy for prostate cancer. The next generation came quickly: Intensity-modulated radiation therapy (IMRT). As good as three-dimensional radiation planning was, radiation oncologists found it had certain limitations—particularly on how finely the radiation dose could be shaped to fit (or avoid) key structures in the radiation field. For instance, the radiation could be shaped to approximate a cube around the prostate, but it couldn't reproduce the actual shape of the gland. Imagine, on a much grander, more sophisticated level, attempting to trace an erratic, curved line with an Etch A Sketch. This meant unavoidably including some normal tissue within the high-dose area. Ideally, because the prostate generally has an irregular shape to start with, and because, like a snowflake, each man's prostate is unique, each treatment should be customized to each man's prostate and body. Also, three-dimensional planning still resulted in uneven coverage, with unavoidable "hot" and "cold" spots within the targeted tissues.

IMRT is the difference between using an Etch A Sketch and a paintbrush. Taking advantage of still more powerful computers and even newer radiation technology, it creates a much more sophisticated treatment plan. Instead of using four beams to treat the prostate, it uses multiple beamlets—sometimes hundreds—generated at multiple angles to "paint" the radiation dose to the prostate while avoiding surrounding tissues, especially the rectum. This approach relies on as many as sixty pairs of movable tungsten "leaves"—slim, rectangular-shaped plates that open and close like little shutters. These allow the machine to sculpt the radiation beam, molding it to fit the individual contours of each man's prostate and pelvic region. (See fig. 9-1 for a visual comparison of IMRT and 3-DCRT).

IMRT treatment planning, like all radiation therapy, is a team effort. Together, the radiation oncologist and physics staff use complex computerized algorithms to fine-tune the treatment and, working with thousands of possibilities, craft the optimal plan out of thousands of possibilities.

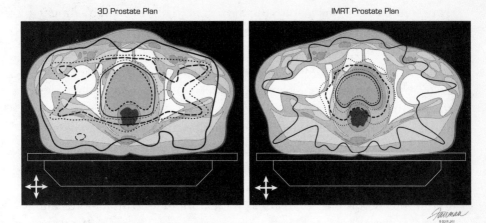

**FIGURE 9-1　A Side-by-Side Comparison of 3-DRT and IMRT Plans**

Like a topographic map, the patterned lines show areas receiving different doses of radiation. Note how the IMRT plan spares the rectum and more closely matches the shape of the prostate, keeping to a minimum the normal tissue contained in the high-dose region. The versatile tungsten leaves, a breakthrough in radiation technology, also block the radiation—much like the lead drape you wear in the dentist's office when you get an X-ray—from areas that aren't supposed to receive it.

## Proton-Beam Radiation Therapy

A unique type of radiation treatment is proton-beam therapy. This uses charged particles instead of electromagnetic waves. The difference here is that the proton beam shoots in a straight line, but it penetrates through tissue with very little effect until it reaches a predetermined distance, at which point it suddenly "detonates," discharging all of its tumor-killing energy. Precise targeting (discussed below) is crucial when using proton-beam therapy. "The effects of proton-beam radiation on tumors are not significantly different from the much more common photon radiation beams used at most centers," notes Song, "but the cost of building a proton facility is much higher, which is why it is not in widespread use."

## What to Expect During Radiation

In all conformal approaches, preparation is key. Like generals masterminding a strategic attack, the radiation oncologists who design your treatment begin by studying the terrain. This is called treatment planning, and it begins several weeks ahead of time, with a series of CT images that give enough cross-section views of the prostate, seminal vesicles, and surrounding territory (including the bladder wall, rectal wall, small bowel, bony structures, and skin) to create a detailed, three-dimensional map of your pelvic region.

Dosage, and the area over which it will be distributed, can be calculated and varied plane by plane, millimeter by millimeter. Each radiation beam—the IMRT approach allows more segments of treatment than traditional external-beam therapy—is automatically shaped by a computer so the energy focuses on the tumor alone (in the prostate as well as tissue outside the gland to which cancer has spread), rather than on its entire neighborhood. This is important, because again, when it comes to dosage, more is definitely better. It takes high doses of radiation to kill prostate cancer—higher doses than used to be possible in the years before these newer techniques evolved. But delivering more radiation usually means triggering more side effects and makes it more challenging to achieve the right balance—killing the cancer but *not* killing healthy tissue right next to it, thereby keeping side effects to a minimum. Here's where the tungsten leaves come into play with the intensity-modulated approach, allowing higher-than-ever levels of radiation to be delivered safely to targeted areas while sparing as much of the surrounding tissue as possible. The advanced technology has allowed doctors to increase the standard dose of radiation, measured in units called gray (abbreviated Gy and named in honor of Louis Harold Gray, an English radiobiologist), from about 65 Gy to about 81 Gy. After-the-fact or instantaneous dose checks then verify that the radiation went to the right spot for the right length of time to help guarantee the most successful treatment possible.

The precision of conformal radiation would be reduced, however, if the patient couldn't keep perfectly still—and frankly, nobody can keep *that* still. Imagine, one good sneeze, for instance, or a coughing fit, or even a case of nervous fidgets. Oops! The bladder gets more radiation than planned, while the prostate gets less. As one means of avoiding this, patients are fitted for their own custom-built body casts, which keep the pelvis immobilized on the table for the few minutes it takes to receive the daily dose of radiation. The cast also makes sure that a patient's body position can be reproduced every time.

## IGRT

This is also an area where the newest advance in radiation oncology, image-guided radiation therapy (IGRT), comes into play. Even if you were able to lie in exactly the same position every day, there is no guarantee that your prostate would cooperate and do the same. This is because the prostate is not fixed to your skin, pelvic bones, or external body contours—the traditional signposts used to align patients for their daily treatment. Research has shown that the prostate can move within the pelvis up to a centimeter or more, says Song. "The location of your prostate during the treatment planning session represents only a snapshot image of its location during that particular session. When you come back for your treatments, the prostate may have moved slightly due to changes in the contents of your bladder or rectum." At many facilities, patients are told to come for treatment with a full bladder and an empty rectum (a full bladder, so that more of the bladder stays away from the prostate; an empty rectum, because it is the most reproducible position). However, even then, the prostate can vary enough to cause occasional errors in targeting. Here is where IGRT can help. Song adds, "Using IGRT, we check the location of your prostate every day after you are placed in the treatment position. Small adjustments can be made based on the location of the prostate *that day*, ensuring that the entire prostate receives the intended treatment—and also that the normal tissues are not in the way."

There is more than one way of performing IGRT. One method is to incorporate a linear accelerator and CT scanner into one machine. The patient lies on the table, a scan is performed, and the images are reviewed and compared with the original CT scan (see figures 9.2a and 9.2b).

If, as the images are scrutinized, someone notices a tiny change and the prostate is in a different position, the patient's position is adjusted before treatment ever starts. Another method uses a handheld ultrasound device to view the prostate through the abdomen while the patient is on the treatment table. A small amount of lubricating jelly is placed on the abdomen, and an infrared laser system tracks the position and orientation of the ultrasound probe as the therapist moves it around to visualize the prostate. The images of the prostate

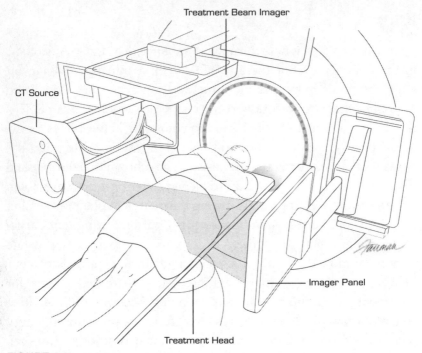

**FIGURE 9.2a**

A patient undergoes scanning on the linear accelerator just before treatment. This unit contains components for both CT scanning (shown with the beam passing through the man's pelvis) as well as high-energy treatment beams (shown underneath the patient). These components rotate around the patient during scanning and treatment. (adapted from D. Bolinsky)

are then converted into three-dimensional space and correlated to the images from the planning CT. Adjustments in the position of the treatment table are made as needed.

A third approach is to place small metallic markers or coils into the prostate (usually, these are made of gold), which are then visible on X-rays taken in the treatment room. The markers appear as beacons, spotlighting the position of the prostate. One particularly well advertised system, the CyberKnife, uses implanted metal markers in conjunction with a pair of cross-firing X-ray imagers for visualization and real-time tracking of the tumor. A small linear accelerator on a robotic arm is used to follow the tumor as it moves because of breathing motion or other organ movement. Although this is technically elegant and appealing, the downside is that it's also slower;

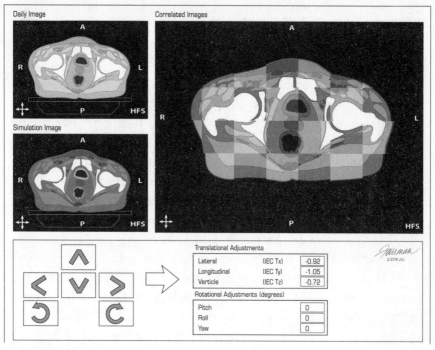

**FIGURE 9.2b**

Images taken during the CT scan on the day of treatment are "fused" with those from the initial planning CT and compared. Then, the position of both the patient and the table may be shifted slightly so that the treatment is delivered precisely where it needs to go, and healthy, normal tissue is protected.

the output of the linear accelerator is relatively low. This means a much longer time lying on the treatment table (up to two hours instead of fifteen to twenty minutes). Also, some evidence suggests that such prolonged doses of radiation may be less effective. Another unique aspect of this treatment machine is that hospitals using it tend to limit treatment to no more than five sessions. (This is likely related to the length of time required for each treatment session as well as to an odd Medicare rule that decreases the hospital's reimbursement if more than five treatment sessions are given with this particular machine.) Although experience with this technology is growing, it remains to be seen whether the prolonged individual doses and severely contracted dose schedules used with it are effective or, for that matter, safe. There is new scientific interest in using shortened treatment courses, but most clinical trials have employed four- to six-week courses of therapy, not five days (see Hypofractionated Radiation Therapy below).

"A good way to think about IMRT and IGRT," explains Song, "is that IMRT allows the high-dose region to be individually shaped to 'fit' the prostate, while IGRT enables us to direct that high dose of radiation precisely to the intended location." Ideally, he adds, both techniques are used to achieve the best outcome with the least toxicity.

Although many centers advertise that they offer these technologies, when you're deciding where to undergo radiation therapy—or any treatment, for that matter—it is important to consider the physician's level of experience and the volume of prostate cancer patients treated at that facility. Song puts it this way: "You wouldn't consider two surgeons equal just because they happen to use the same instruments. Yet, some people believe that one radiation oncology center is equivalent to another if they are using similar technology." Centers that treat a high volume of patients will be most familiar with the technology and methods and how to use them most effectively. More advice: Doing it right is not a quick, flyby experience. "It often takes us more time to devise a treatment plan with modern techniques, and you should feel comfortable that your treatment team will take the necessary time and effort to create an optimal plan," cautions Song. So much work goes on behind the scenes—on the part of the radiation oncologist, medical physicists (physicists specially trained in the use of radioactive materials and technology), and medical dosimetrists (people trained in the use of treatment-planning software). They don't just plan the treatment; they monitor it exhaustively along the way, performing many checks and double checks, making sure that the treatment you're receiving each day is correct and accurate. Your goal here is to cure the cancer. As we discussed in chapter 8, taking a few weeks or even months to find the right doctor and center to cure your prostate cancer is not going to mean that you miss your window for being cured. The cancer has been in there for years. Taking a little extra time now to seek therapy at centers with significant expertise, a high volume of patients, and high-end technology may well be the best investment you ever make.

## WHAT IF I'VE HAD A TUR PROCEDURE FOR BPH?

Your predicament is the same as that of men who are going to have a radical prostatectomy—you've got to wait for the swelling and inflammation to go down, generally about eight to twelve weeks, before you can undergo any new treatment. This waiting period, though it may seem agonizingly long, is critical. It helps minimize your risk of becoming incontinent or developing scar tissue around the urethra from radiation damage to not-yet-healed tissue. (For more on this, see chapter 8.)

## Complications

For the first few days or even the first couple of weeks of external-beam radiation therapy, patients may feel nothing out of the ordinary; it takes a while for the cumulative effect of radiation to manifest itself. They can continue all of their normal activities—driving, working, exercising, and having sex. (Unlike seed implantation, discussed below, this form of radiation does not make men radioactive). But by the third to fifth week, many men react with symptoms that can range from mild to severe—although in most cases, these symptoms, called acute symptoms, are mild. Acute symptoms generally go away on their own, days to weeks after the course of treatment is over.

### Fatigue

This is the most common complication and is usually mild to moderate. Most men with full-time jobs are able to keep right on working eight hours a day; rarely does the fatigue become severe enough for them to take off work completely. Exercise on a moderate basis, for men already accustomed to it, may help with radiation-induced fatigue; Johns Hopkins scientists are currently studying this.

### Urinary Symptoms

During radiation treatment, men may experience an increase in nocturia (waking up from sleep at night to urinate). They may also need to urinate more frequently during the day or experience urinary urgency (inability to suppress the need to urinate). Although these symptoms of urinary tract irritation are temporary, in 25 to 30 percent of men, they become acute enough to require medication, such as Hytrin (terazosin), Cardura (doxazosin), Uroxatral (alfuzosin), or Flomax (tamsulosin), during the treatment course.

### Rectal Symptoms

Fortunately, with the use of IMRT and IGRT, these have become much less common and are much less severe. About one-third of men experience a mild increase in the number of daily bowel movements (usually two to three per day) and/or experience more loose stools than normal. Diarrhea is rare. If needed, a doctor may suggest a reduced-fiber diet or medications such as Imodium (loperamide) or Lomotil (diphenoxylate).

### Late Symptoms

Sometimes, men develop what are called late symptoms six months or more after treatment. In one study of 1,100 men, about 1.5 percent of men needed minor surgical intervention for urinary symptoms—primarily urethral stricture or bladder neck contracture. Urethral strictures seem to develop mostly in men who had previously undergone a transurethral resection (TUR) procedure for benign prostatic hyperplasia (BPH). A bladder neck contracture can be reopened in an easy outpatient procedure as a urologist, using a cystoscope, makes a few tiny cuts to relax the tight scar tissue. Most urethral strictures respond well to dilation—stretching the urethra in one or two sessions—but stubborn strictures also may be treated with tiny incisions, like those done to ease bladder neck contractures.

In another analysis, researchers at Fox Chase Cancer Center in Philadelphia administered quality-of-life questionnaires to 139 patients three to six years after treatment with 3-DCRT. They found that 2 percent of the men were wearing a daily pad because of stress incontinence and that 2 percent considered their "urinary bother" to be a big problem. No man, however, was totally incontinent. Thirty-one percent of the men reported that they had rectal urgency (the sudden need to have a bowel movement and difficulty making it to the bathroom in time); 20 percent felt that their "bowel bother" was moderate, and none of the men considered their bowel bother to be a big problem.

The use of IMRT improves on these results. In the study of 1,100 men noted above, just a little over 2 percent of the men experienced moderate to severe chronic rectal problems, including rectal inflammation, diarrhea, rectal bleeding, or development of an anal stricture (tight scar tissue that can interfere with bowel movements). The good news is that men who had IMRT had significantly fewer late rectal complications than did men who were treated with 3-DCRT. The rate of rectal toxicity (bleeding and diarrhea) requiring surgical or laser intervention was 0.5 percent in men treated with IMRT, compared with 2 percent in men treated with 3-DCRT.

## Sexual Function

Radiation can take a gradual toll on a man's ability to achieve an erection. This is thought to be a result of damage to the small blood vessels that control erection, causing them to shrink or become scarred over time. "Recent research suggests that radiation-induced impotence is due to the dose to the penile bulb, which sits just below the lower portion of the prostate and may be inadvertently included in the treatment field," notes Song. In the Fox Chase study, in men younger than sixty-five, 73 percent were potent at three years, and 59 percent were potent at five years. Another study surveyed 1,187 men five years after they were treated with either surgery or external-beam radiation. Overall sexual function declined in both groups to approximately the same level, but erectile dysfunction was slightly more prevalent in the radical prostatectomy group than in the external-beam radiotherapy group (79 percent compared to 63 percent). Sexual potency is difficult to measure; age, stage of disease, and a man's sex life before treatment all play a role in his ability to have an erection afterward. Men younger than sixty who are sexually active and who are treated when the cancer is in the earlier stages (confined to the prostate) are most likely to remain potent after radiation treatment. However, many men treated with radiation are older and more likely to have problems with impotence anyway—either because they're taking medications that can interfere with sexual function or simply because of their age. (This is discussed in detail in chapter 11.)

One fact you should know about radiation therapy is that its effect on potency is slower and much more incremental than radical prostatectomy's more immediate impact. Radiation seems to cause a man's ability to have an erection to diminish over time (months to years); about half the men who receive it are impotent at seven years after radiation treatment. This is probably because of radiation's effect on the blood vessels, resulting in an eventual decrease in blood flow to the penis. One Australian study found that 62 percent of 146 men who were potent before they began radiation therapy were potent one year afterward; but by two years after treatment, this number had dropped to 41 percent. (Note: This doesn't mean a man who undergoes radiation therapy can't still have a normal sex life. Viagra and other erectile dysfunction drugs can improve sexual function in men after radiation therapy, particularly in men who can achieve partial erections. See chapter 11.)

## Adding Hormonal Therapy to Radiation

It used to be that doctors would give a man a full radiation treatment and then—only if the treatment was not successful months or years down the road—start hormonal therapy (shutting off his supply of the male hormone testosterone; this is discussed in detail in chapter 12). But what if a man takes a temporary course of hormones—for two or three months—and *then* begins radiation? This idea, called neoadjuvant hormonal therapy, has been shown to be beneficial in several studies, although the details are still being worked out. For example, how much hormonal therapy, also called androgen ablation, does a man need—how long should he take the hormones before starting the radiation? Does hormonal therapy somehow make the cancer more responsive to the radiation? And will the short-term promise hold up in long-term studies? The answers are not yet clear. One study performed by the Radiation Therapy Oncology Group compared six months of hormonal therapy with two and a half years of hormonal therapy, with both groups of men receiving radiation. They found that the men who received the hormones longer had better results on subsequent PSA tests, but there was no difference in overall survival. This may be because there were more cardiac complications in the patients given long-term hormonal therapy; however, these heart problems may have been more prevalent in that group before the treatment began.

What is it about hormones that makes radiation more effective? For one thing, they shrink the volume of the prostate, which means that radiation has less ground to cover—and this, in turn, can mean less toxicity (and risk of side effects) to nearby normal tissue in the rectum and bladder. For another, hormones seem to make radiation more efficient. Experimental studies have shown that with hormonal treatment, a lower dose of radiation (fewer Gy) is needed to kill the cancer, in part because the prostate is smaller and in part because there are fewer cancer cells that need to be killed. Together, hormones and radiation seem to encourage a process called apoptosis—basically, suicide of cells, in this case, cancer cells (this process is discussed further in chapter 12). This combination of hormones and radiation also shifts cells from an active to a resting phase, making them much more like "sitting ducks" and easier to kill.

In brachytherapy (treatment with implanted radiation seeds), when hormones reduce the size of the prostate, it's easier to place the seeds accurately and to make sure they're reaching the entire gland. (This is not always an easy task in men in whom the prostate is so large that it extends under the pubic arch.) Taking a three-month course of hormones before brachytherapy also may reduce the likelihood of complications such as urinary retention or incontinence in men with large prostates.

The first study that provided encouragement was reported in the *New England Journal of Medicine*. Researchers found that men with locally advanced prostate cancer who received conformal radiation therapy plus hormonal therapy were more likely to be disease-free at five years than were men who received radiation alone. The men received monthly hormone-suppressing injections for three years. In this study, 85 percent of the men in the combined-treatment group were free of disease at five years, compared to 48 percent of the men in the radiation-only group. These are impressive results, although once again the researchers' definition of failure was not as stringent as it could have been. Here, PSA failure was defined as a PSA level greater than 1.5 ng/ml and increasing on two consecutive measurements. Most important, this study showed an improvement in survival rates—how long patients lived. However, some physicians have begun to ask whether hormones alone would have provided this improved outcome. In a study now under way, scientists are looking at hormonal therapy alone versus radiation plus hormones for patients with locally advanced (high-risk) prostate cancer. Until we know the results of that study, there will always be the argument that the hormones by themselves are prolonging life rather than augmenting the effect of radiation.

However, several studies suggest that the dose of radiation does play an important role in patients with intermediate- or high-risk prostate cancer—the men currently treated with combined hormonal therapy and radiation. Results combined from four Radiation Therapy Oncology Group studies showed that among men with high-grade (Gleason 8 to 10) disease, receiving a higher dose was significantly associated not only with better PSA control but also with a better overall survival rate. Another recently published study from Spain evaluated men who had all received hormonal therapy and radiation at different treatment centers. Men with high-risk cancers treated with higher radiation doses to the prostate were less likely to have a recurrence of PSA than the men who had received lower doses. Recently, doctors at M.D. Anderson compared the effects of using 70 versus 78 Gy of radiation on patients with a PSA level greater than 10 ng/ml. In this randomized study, the men who received higher doses not only had better PSA control but were less likely to have distant metastases.

At the heart of the discussion regarding the importance of radiation in men with high-risk prostate cancer is whether the disease is contained within the prostate, or whether tiny bits of cancer have already spread elsewhere (these are called micrometastases), beyond the local area. Research from Harvard analyzing the relationship between local control and distant metastases sheds some light here. In a study of more than 1,400 men treated with radiation, local (within the prostate) failure was the strongest predictor for having future distant metastases. This study had a very interesting finding: the risk of developing distant metastases increased with time *after* local failure occurred—suggesting that these metastases were not present at diagnosis, but that they occurred because of the local failure. As we'll discuss in chapter 12, hormones alone cannot cure prostate cancer. For now, the standard of care for patients with intermediate- or high-risk prostate cancer consists of both radiation and hormones, not hormones alone.

Other recent studies have investigated the influence of hormones plus radiation. Although no study has shown across the board that all patients benefit from the addition of hormones, with most studies, there have been subsets of men who seemed to do better—particularly men with positive lymph nodes and high Gleason scores. Thus, it is now generally accepted that if a man with advanced disease (for example, a bulky T3 tumor), a high Gleason score, or positive lymph nodes is going to be treated with external-beam radiation therapy, he should also receive hormonal therapy for at least two or three years. There is also some evidence that short-course hormonal therapy, given just around the time of radiation therapy, may benefit men with smaller tumors. One randomized trial from Harvard specifically addressed the question of whether men with a Gleason score of 7 or higher or a PSA level of 10 ng/ml or higher should receive a short course of hormonal therapy before and during radiation treatment. They found that after five years, there was not only an improvement in cancer control but also a 10 percent improvement in overall survival in those who had hormonal therapy in addition to radiation. This study has led to the widespread use of short-course hormonal therapy in this group of patients.

## Should You Receive Hormonal Therapy?

Before you make any decision, you should consider another very important issue—quality of life. There are some definite downsides to the long-term use of hormone-suppressing drugs. In some men, testosterone production doesn't always return promptly after these drugs are stopped. The side effects of hormonal therapy can be profound. Even with short courses (two or three months), men experience the loss of libido and potency, plus "hot flashes" and weight gain. With long-term treatment, there are the additional risks of osteoporosis (and fractures that result from this bone degeneration), anemia, fatigue, loss of muscle mass, and depression. Depending on the particular kind of hormone suppressors used, this treatment can also be very expensive. (A detailed discussion of hormonal therapy can be found in chapter 12.)

## RADIATION PLUS TEMPORARY HORMONAL THERAPY: WHICH MEN COULD BENEFIT?

Here's a statistic: about half of American men with prostate cancer are treated with some form of radiation therapy. But after that, it's a bit harder to generalize and more complicated to determine which men will need additional treatments in combination with the radiation. For most men—those diagnosed with early-stage, low-risk cancer—radiation therapy alone is enough, says the Johns Hopkins radiation oncologist Ted DeWeese. "These men rarely experience a clinical recurrence of cancer after treatment. But some men are diagnosed with more aggressive disease and are at greater risk for recurrence."

Which men, then, are at extra risk? The Partin and Han tables, which are based on the course of prostate cancer in thousands of men, can predict the likelihood of cancer recurrence with 95 percent accuracy. One surprising revelation of such tables, says DeWeese, is that "a substantially greater number of patients than we previously believed actually have cancer that is already outside the prostate at diagnosis—even though it is not able to be detected by physical examination or scans." With the help of such data, "we can group patients into low-risk, intermediate-risk, and high-risk groups for tumor recurrence," he adds. This is very important, because at five years after treatment, men with intermediate-risk disease have a likelihood of biochemical recurrence—the return of PSA—of about 40 to 50 percent. The odds of recurrence for men with high-risk disease is 65 to 75 percent. "Clearly, for patients with intermediate- and high-risk disease, we need better therapeutic approaches."

One approach that immediately suggests itself is based on prostate cancer's sensitivity to hormonal therapy (suppressing the male hormones, or androgens). Can hormonal therapy make radiation treatment more effective for men with localized prostate cancer? For men at high risk of recurrence, "a number of studies have been conducted to test the benefit of this combined treatment," comments DeWeese, "and each trial has shown a significant advantage in improving cancer outcome." This includes controlling the cancer in the pelvis, limiting the risk of developing metastatic disease, and in one trial, prolonging life. These studies "strongly argue" for the combined approach in high-risk men.

But what about the men with an intermediate risk of recurrence? These men have stage T1b–T2b disease, with a Gleason score of 7 or a PSA level between 10 and 20 ng/ml. Can the combined treatment help them as well? The latest evidence signals a hearty "yes" to temporary androgen suppression for these men, too. In a recent study reported in the *Journal of the American Medical Association*, men with primarily intermediate-risk cancer were treated with either a short course (six months) of androgen suppression in addition to radiation therapy or with radiation therapy alone. "This study is very important," says DeWeese, "because it is the first trial to demonstrate that men with intermediate-risk disease who receive a short course of androgen-suppressive therapy plus radiation achieve a significant increase in overall survival when compared to men treated with radiation therapy alone."

However, DeWeese notes, "the radiation doses used in this study were relatively low by today's standards. At Johns Hopkins, we routinely administer higher radiation doses to the prostate and areas around it," using techniques such as IMRT to deliver these higher doses safely. "This is more likely to eradicate prostate cancer cells and to improve control of cancer. So it might be that the low radiation dose used in this study could have resulted in lesser control of cancer than if higher doses had been used." It is not clear how higher doses of radiation affect hormonal therapy. Could this also mean that hormonal therapy is only helpful with lower doses of radiation? "While this is a possibility, it cannot be easily answered with one or even several studies," says DeWeese. "We will continue to use higher radiation doses along with androgen suppression in men with intermediate-risk disease, because it has been shown to be beneficial and to increase survival."

However, DeWeese adds, the field of radiation therapy is constantly evolving. "As we are able to deliver significantly increasing doses of radiation with unprecedented accuracy and precision, whether all patients will ultimately require hormonal therapy is not clear."

## Interstitial Brachytherapy
## (Implanting Radioactive Seeds)

Brachytherapy is basically hand-to-hand combat, implanting tiny sources of radiation directly in the cancerous tissue instead of launching missiles from a distance. (The term *brachy* comes from the Greek word for short, as in a short distance away from the malignancy. Confusingly, doctors often use the terms "brachytherapy," "interstitial radiotherapy," and "seeds" interchangeably.) The concept is not new. Pierre Curie thought of it nearly a century ago, even before external-beam radiation treatment came onto the scene, and doctors in New York tried it several years later; they inserted thin glass tubes containing a radioactive substance called radon directly into tumors. The treatment killed tissue, but the results were uneven; some of the targeted tissue was devastated, while other tissue remained unscathed. In the next decades, scientists improved the technique, but its popularity waned as hormonal treatment developed and external-beam radiation therapy improved (see above). In the 1950s and 1960s, however, improvements in dosages and radioactive materials helped foster a comeback for brachytherapy: doctors implanted radioactive gold "seeds," or tiny chunks of radioactive material, in men with prostate cancer. This was combined with external-beam radiation therapy. A few years later, doctors began using radioactive iodine seeds to fight prostate cancer.

Over the years, several other radioactive materials, including palladium, have been tested, and the means of implanting them have evolved from a subjective, freehand technique (which requires surgery to give the doctor access to the prostate) to state-of-the-art, ultrasound- and CT-guided systems involving templates. Doctors have become highly sophisticated in targeting and placing these tiny pellets—4.5 millimeters long, they're the size of a grain of rice—and monitoring the dosage.

### Who Should Get This Treatment?

Brachytherapy alone (the use of seeds without something else, such as external-beam radiation therapy) is not ideally suited for men with a large, bulky tumor, a high-grade (Gleason score 8 or above) tumor, or lymph node metastases. Most implantation regimens don't include the seminal vesicles or tissue outside the prostate, so if there's the slightest risk that cancer has spread to these areas, implanting radiation seeds *within* the prostate won't do anything to fight the cancer *outside* it. (Although, because the radiation dose can extend a few millimeters beyond the wall of the prostate, some men with extracapsular penetration may be candidates for brachytherapy.) If there is a risk that cancer has spread beyond the prostate, men are also treated with supplemental external-beam radiation therapy.

The clinical research committee of the American Brachytherapy Society and the Prostate Brachytherapy Quality Assurance Group recently published recommendations for selecting patients who are best suited to brachytherapy alone, brachytherapy plus external-beam radiation therapy, and brachytherapy in conjunction with hormonal therapy. *Radiation seeds are not recommended for men who have had a previous TUR procedure.* For one thing, because they've had significant amounts of tissue around the urethra removed to alleviate their BPH symptoms, there's not a lot left to hold the seeds in place. Men who have had a TUR are also much more likely to develop urinary problems such as urethral stricture and incontinence from this therapy. Men with urinary problems (who score higher than a 14 on a symptom score questionnaire such as the one in chapter 2) are not ideal candidates for brachytherapy. Also, men who are in otherwise poor health, men who have a life expectancy of less than five years, and men with distant metastases should not undergo this procedure.

The American Brachytherapy Society also cautions that some men who are not ideal candidates for brachytherapy can be implanted successfully if the procedure is performed by a physician with expertise in handling cases that present "technical difficulties." The problem here is the risk that the radiation coverage may be inadequate or uneven. Men in this group include men with prominent median lobes of the prostate (detected by ultrasound), men with severe diabetes, men who have had previous pelvic surgery or radiation treatment, and men with obstructive urinary problems resulting from BPH. Men with very large prostates (greater than 60 cubic centimeters) are not ideal candidates for brachytherapy. This is because the larger the prostate, the more seeds it takes to kill the cancer, and the greater the likelihood of complications and the larger expanse of rectum exposed to radiation; also, the prostate may intrude on anatomical structures, such as the pubic bone, which may interfere with seed placement. But as we discussed above, some men with large prostates may be able to have this treatment if they have a course of hormonal therapy first (lasting about three to six months) to shrink the prostate.

## The Ideal Patient for Brachytherapy Alone

The ideal patient for this treatment is a man with localized disease who is also ideally suited for external-beam radiation therapy and radical prostatectomy—early-stage cancer (T1 to T2a), low-grade Gleason score (2 to 6), and a PSA level less than 10 ng/ml. Men with stage T2b and higher, with Gleason scores of 7 or higher, or a PSA level greater than 10 ng/ml will likely be given external-beam radiation therapy, too, as a "boost" to brachytherapy.

As with conformal external-beam therapy, the technology here is continually improving. Before the development of sophisticated guidance systems, major problems arose from seeds being either too far apart or too close together, resulting in an uneven distribution of radiation throughout the prostate; some cancer cells were killed, but some weren't. In many cases, the cancer returned or never completely went away in the first place. Better placement, thanks to three-dimensional scans like those used to design conformal therapy, may change this picture.

As a treatment choice, brachytherapy has many attractive features, DeWeese adds. For one thing, there's no hospitalization; it's a simple outpatient procedure. There's hardly any recovery time and no lengthy time away from work or normal activities. "Very high doses of radiation can be concentrated within the prostate, with hardly any damage to surrounding tissue."

## What to Expect

Before beginning interstitial brachytherapy, you should undergo an extensive physical examination and digital rectal examination. The physician will estimate the size of your prostate based on the examination as well as other studies, such as a CT scan or the ultrasound performed at the time of biopsy. You may need to undergo a cystoscopy (in which a tiny, lighted tube is inserted through the anesthetized penis and threaded through the prostate and into the bladder to check for abnormalities) to evaluate your particular anatomy (especially to see whether your prostate has a large middle lobe that protrudes into the bladder) and make sure the cancer is contained within the prostate. Next is the treatment-planning session, which is usually performed several weeks before the procedure (but it can also be done during the procedure; this is called intraoperative treatment planning). With the help of transrectal ultrasound, CT scans, and a computerized guidance system, doctors can establish the volume of your prostate, create a template that marks exactly where the seeds should go, plus determine how many seeds you need, how deeply they should be inserted, and how strong their radiation should be. You may need other tests to make sure your body can tolerate anesthesia; these may include blood tests (to check for bleeding problems), an electrocardiogram (EKG), or a chest X-ray.

## To Prepare

Starting two days before the procedure, eat a low-fiber diet (fiber is found in fruits and vegetables and in whole grains such as oatmeal and most cereals). After midnight, drink clear liquids only, and try not to drink anything for six hours before the procedure. Note: If you are on medications that must be taken regularly or with food, or if you have other dietary needs, don't worry; this is very common. Plan ahead by discussing this problem with your doctor. Do *not* simply stop taking any medication just because you're not supposed to eat or drink anything. Because it's essential that the bowels are clear (so that nothing blocks or interferes with the ultrasound image of your prostate), you will be asked to give yourself an enema on the morning of the procedure.

## During the Procedure

A combination of antibiotics (to minimize the risk of infection) will be administered intravenously. Anesthesia varies; you may be given general or regional anesthesia. At Johns Hopkins, general anesthesia is usually preferred because the patient is asleep and less likely to move during the procedure. In spinal anesthesia, a tiny needle is used to inject a local anesthetic into the small of the back through the dura, the membrane lining the spinal cord, and into the spinal fluid. Within minutes, patients feel numb, relaxed, and heavy from the waist to the toes. Afterward, the patient will be asked to lie flat in bed until the numbness goes away and he can move his legs again. Epidural anesthesia is like having an intravenous (IV) tube hooked up to the back instead of to a vein in the arm. A local anesthetic enters the body through a tiny plastic tube inserted between the vertebrae of the spine, near the small of the back. The epidural anesthetic bathes the area outside the membrane lining the spinal cord, temporarily numbing the nerves in the lower body. Unlike spinal anesthesia, which comes in one dose, epidural anesthesia can be given continuously. The area of numbness can be adjusted; so can the degree of pain relief.

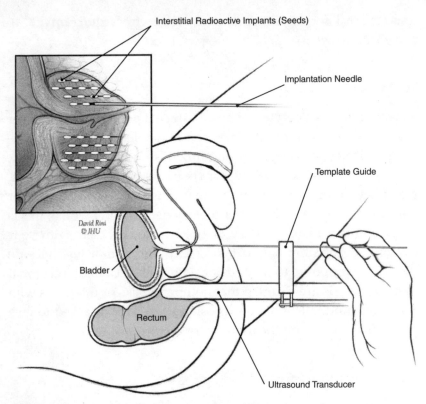

**FIGURE 9.3 Implanting Radioactive Seeds (Brachytherapy)**

Radiation oncologists use advanced-guidance ultrasound systems, three-dimensional treatment planning, and templates to ensure the precise placement of seeds. This also helps guarantee an even distribution of radiation throughout the prostate.

The procedure is performed with the patient on his back in the lithotomy position—which gives the best access to the perineum, the area between the rectum and scrotum—with his legs raised in knee stirrups, hips elevated, and buttocks at the end of the table (see fig. 9.3).

Your doctor will probably use transrectal ultrasound during the procedure to guide seed placement and stabilizing needles to help keep the prostate as still as possible. Depending on the size of your prostate and the radioactive material your doctor is using, you will probably receive between fifty and eighty seeds. At some centers, the needles are inserted under CT or magnetic resonance imaging (MRI) guidance; some centers also use fluoroscopy (an X-ray image that appears live on a TV screen instead of as a still photograph). The choice of radioactive isotopes (seed material) also varies; some doctors prefer iodine, others palladium. Palladium has a shorter duration of effect but puts out a higher initial dose of radiation. Its half-life (the time it takes for half of the material to disintegrate) is seventeen days; the half-life of iodine is fifty-nine days. Because these isotopes emit energy in different ways, the doses of iodine and palladium used are different (slightly lower with palladium).

Innovations in imaging have helped doctors do a better job of spacing both kinds of seeds to avoid creating "hot spots," areas receiving too much radiation—particularly around the urethra—and "cold spots," where cancer is not treated. A refined technique called the modified peripheral loading method also helps keep dosage even. The American Brachytherapy Society looks forward to the development of real-time, on-line dosimetry, which would provide immediate feedback during the procedure, in the near future. At Johns Hopkins, radiation oncologists and urologists are working with engineers to fine-tune such a system so that the precise dosage of each seed can be seen during the procedure and the treatment plan updated on the spot (see below).

### Afterward

You will be taken to a recovery room for about two hours; an ice bag may be placed between your legs to help keep swelling down in the perineal area. When you have regained feeling in your legs (and are able to walk to the bathroom), the urinary catheter will probably be removed. (In some men, the catheter may be left in overnight.)

You will probably be given a round of antibiotics to take for about five days and some form of pain medication and anti-inflammatory medication, although the vast majority of men do not feel the need to take any pain medication. If you do require medication, an over-the-counter drug such as ibuprofen (Motrin, Advil) or acetaminophen (Tylenol) works well; however, if you are in severe discomfort, your doctor may prescribe a stronger medication (one containing codeine or morphine).

Although brachytherapy is an outpatient procedure, you may feel some fatigue and drowsiness afterward due to lingering effects of the anesthesia. Plan on having someone drive you home, and don't try to drive for at least twelve hours afterward. Note: *Most doctors will refuse to perform the procedure or may want you to stay in the hospital overnight if you do not have a ride home.*

There are no dietary restrictions; after you are out of the recovery room, you can eat and drink whatever you wish. For the first two days, avoid heavy lifting or strenuous exercise. To minimize the risk of blood clots, avoid sitting or standing in the same position for a prolonged period. Drink plenty of fluids (at least six to eight large glasses' worth) to keep your urine clear; eat extra servings of fruits and vegetables (to help prevent constipation), and take it easy and rest often. Because men are basically radioactive after brachytherapy, you will probably be advised to avoid close contact with children (letting them sit on your lap or come within 2 feet of you) and pregnant women for a few weeks to months after the implantation, until the radioactivity wears off (the length of time depends on whether you have received iodine or palladium).

Guidelines vary, but you will probably be told that it's okay to sleep in the same bed as your spouse or partner. Studies have shown that people living in Denver, Colorado, for a year receive more radiation (from solar radiation) than the partner of a man who has had brachytherapy. There has never been a published account of a man ejaculating a seed into his partner, and the risk of radiation damage from a single seed is minimal. But to be on the safe side, some doctors advise men to abstain from intercourse for as long as two months and to wear condoms for a similar period of time. There is also a minimal risk that a seed might migrate to the lung. Although this does not cause any symptoms or harm to the lung, you may be scheduled to have a chest X-ray at your first follow-up visit. Some doctors perform cystoscopy after surgery to remove any blood clots and stray seeds from the bladder or urethra.

### Call your doctor immediately if:

- You pass blood clots larger than a dime, either through your penis or rectum;
- You are unable to urinate within four hours of drinking two large glasses of liquid;

- You have a temperature greater than 100.5 degrees Fahrenheit or shaking chills;
- You are in pain, and pain medication doesn't help; or
- Your Foley catheter falls out of your bladder.

## Complications

In the past, evaluating the complications of brachytherapy was confusing for doctors as well as patients, mainly because there were studies whose results and criteria vary widely. Some reasons for this are that different brachytherapists have different techniques and, frankly, levels of expertise; that some doctors implant seeds in patients who would be ruled out for this treatment by other doctors; and that some doctors leading various studies may not specify, may lump in different categories, or may not even be aware of all the complications their patients have had. Over the years, however, efforts by the American Brachytherapy Society and others have led to increasing standardization in how brachytherapy is performed. They have made recommendations on issues including how the radioactive material is calibrated, how the dose to the prostate and surrounding tissues is specified, and how the results should be evaluated. Much has been added to the medical literature, as well; for example, understanding the factors that can help predict postbrachytherapy toxicity has helped radiation oncologists become more effective in selecting patients for treatment.

Remember, any form of radiation—or any treatment, for that matter—is operator-dependent. In other words, it's only as effective as the doctor performing it. Seed implantation takes skill and practice. If you choose to undergo brachytherapy, you should have it done at a center where at least several procedures are performed a month. In addition, make sure that your radiation oncologist performs a CT scan or some other form of imaging "quality check" after the procedure. Your doctor should also follow the course of brachytherapy patients afterward to check for any side effects or complications. Knowing what happens to you is (at least, it should be) essential for your doctor and treatment team. It gives them valuable feedback and can help them fine-tune their methods to achieve the best results. Unfortunately, there are still some centers that do not perform these necessary quality-assurance tasks.

One major consideration to keep in mind when evaluating complications of brachytherapy is that the placement of the seeds has changed dramatically over the last decade. Early pioneers of brachytherapy generally used the uniform-loading approach; they placed seeds fairly evenly throughout the prostate. However, this often resulted in very high doses to the urethra, because the center of the prostate received radiation from all directions—and the poor urethra was completely surrounded by seeds. This meant that in some cases, the urethra got three or four times the prescribed dose to the prostate, and the rate of urethral complications was, understandably, much higher. In recent years, with better understanding of dosimetry and with the help of ultrasound imaging, physicians have begun placing the majority of the seeds toward the periphery of the prostate rather than uniformly throughout. With this technique, called peripheral loading, the center of the prostate still receives adequate radiation, but the dose to the urethra is no longer overwhelming. "Much of the earlier published literature on complications after brachytherapy was done on patients who received uniformly loaded rather than peripherally loaded implants," notes Song.

Here are some of the complications you can expect from the implantation of radioactive seeds: the risk of death is extremely rare and generally is linked to anesthesia (either general or spinal anesthesia may be used, although at least one center uses only local anesthesia). There is a great variation in the incidence of late (not immediately after seed implant) complications—ranging from zero to 72 percent—depending on which study one chooses to quote; the most common range is from 5 to 10 percent.

## Urinary Retention

The major acute (immediate) complication of brachytherapy is urinary retention, the inability to empty the bladder completely. This happens when the tissue surrounding the implants begins to react—with bleeding, swelling, and inflammation—to the trauma of having a needle stuck in it repeatedly (just as, on a smaller scale, the prostate swells after a biopsy). Most but not all men will experience some degree of urinary retention during the first few days after seed implantation. Some radiation oncologists start all of their patients on alpha-blockers such as Cardura (doxazosin), Hytrin (terazosin), Uroxatral (alfuzosin), or Flomax (tamsulosin) prior to the implantation. Patients may continue to take them for two or three months after the procedure and then taper them gradually as the symptoms resolve. Other radiation oncologists also administer low doses of steroids as a preemptive strike before and during the procedure to combat swelling of the prostate. Urinary retention may have a delayed onset as well, peaking between two weeks and three months after brachytherapy. The symptom is the same, but the cause is different—irritation in the urethra and prostate, which develops as the radiation's effects begin to be felt. This, too, is only temporary; it gradually improves and usually goes away within about two months. In the most severe cases of urinary retention, some men (about 5 percent) may need an indwelling Foley catheter (usually for a week or so) or may choose to insert a catheter several times a day to drain the bladder. Rarely, men may need a TUR of the prostate, if urinary retention does not improve with time. Several studies have found a high rate of incontinence in men who have had a TUR *before* receiving the seeds (see below). There is less information on the risk of incontinence in men who undergo a TUR *after* seed implantation, but the risk may be as high as 17 percent; it is probably lower if a more conservative TUR is performed.

**Bowel Problems**

Brachytherapy, in theory, has better rectal-sparing properties than external-beam radiation. Overall, about 10 to 15 percent of men experience rectal symptoms, including loose stools, diarrhea, rectal bleeding, or rectal urgency after seed implantation. A study of 825 men treated at Memorial Sloan-Kettering Cancer Center with brachytherapy (140 also received some external-beam radiation) found that 9 percent of men reported mild rectal symptoms that didn't require medication or treatment, and 7 percent had symptoms that did require medication, such as suppositories or steroid enemas. Symptoms tended to peak in incidence at eight months and had resolved in all patients by three and a half years. In other studies, rectal bleeding has been reported in between 5 and 20 percent of men. Men treated more aggressively (for example, men with larger stage T3 or T4 tumors who also got external-beam radiation) or men who had larger tumors (and therefore got more seeds or a higher dose of radiation) tended to develop more severe rectal problems, such as ulcers. Stool softeners, steroid enemas, and anti-inflammatory drugs may help rectal ulcers go away, but more serious ulcers that destroy tissue may require further intervention. In the Memorial Sloan-Kettering study, four patients (0.5 percent) developed rectal ulceration identified on colonoscopy, but in three of the men, this went away on its own. None of these men required hospitalization or surgical intervention. In many cases of rectal bleeding, healing eventually occurs with time and supportive care such as steroid enemas, but if the bleeding is persistent, further measures may be needed. New evidence suggests that argon plasma coagulation or hyperbaric oxygen therapy (this involves sitting in a pressurized oxygen chamber for several sessions) may be effective treatment for rectal ulceration caused by radiation. Note: If you have rectal bleeding after brachytherapy, there is also the chance that it is caused by something else—perhaps colonic polyps or colorectal cancer. See your doctor; you may also need to be examined by a gastroenterologist to rule out other causes.

## Prostatitis

In one study of 115 patients who had radioactive seeds implanted, five men developed prostatitis (for more on prostatitis, see chapter 2) and reported severe irritative urinary symptoms. The investigators suspected that in these men, the seeds became infected.

## Urinary Problems

From 10 to 37 percent of men in several studies had urinary problems including urethral stricture, bladder neck contracture, and damage to the urethra that caused irritative urinary symptoms. Most of these occurred in men who had already experienced such problems (from BPH, for example) or who had undergone a TUR procedure. For example, incontinence, which occurred in 5 percent of men, was not a problem for men who had not had a TUR. As many as half of men who have had a TUR who undergo brachytherapy develop incontinence, sometimes months after the procedure. In rare cases, severe, prolonged bleeding may also occur, requiring treatment with hyperbaric oxygen (see above). As we discussed earlier, a major factor in the development of urinary problems seems to be placement of the seeds. In the past, trouble was more likely to develop when seeds were implanted too close to the urethra. Such complications have become less common as doctors have moved to the peripheral loading approach and as brachytherapy has been increasingly ruled out in men who have undergone a TUR or other surgical intervention in the urethra.

There have been several patient-reported studies comparing urinary function after radical prostatectomy and after brachytherapy. In one study from the University of Virginia, at six months after treatment, there was no significant difference between the two groups on the issues of "bothersomeness," or impact on quality of life. In a study from the University of California, Los Angeles, at one year after treatment, brachytherapy patients had worse obstructive symptoms and were more bothered by urinary and bowel problems, while prostatectomy patients had worse urinary leakage. In more recent research, scientists evaluated questionnaires from 248 men who were treated using the peripheral-loading approach. Urinary symptoms and quality of life were assessed before and after brachytherapy (at a minimum of eighteen months after the procedure). There were no significant differences between pretreatment and post-treatment scores for any of the categories, except for small but significant increases in urinary urgency and weakened stream. Interestingly, men who had experienced urinary symptoms before treatment actually showed long-term *improvement* by 31 to 58 percent.

## Sexual Problems

The major sexual side effect is impotence, although ejaculatory pain, pain in the testicles, and blood in the semen may also occur. In several studies, impotence was found to affect at least 40 percent of men—although not immediately after implantation. A man's ability to have an erection appears to diminish over time, finally reaching a plateau, just as it does in men who get external-beam radiation treatment, probably because of gradual damage to small blood vessels. (This can be helped by erectile dysfunction drugs such as Viagra, which are discussed in chapter 11.)

Much of the information on the recovery of sexual function after brachytherapy is anecdotal. However, a recent study from the University of Pennsylvania used a validated quality-of-life questionnaire in men who underwent seed implantation between 1992 and 1998. In general, the patients were older than men undergoing radical prostatectomy; the average age was sixty-nine. Before treatment, eighty-one men said that they had erections sufficient for intercourse. Two years after treatment, 49 percent of these men remained potent. As with every form of treatment for prostate cancer, younger men fared better: 52 percent of men younger than seventy remained potent, compared with only 45 percent of men over age seventy. The study also found that short-term (for three to six months) treatment with hormones before brachytherapy did not increase the likelihood of erectile dysfunction. More favorable results have been reported by others who noted that at three and six years, 80 and 60 percent, respectively, were potent. The major factors that influenced this were a high implant dose and whether sexual function was normal or marginal before treatment. A large study of 992 men compared brachytherapy with external-beam radiation. Men who received brachytherapy reported greater sexual function and the least change in sexual function overall, and those who had both external-beam radiation and brachytherapy reported the greatest decline in sexual function.

Despite the fact that most men have infertility (from either partial or complete loss of semen) after brachytherapy, there has been a report of three patients impregnating their partners. To be on the safe side, it is advisable to use contraception while the seeds are still active as well as two to three months afterward, to minimize the potential risk of conceiving with sperm affected by radiation.

### Temporary Seeds: High-Dose-Rate Brachytherapy

A variant of brachytherapy, usually given along with external-beam radiation, is high-dose-rate (HDR), or temporary, brachytherapy. As its name suggests, the seeds don't stay in; they're removed at the end of each treatment session. These seeds, used more frequently in Europe and at a few centers in the United States, are made up of highly radioactive iridium-192. They are inserted (and then removed) with the help of a robotic arm through plastic tubes, or catheters, at precise locations throughout the prostate. Most centers performing HDR brachytherapy use several treatment sessions. Typically, after the catheters are placed, two or three treatments are delivered, with at least six-hour intervals in between treatments. Patients are usually admitted to the hospital while they wait between treatment sessions, and pain medication is given to minimize discomfort from the catheters. At some centers, the catheters are removed, and the men go home and then come back a few weeks later for another round of treatment (which requires another visit to the operating room for catheter placement). In general, temporary brachytherapy has been used for men with more aggressive cancer or with cancer that extends slightly beyond the prostate. Most studies have evaluated the use of HDR as a boost during or after external-beam radiation, a means of getting higher doses of radiation to the prostate. The results of these studies are somewhat difficult to interpret because of significant variations in the characteristics of the patients treated, but when compared with the results of external-beam therapy alone, the cancer control rates are about the same or better. No randomized studies have been performed comparing HDR treatment with high-dose external beam radiation. Recently, investigators in Detroit have been using HDR alone as monotherapy for low-risk prostate cancer, giving six doses over two separate catheter implant sessions. The long-term results of this method are not yet known.

## Hypofractionated Radiation Therapy

As we discussed earlier in this chapter, radiation oncologists have long believed that the best way to balance killing tumor cells with protecting normal tissues is to spread the radiation dose out over many weeks; this idea is called fractionation. However, new laboratory and clinical evidence suggests that this may not necessarily be true for prostate cancer—that prostate cancer may be particularly vulnerable to larger daily doses of radiation, much more so than other tumor cells. As a result, there is a growing interest in hypofractionated radiation, in which higher doses of radiation are delivered over a shorter time period—in four to five weeks, for instance, instead of eight weeks. In the past, giving such large doses of radiation on a daily basis would have increased the risk of damaging normal tissues. However, with today's new targeting and treatment-planning methods, it is possible that hypofractionated radiation can be safely administered. In preliminary clinical results from one study, scientists compared one hundred men who were randomly assigned to receive either standard treatment (2 Gy per day to 76 Gy total) or hypofractionated treatment (2.7 Gy per day to 70.2 Gy total). They found that the men in the hypofractionated group had slightly more gastrointestinal side effects. Another study of one hundred men, done by scientists at M.D. Anderson, had a longer follow-up (an average of sixty-six months). The study showed that the men in the hypofractionated group had rectal and urinary side effects that were comparable to those found in men who received standard radiation, but they had better rates of PSA control. Although these results appear promising, for now this approach should be performed only in clinical trials. It will take many years or even decades to make sure that this treatment is safe and to know how effective it is. Some of the side effects that could occur from these higher daily doses may take months or even years to manifest themselves. Thus, men in these clinical studies must be followed for long periods of time.

## Cryo/Thermal Ablation (Freezing or Heating the Prostate)

These techniques are enthusiastically endorsed by their advocates, who point out that because they require no surgery, they offer a minimally invasive outpatient treatment with few side effects. What could be better?

Well, actually, what could be better would be radiation and radical prostatectomy, and the reason is the urethra. The prostate, as we learned in the beginning of this book, is strategically located between the urethra and the bladder. When it is removed surgically, the bladder is mechanically reconnected to the urethra. With radiation therapy, although the cancer cells are eliminated, the shell of the prostate remains behind, like the ribs and timbers of an old shipwreck, as a scaffolding to link the bladder and urethra. With cryoablation (also called cryotherapy, cryosurgery, or cryosurgical ablation) or thermal ablation, the prostate is physically heated or cooled to extreme tem-

## *"BETTER MOUSETRAPS" TO MAKE BRACHYTHERAPY EVEN MORE PRECISE*

**B**rachytherapy has come a long way since the 1970s, when doctors made an incision in the prostate and tried to space the seeds evenly through a freehand approach. Over the last decade, with the use of CT scans and ultrasound guidance to place the seeds through the perineum and the development of dosimetry—precise placement of the seeds to kill prostate tissue, but avoid harming nearby organs, such as the bladder and rectum—brachytherapy has become much more effective. This is particularly true as more men, with the help of regular PSA screening, are diagnosed with early-stage prostate cancer, where the cancer is still confined within the prostate.

The goal is perfection—curing prostate cancer with minimal side effects—and as good as brachytherapy has become, radiation oncologists and colleagues are working to improve it. One challenge is that there is no "regulation" prostate—no standard in size, shape, or tissue consistency. Every man's prostate is different. This means that "the highest level of precision is sometimes difficult to achieve, even for the most experienced physicians," says the Johns Hopkins radiation oncologist Danny Song. Sometimes, for example, dense prostate tissue slightly bends the needles used to place the seeds, and the implanted seeds don't always end up exactly where they are supposed to be. In addition, "although we use ultrasound to view the prostate during the procedure, seeds cannot readily be seen on the ultrasound image once they have been placed. This means that the results are not always exactly what was intended—and yet, this cannot be identified and corrected in the operating room."

***Treating a Moving Target:*** Even with preplan (a map and radiation dosage guide drawn up before the procedure) and intraoperative, real-time dosimetry, "the treatment plans are based on a fixed organ," says the Johns Hopkins urologist and pathologist David Chan. "In reality, the prostate gland is mobile. As it is pierced with needles, the prostate gland can move, rotate, and swell. The radioactive seeds can also move, shift, and migrate during the procedure." (This frustrating movement of the prostate, by the way, can also happen during a needle biopsy done to look for cancer and is why doctors now take a dozen samples instead of just a handful.)

What's needed, continues Chan, is "a better mousetrap"—improved dosimetry. And for help with this, the radiation oncologists have two promising models on the horizon. One is the brainchild of Dan Stoianovici, an engineer and the director of the Brady Robotics Laboratory at Johns Hopkins. He has been developing a computer-driven robot that can place seeds into the prostate, guided by continuous, real-time MRI imaging. "The concept," explains Chan, "is that as the seeds are placed, the prostate gland is constantly imaged and evaluated for adequate dosimetry. If a seed shifts, a 'cold spot' would be recognized and treated. This is not possible with current techniques." Another benefit: "The automatic implant device will make the success of treatment independent of the operator," adds Chan. "Dr. Stoianovici's work is revolutionary."

Another approach involves a device created by Gabor Fichtinger and colleagues in the Johns Hopkins School of Engineering. "This device links an X-ray machine, which is capable of viewing the seeds but not the prostate, to an ultrasound, which can view the prostate but not the seeds," says Song. Like the storied Jack Spratt and his wife, the X-ray and ultrasound complement each other. "The concept," explains Chan, "is that as the seeds are placed, the prostate gland is constantly imaged and evaluated for adequate dosimetry. If a seed shifts, a 'cold spot' would be recognized and treated. This is not possible with current techniques." The result: "An ideal seed distribution," says Song.

The next step is to prove that these "better mousetraps" work as well as the Hopkins scientists expect. With the help of funding from the Prostate Cancer Research Program of the Department of Defense, Song and colleagues will conduct a randomized study, comparing men treated with standard brachytherapy techniques to men treated with the new system. If shown to be effective, this technology will rapidly be made available to all physicians who are using brachytherapy to treat prostate cancer.

peratures, causing all of the cells to die. If this truly happened and the entire prostate were destroyed, the urethra would be zapped right along with it. Then there would be no connection between the bladder and the distal urethra (the part of the urethra on the other side of the prostate), and you could not urinate. Instead, the urethra is protected, kept at a normal temperature while the surrounding prostate is either frozen or cooked. With cryotherapy, the urethra and surrounding tissue (called the periurethral tissue) are heated; and with thermal therapy, these tissues are cooled.

But this is where the multifocal nature of prostate cancer, which we've talked about earlier, presents a problem. A study from the Mayo Clinic found that 66 percent of prostate cancers were located within 5 millimeters of the urethra; 45 percent were within 1 millimeter; and 17 percent actually touched the urethra. *This means, theoretically, that as many as 83 percent of men could have their cancer spared right along with the urethra.* Any man with localized prostate cancer who is otherwise healthy and can expect to live for many more years should consider this fact very carefully before choosing cryoablation or thermal ablation.

## Cryoablation

Who is a candidate for cryoablation? If you ask the doctors who perform this treatment, they will tell you that the ideal candidate is a man with a high-grade or high-volume tumor who is not potent or interested in maintaining potency, or a man whose cancer has returned after radiation therapy. In addition, cryoablation is also being offered to men with localized prostate cancer, especially men who are not candidates for radical prostatectomy because of obesity, cardiac disease, or inflammatory bowel disease. Further, cryoablation advocates believe that any man who has no evidence of metastatic disease and at least a ten-year life expectancy can be considered a candidate, as well—if, after reviewing all the information, he believes that watchful waiting, radical prostatectomy, and radiation therapy are not options for him.

Who is probably not a candidate? Men who have undergone a TUR procedure for BPH (especially if a lot of tissue was removed), men with a very large prostate, and men who do not have a rectum or whose rectum is not easily accessible because of rectal stenosis or other major rectal problems. Men who have had a TUR are more likely to develop sloughing of the urethra (passing bits of dead tissue during urination) and urinary retention; for men with prostates larger than 50 cubic centimeters, the pubic bone may interfere with complete freezing of the prostate. (However, a short course of hormonal therapy may shrink the prostate to a more treatable size.)

The technology for cryoablation has come a long way since the 1960s, when freezing was accomplished through the urethra. Today, the third-generation cryoablation technique involves the placement of multiple 17-gauge (1.5-millimeter) needles, through which pressurized argon gas is used to freeze the prostate and helium to thaw it. The placement of the needles varies, but the physician, using a template—

similar to that used in brachytherapy—places eight to twenty-five needles into the prostate through the perineum, without making an incision. This is done under anesthesia, with the patient placed in the dorsal lithotomy position (as in brachytherapy), with his legs in stirrups. Transrectal ultrasound helps guide the needle placement and also helps the doctor monitor the degree of freezing until an "ice ball" has been created. Multiple thermocouples (temperature change–measuring devices made up of two different metals) are placed throughout the prostate—at the sphincter, over the rectum, and adjacent to each neurovascular bundle. The thermocouples at the external sphincter and rectum are sentries, on guard to minimize the risk of causing incontinence or a fistula (a hole in the rectum). The thermocouples in the middle of the gland and near the neurovascular bundles are there to make sure that the temperature goal of –40 degrees Celsius is reached. But even if the target temperature is not reached, the freezing process is stopped when the edge of the "ice ball" has extended just beyond the capsule of the prostate.

Before the freezing begins, a urethral warming catheter is placed through the urethra into the bladder. Heated (to 43 degrees Celsius) saline is continuously circulated through this catheter by a water pump. Your doctor will probably perform two ten-minute freezing sessions, allowing the prostate to thaw passively between sessions. After these freeze-thaw cycles, the urethral warmer will be left in place for a few minutes to minimize the risk of urethral sloughing. And then it's over. The needles are removed, pressure is applied to the perineum, the urethral warmer is removed, and a Foley catheter is inserted; this catheter will be removed in two or three days. You may be allowed to go home that same day, or you may spend the night in the hospital. You will probably take antibiotics, an oral pain medication, and an alpha-blocker for several days.

Potential complications of cryoablation include urethral sloughing, urinary retention, urgency or stress incontinence, pain in the penis, pelvic pain, swelling of the scrotum, impotence, and development of a fistula between the rectum and urethra. These complications have decreased significantly over the last few years, with better urethral warming and the third-generation, small-diameter needles.

Previously, in theory, doctors thought that all men should be impotent after cryoablation because, in an attempt to destroy all the cancer, the prostate tissue closest to the neurovascular bundles was deliberately frozen. (For more on these neurovascular bundles, see chapter 8.) In practice, however, because these nerve bundles have an abundant blood supply, it was more difficult to reach a low temperature in this region. Recently, some doctors have worked to limit the amount of freezing in a technique known as a "male lumpectomy"—in which the prostate is frozen only on one side or even in just a few spots. Recognizing that there is no good imaging technique that can accurately pinpoint cancer in the prostate, doctors who use this technique perform an extensive needle biopsy, which they call a three-dimensional prostate mapping biopsy. This is carried out under sedation in a surgical center and is similar to the ultrasound-guided procedure done before brachytherapy, using a detailed grid. Tissue samples are taken every 5 millimeters throughout the prostate, and the location of each one is labeled on the grid—so that a positive biopsy can be correlated with its exact location in the prostate, and the doctor can use this to decide which areas to freeze. As yet, there are no reliable reports on whether this is effective. Physicians using this approach note that if there is a recurrence of cancer, they can always go back and refreeze the prostate.

Third-generation cryoablation is still too new for us to have long-term results, and short-term results aren't terribly plentiful. However, in a multicenter trial of 122 men who underwent treatment with third-generation cryoablation at eight institutions between 2000 and 2002, tissue sloughing occurred in 5 percent. Three percent of men had incontinence that required the use of pads; 5 percent experienced urgency incontinence, and 2.6 percent had rectal discomfort. None of the men developed a fistula, and none had an infection; 87 percent of men who previously had been potent were impotent.

## Thermal Ablation

It's the opposite approach taken in cryoablation—applying heat instead of cold—but the idea is the same. Tissue-destroying heat is delivered to the prostate, and the urethra is cooled to protect it. Currently, doctors are exploring several different sources of heat, studying their potential to eradicate the tumor, minimize complications, and shorten recovery time. These include:

- High-intensity focused ultrasound (HIFU),
- Photodynamic therapy (PDT),
- Microwave energy, and
- Radio frequency interstitial tumor ablation (RITA).

Currently, the most popular technique uses the Sonoblate system and the Ablatherm HIFU device. During this procedure, done with a man under general or spinal anesthesia, an ultrasound probe is placed in the rectum, inside a balloon-shaped latex cooling device that keeps the temperature of the rectal wall at less than 37 degrees Celsius. Guided by ultrasound imaging, the doctor determines the boundaries of the treatment area and marks the distance between the rectum and the wall of the prostate. The procedure itself sounds like an artillery drill: Once the coordinates have been set, the computer places the firing head in the target region, and treatment begins automatically. A beam of focused ultrasound waves is emitted intermittently. Each shot lasts three to five seconds, with a gap in between. The treatment continues, layer by layer, until the entire area is covered. It takes less than three hours to treat a small prostate. Men with large prostates, as in the case of cryoablation and brachytherapy, may undergo hormonal therapy ahead of time to shrink the prostate.

Data on HIFU is sparse, but incontinence rates of 7 to 15 percent have been reported, along with development of a fistula between the rectum and urethra in 1 percent of men. Rates of erectile dysfunction range from 22 to 70 percent. These complications were reported in men who underwent a limited TUR before the thermal ablation. In another series of men who did not undergo a TUR, men needed a catheter for an average of fourteen days, 24 percent of patients developed a urethral stricture, 2 percent required a TUR for prolonged urinary retention, 2 percent had some problems with incontinence for a month, and 2 percent developed a fistula between the rectum and urethra. Twelve percent of the men who were sexually active before the procedure experienced erectile dysfunction, and three of these men were helped by erectile dysfunction drugs.

Most of the other thermal ablation techniques are still investigational. PDT involves administering a photosensitizing drug intravenously and then shooting light at a certain wavelength at the targeted area. This causes a photochemical reaction that is highly toxic to tissue. The trick here is to produce enough illumination to penetrate the prostate.

With microwave therapy, the aim of treatment is to heat the entire prostate to between 55 and 70 degrees Celsius without damaging the rectum. This form of treatment has been shown to be safe and effective in helping men with BPH. Recently, it has also been used in men whose prostate cancer has come back locally after radiation therapy.

The newest of these approaches is RITA, which involves heating the prostate to 100 degrees Celsius with radiofrequency energy. Heat is produced by molecular agitation; the molecules in the electrical field collide, resulting in the death of tissue.

In theory, all of these modalities—although promising and effective in treating BPH—suffer from the same problem as cryoablation. In an effort to preserve the urethra, the central core of the prostate must be cooled. But sparing even some prostate tissue means that some cancer cells may be spared as well. Also, the nature of the prostate—its irregular shape and its proximity to vulnerable structures just a few millimeters away—provides further challenges. How can a physician eliminate the prostate's peripheral zone, where cancer often grows, without injuring the rectum, the neurovascular bundles, or other important organs? None of these procedures has been tested widely or evaluated with long-term PSA follow-up. But what about the long-term outlook, and the biggest question of all— has the cancer been controlled? For a detailed discussion of the results of all forms of treatment for localized disease—surgery, radiation, and cryo/thermal ablation—see chapter 10.

# 10

# HOW SUCCESSFUL IS TREATMENT OF LOCALIZED PROSTATE CANCER?

▶▶▶ **READ THIS FIRST**

Will my cancer be cured forever? Out of a massive amount of information about a complicated, confusing, infuriating disease, we have only two incontrovertible facts about cure. If you are going to be cured of prostate cancer, your disease must be diagnosed at a stage when it is curable, before the cancer has escaped to a distant site. And the treatment has to work.

What's the best form of treatment for localized disease? This is a major dilemma, because it's a moving target. There are multiple options: retropubic, perineal, and laparoscopic/robotic radical prostatectomy; many forms of radiation therapy—3-D conformal, intensity-modulated, image-guided, proton-beam, plus brachytherapy with or without external-beam radiation, and all of these with or without hormonal therapy. Worse, there are many definitions of success, and study results can vary widely, depending on the stage of the disease when a patient is treated.

However, we can say with confidence that there is good news. Although no one form of treatment is best for everyone, there are two good options for the cure of localized prostate cancer: surgery and radiation. We have followed the results of surgery for decades; we'll discuss our long-term findings below. And with recent advances in state-of-the-art imaging and high-dose delivery techniques, it is possible with today's radiation therapy to make certain that all prostate cancer cells will be killed. The next step is up to you. Your task now is to take all of this information, decide on the treatment that is best for you, put yourself in the hands of the right expert, get past this disease, and start living the rest of your life.

## Curing Localized Prostate Cancer

Will my cancer be cured forever? This question is the bedrock of the book, what everyone wants to know, and what every man with localized prostate cancer has the right to expect.

There are two rules here, two home truths that—like proverbs—sound so simple that, at face value, they seem superfluous. And yet, out of a massive amount of information about a complicated, confusing, infuriating disease, these are the only incontrovertible facts. If you are going to be cured of prostate cancer, your disease must be diagnosed at a stage when it is curable, before the cancer has escaped the prostate, and the treatment has to work.

Remember what we've said throughout this book—*prostate cancer is multifocal*. It's not like an isolated dandelion that springs up and (if the seeds haven't blown elsewhere in the yard) can be dug up and eliminated. It's more like clover, which crops up in more than one spot at the same time. Prostate cancer starts in many places throughout the entire prostate, simultaneously. The same factors that cause cancer in one area of tissue cause it to develop a few millimeters away, and a few millimeters away from that. *The average number of separate tumors in prostates removed in surgery is seven.* This is why surgeons must work very hard to remove the entire prostate and avoid positive surgical margins and why radiation oncologists have learned that it is necessary to deliver high doses of radiation precisely to the prostate. It also explains the Achilles heel of cryo/thermal ablation—because, in order to protect the urethra, it is very difficult to achieve the goal of total prostate coverage.

Now, how do we know when we've scored a bull's-eye? Which forms of treatment mark a direct hit in the target, and which land shy, leaving room for uncertainty (and for cancer to return)? Our greatest judge of the success of treatment is prostate-specific antigen (PSA) levels. Thanks to PSA, we have a better idea, first of all, whether a man is curable (by factoring the PSA level with the clinical stage and Gleason score in the Partin Tables). PSA also tells us whether cure has been accomplished.

As we discussed earlier in the book, the advent of widespread PSA testing in the 1990s has enabled prostate cancer to be diagnosed, on average, five years earlier than it used to be. If your cancer was diagnosed by a change in PSA level, be grateful. You've been given a gift of five years over the unfortunate men who used to be diagnosed only when cancer had gotten large enough to be felt in a rectal exam—or worse, when it caused symptoms such as urinary retention, because it had grown big enough to interfere with the urethra; or back pain, because it had already spread to the bone. For men with prostate cancer, PSA testing has been a godsend. This five-year lead time has dramatically shifted the window of curability for most men. Twenty years ago, 75 percent of men diagnosed with prostate cancer had tumors that extended beyond the prostate. And sadly, of the 25 percent of men we thought were curable back then, fewer than half truly were.

Until PSA testing, the possibility of being cured of prostate cancer was unlikely, because for most men, even at the point of diagnosis, it was already too late. Now, thank goodness, *most men who are diagnosed with prostate cancer have potentially curable disease*—all the more reason why it's so important to identify the best way to cure them. Because the disease can be cured, if the treatment works.

## So, What Works Best?

Researchers have been trying to nail this down for decades. Initially, scientists tried to compare the overall survival rates of men who underwent one form of treatment versus another. This didn't work very well. Because most men were older (average age seventy-two) at diagnosis, by the time ten or fifteen years had gone by, most of these men had died from some other cause. Thus, overall survival didn't turn out to be a good measure of treatment success. Next, researchers looked at cancer-specific survival—that is, the number of men who lived for fifteen years and died of prostate cancer. This proved a better, more specific approach, because it asked the question everyone wanted answered: Of the men healthy enough to live ten or fifteen years, how many died of prostate cancer? In how many of these men did cancer progress to the point where it killed them?

Next, taking this one step further, researchers asked, what percentage of men who lived ten or fifteen years had no signs of cancer? That is, they weren't just alive after treatment, but they had never had a recurrence of cancer that required further treatment. Why is this important? It's more than just a technicality. Which would you prefer? To be alive ten years after treatment, even if it meant that your cancer had come back and you then needed additional treatment, such as radiation or hormones, and you were subjected to further side effects? Or to be alive, healthy, with an undetectable PSA level, with the prostate cancer as a significant but temporary blip on the radar of your life, thinking about it only once a year when you get your follow-up PSA test? Although both men count on the plus side as far as statistics go, because they are alive, it's a no-brainer—option B is light-years away from option A in terms of *quality* of life.

But it took ten to fifteen years to reach these answers. During this time, progress in the treatment of prostate cancer dragged on and on, with no one knowing for sure whether any man was really cured and whether any particular form of treatment was better. In the mid-1980s, with the development of PSA testing, we had a new way to tell whether any prostate cells existed in men who had undergone treatment for cancer. Testing PSA levels as a follow-up marker proved very sensitive; after the first elevation of PSA after treatment, we've learned, it can take two, five, or even ten years for a man to develop symptoms of metastatic disease or signs of cancer on a bone scan.

PSA testing also provided a rude awakening in the late 1980s, when we learned that only 10 or 20 percent of men who received radiation therapy had low PSA levels ten years after treatment. In large part, this was because the men who underwent radiation therapy at that time had been adversely selected—they were not considered good candidates for surgery, because it was unlikely that all of the cancer could be cut out of them. But radiation oncologists also realized that there was much room for improvement in the way they were delivering radiation, and they have been trying ever since to do a better job of killing cancer. Since the late 1980s, the field of radiation therapy for prostate cancer has been revolutionized by the techniques (described in chapter 9) aimed at delivering higher doses to the prostate: 3-D conformal therapy, intensity-modulated therapy, image-guided therapy, proton-beam therapy, brachytherapy (alone or with external-beam therapy)—and all of these with or without hormonal therapy.

The other major development in this field over the last twenty years has been the ability to know the extent of prostate cancer and to use this finding to predict the probability of cure. Before 1980, only 7 percent of men with localized prostate cancer underwent radical prostatectomy. Thus, for the vast majority of men treated during those years, we never knew whether the cancer was confined to the prostate or whether it had spread outside the prostate into the seminal vesicles or adjacent lymph nodes. (The only way to know this for sure is for a pathologist to examine the actual prostate and surrounding tissue, and the only way this is possible is for it to be surgically removed and sent to the lab.) For years, we were dealing with a black box: 93 percent of men with what we thought to be localized prostate cancer were all scrambled together—some really were curable, some weren't—and we were using crude end points to gauge success that took a long time to determine.

Then, in 1982, the anatomic approach to radical prostatectomy was developed. Surgeons and patients found this technique more acceptable because it was safer and associated with fewer side effects. Over the next decade, 35 percent of men with localized prostate cancer chose this form of treatment. As a result, we had a lot more prostates to examine, and in many more men, we were able to determine conclusively whether the cancer was confined to the prostate, or whether it had spread outside the prostate to the seminal vesicles or lymph nodes.

These pathologic findings, available only from men who chose surgery, were then correlated with the three things that could be measured in every man diagnosed with prostate cancer—the clinical stage, Gleason score, and PSA level. This led to the development of the Partin Tables. And then we could begin to predict which men were really curable. These findings, initially collected at Johns Hopkins, have been expanded to include more than five thousand men, have proven reliable, and now can tell men and their doctors the most important fact necessary in choosing a form of treatment—the probability of cure.

That's the background. Now, let's examine the success of surgery, radiation, cryoablation, and thermal ablation in curing prostate cancer.

## Cancer Control After Radical Prostatectomy

*There is no better way to cure cancer that is confined to the prostate than total surgical removal.* This is what all other forms of treatment attempt to accomplish. Thus, it's important that you understand the results of radical prostatectomy—just what it can and cannot do—and the fine points in interpreting these results, before you can make an informed evaluation of other treatment approaches.

### Surgical Margins

The first indisputable fact here is that *for any form of treatment to cure prostate cancer, the cancer must be curable in the first place.* Is your disease curable? We can learn almost everything we need to know about where you stand before surgery from the Partin and Han tables—the next best thing to a crystal ball—using your clinical stage, PSA level, and Gleason score. After surgery, other information helps to fine-tune this picture. The pathologist can determine the facts of your cancer—the Gleason score of the *entire prostate*, for example (as opposed to the educated guess made by examining just a few cores of tissue). From the pathologist, we can learn whether the cancer was organ-confined, whether there was capsular penetration with negative surgical margins (also called specimen-confined disease), whether the margins were positive, and whether the seminal vesicles or lymph nodes were involved. All of these factors have a profound impact on predicting the success of treatment.

### What Are Surgical Margins, Anyway?

This is a confusing point for many men. When the prostate is removed, it should be covered by several layers of tissue. It may help to think of the cancerous prostate as a gift in a box (although it's not much of a present) and the tissue surrounding it as wrapping paper. After radical prostatectomy, your prostate goes to the pathologist, who immediately coats the outside of the entire specimen—outlining the wrapping paper—with India ink. The prostate is then put in fixative for twenty-four hours before it is sectioned, stained, and examined under the microscope. The India ink creates a landmark, so the pathologist can figure out exactly how far the cancer has spread. If the cancer is all contained within the box, we call it organ-confined. Even if the cancer penetrates the box (this is capsular penetration), it can still be completely covered with wrapping paper. We call this specimen-confined. In both of these cases, the men are considered margin-negative. If the cancer has penetrated the box and the wrapping paper as well, this is called a positive surgical margin. The pathologist can see cancer cells at the edge of the India ink, and this suggests that there may be cancer beyond the outermost edge, where the surgeon removed the prostate. In chapter 8, we talked about men who had positive margins with organ-confined disease. How does this happen? Imagine, to continue our box image, that the package has been damaged; there is a tear in the wrapping paper and the box. Some of the box may even be missing. This is how a man can have a positive margin even if his cancer is still confined inside the prostate.

## When Surgical Margins Are Positive or Too Close to Call

In an ideal world, the pathologist would immediately send a triumphant report to the surgeon: "I've looked at the prostate tissue you removed from Mr. Jones, and all of the edges are clear. Congratulations! You've removed all the cancer!"

Fortunately, it often happens that way. At Johns Hopkins, fewer than 10 percent of the patients are found to have cancer at the margins, the edges of the removed tumor. Sometimes, however, the pathologist's report is more ambiguous. The report states that the margins are close, meaning that cancer is just a hairbreadth away from the edge of the specimen.

The expert pathologist Jonathan Epstein, of Johns Hopkins, has good news about these margins:

## Close Margins Are Almost Always Negative

Epstein studied men whose tumors were particularly close—less than 0.2 millimeter—to the surgical margin. Even though there wasn't a comfortable cushion of tissue between the tumor and the edge of the prostate, "those patients do just as well as if there's more separation between the tumor and the margin."

Even if the surgical margins are positive, this does not necessarily mean that cancer is left behind. How can this be? "There are several different explanations why, when the margins are positive, the tumor may still be cured," says Epstein. "One is that literally, you cut across the last few tumor cells"—and what appears to be remaining cancer is actually a cross section of the perimeter of the tumor. "Even though it looks like it's a positive margin, there's really no cancer left in the patient."

Another explanation is that the act of surgery itself finishes the job, killing any remaining cells. No cut or injury to tissue happens in a vacuum; the area around the cut is affected, too. (Think of lightning striking a tree; the tree dies, but so does a ring of grass around it.) "When the surgeon cuts across tissue, the blood supply is cut off, there's dead tissue, and that can kill off the last few tumor cells that might have been left behind," Epstein says.

There's also the potential, "and this probably accounts for a lot of cases," that it's an "artifact"—basically, a false positive margin. Sometimes, "since there's so little tissue next to the prostate, when the surgeon tries to dissect it from the body and hands it to the nurse, and then the nurse hands it to the pathologist, everyone's touching the gland. If you're talking about 0.2 millimeter of tissue, that tissue can be disrupted very easily. It can appear that the tumor is at the margin—but in fact, there was some additional tissue there that just got disrupted during all the handling." In other words, a few good buffer cells got rubbed off.

### And Then There's the Sticky Cell Phenomenon

When cancer reaches beyond the prostate to invade nearby tissue, it produces a dense scar tissue that acts like glue. As a surgeon removes the prostate, this thick scar tissue sticks to the surrounding cancer cells—picking them up like a lint brush. So in some cases, although the pathologist may see cancer cells at the margin and make a judgment of positive surgical margins, there are no cancer cells left inside the patient. The sticky scar tissue took them all away.

Epstein has extensively studied instances in which the surgeon removed the prostate, looked at it, suspected that some cancer cells were left behind, and went back and cut out more of the surrounding tissue. "In pathology, we got two separate specimens," says Epstein. "One was the prostate, one was this extra tissue, the neurovascular bundle that the surgeon was thinking of leaving in the patient but decided to remove." Even when there appeared to be a positive surgical margin at the edge of the prostate, in 40 percent of these patients, there turned out to be *no cancer left behind* in that adjacent tissue.

## PSA After Radical Prostatectomy

The best way to determine whether all the cancer has been removed in a radical prostatectomy is to check for the presence of PSA. Many men are surprised by this; they reason—and rightly so—that if the prostate has been removed, there should be no PSA. Indeed, after a radical prostatectomy, the PSA level should be undetectable. If it is not, this suggests that some prostate cancer cells managed to escape the prostate before it was removed.

But don't have your PSA tested too soon. PSA has a lengthy half-life in the bloodstream (two or three days)—which means it takes quite a while for PSA levels to go down after a radical prostatectomy. For example, if your PSA level before surgery was 10 ng/ml, it would take seven half-lives before the PSA fell into the undetectable range (less than 0.1 ng/ml). If you had your blood tested the day after surgery, your same level of PSA would pop right up, suggesting that the operation hadn't done any good. This is misleading, of course. But to avoid having to deal with such unnecessary stress, you should not have your PSA tested until about eight to twelve weeks after surgery—when PSA should be at rock bottom. After this point the PSA level should be tested every six months in men with positive margins, seminal vesicles, or lymph nodes. For most other men, a PSA measurement is only necessary once a year.

What kind of PSA measurement do you need? A simple, total PSA. You don't need a free PSA test. Also, we do not advise getting one of the ultrasensitive tests. (See PSA Anxiety: The Downside of Ultrasensitive Tests below.)

Do you need any other tests? No. PSA is extremely sensitive—so much so that, if your PSA is undetectable, there is no other test—a bone scan, computed tomography (CT) scan, magnetic resonance imaging (MRI), other blood tests, or a rectal examination—that could find any residual tumor. For many men, this is good news.

If PSA is undetectable after surgery, there is no need for a rectal exam: And here's more good news. Men hate the digital rectal examination—so much so, in fact, that the desire to avoid it may lead men to put off follow-up visits to the doctor after radical prostatectomy. From a medical standpoint, in turn, the rectal exam is only as good as the physician performing it. Similarly, another test often used in the follow-up monitoring of prostate cancer patients after surgery, the radionuclide bone scan, is expensive and also may lead to further tests if the findings are inconclusive.

Is there a better way? A Johns Hopkins study led by the urologist Charles R. Pound found that PSA is such a sensitive marker of prostate cancer that if PSA is undetectable, men don't need a digital rectal examination or further imaging studies *at that time*. In other words, they're off the hook. (However, men with a low PSA level still need careful follow-up with a PSA test every year, because it is possible for PSA levels to go up in the future.)

In the investigation, whose results were published in the *Journal of Urology*, scientists studied the medical histories of nearly two thousand men who underwent radical prostatectomy at Johns Hopkins over a fifteen-year period—a study of more than ten thousand patient-years of follow-up. Of these men, 56 developed a local recurrence of cancer, and 118 developed distant metastases. For some of these men, it took several years for cancer to return—which is why men need to keep getting regular PSA tests, even several years after surgery—but no man with an undetectable PSA had evidence of local recurrence or distant metastases at that time.

### For How Long Do I Have to Keep Getting My PSA Tested?

When the first PSA test comes back "undetectable," many men feel that they are "home free" from prostate cancer for good. Unfortunately, that is not the case. With some cancers, the magic number is five years; if the cancer hasn't come back by then, it never will. Prostate cancer, as always, is a bit more difficult. If some cancer cells escaped the prostate before it was surgically removed, these tiny offshoots of cancer can exist at very low levels, growing very slowly for years before they reach a size that will produce enough PSA to be detected in the blood. The good news is that almost all men who develop a recurrence of PSA have it within ten years of surgery. Almost. For a very few men, however, prostate cancer can rear its ugly head again between ten and fifteen years after surgery (the good news here being that the longer it takes for PSA to return after treatment, the better the likelihood that it will respond to a second go-round of treatment; see below).

In a study carried out by Mohamed Allaf, we evaluated nearly 3,500 men who underwent a radical prostatectomy at Johns Hopkins, some of them for more than fifteen years. Surgery cured the vast majority of these men. At twenty years, 71 percent had an undetectable PSA level. Of the men who eventually developed an elevated PSA level, it went up in the first five years in 58 percent; between five and ten years in 42 percent, and beyond ten years in 10 percent. In men who were at the lowest risk for recurrence (PSA level less than 10 ng/ml, stage T1c or T2a disease, and a Gleason score of 6 or lower) recurrences came later: only 16 percent by five years, 74 percent between five and ten years, and 10 percent after ten years. Thus, although 90 percent of men who will eventually fail treatment do so within ten years, the safest bet is for you to keep having a yearly PSA test for the rest of your life.

## Results of Radical Prostatectomy at Johns Hopkins

How successful is radical prostatectomy? Base your information on facts, and take any scary news reports (and there is always at least one circulating out there) with a large grain of salt. For example, one retread we see every now and then says something like this: "One-third of men who undergo radical prostatectomy will have a recurrence requiring treatment within five years." This is misleading, and it terrifies many men who rightly believe they have been cured. In fact, this statistic refers to men who are either not curable at the time of surgery or who underwent surgery that did not completely remove their prostate. It does not refer to men with specimen-confined prostate cancer, the ideal men who should be having this procedure and the men selected for this procedure by the Partin Tables. Some men can still benefit from surgery, such as younger men with cancer in their lymph nodes (although surgery is unlikely to cure prostate cancer in these men, it reduces many complications of advanced disease and may prolong survival; see below). But the overwhelming majority of men who undergo radical prostatectomy today have curable disease. Thanks to PSA testing, cancer is being caught earlier than ever before. When did the "one-third of men who have a recurrence" undergo surgery? If it was in the 1980s, as we discussed above, many men weren't even diagnosed until the disease was difficult to cure. Because of this, their long-term probability of having an undetectable PSA level is far worse than that of men who were treated in the 1990s.

So, how do we measure the success of radical prostatectomy? What is failure? Surgeons like their evidence in black and white. Therefore, we have a strict cutoff: After radical prostatectomy, we believe that the PSA level should be undetectable—less than 0.2 ng/ml, although some urologists use a cutoff of 0.4 ng/ml. (Avoid the ultrasensitive PSA tests; they're often more trouble than they're worth—see PSA Anxiety: The Downside of Ultrasensitive Tests below.)

At last, we have truly long-term results on a large number of men who have been followed for more than twenty years. *In all of these patients, the probability of maintaining an undetectable PSA at five, ten, fifteen, and twenty years was 90 percent, 82 percent, 78 percent, and 71 percent, respectively.* Furthermore, by twenty years, only 6 percent of the men had developed a recurrence of cancer at the surgical site. Thus, radical prostatectomy was very effective at controlling local disease, and the reason the other men had a recurrence was that the cancer had spread to distant sites (like bone) before surgery, in the form of invisible, impossible-to-detect, distant metastases.

These results have been reported by other centers as well, and they may well be used as the gold standard by which all other forms of treatment should be compared. And yet, these results are not the final answer, and ultimately, they won't even turn out to be the gold standard. Better results are on the way. How can this be? Because five hundred men in this study were diagnosed in the pre-PSA era (before 1989), when cancer was not usually detected early. In these men, it was much more likely that microscopic flecks of cancer had already left the main tumor, even before diagnosis, casting themselves into the bloodstream like dandelion seeds in the wind, taking root elsewhere in the body. These invisible motes of cancer are called micrometastases. In 1980, only 30 percent of men who underwent a radical prostatectomy at Johns Hopkins had specimen-confined disease. But today, 80 percent of the men who undergo radical prostatectomy at Johns Hopkins have specimen-confined cancer. It stands to reason, then, that in men diagnosed today, the fifteen-year probability of an undetectable PSA level would be better than 66 percent. And indeed, it is.

In a later study, we compared five hundred pre-PSA–era men, who underwent surgery between 1982 and 1988, to men who underwent surgery between 1989 and 1998. The picture keeps getting better: at ten years, the likelihood of having an undetectable PSA level for men who underwent surgery between 1982 and 1988 was 67 percent. But in men who underwent surgery between 1989 and 1992, it skyrocketed to 80 percent. And once we have ten-year data on the men who underwent surgery in the 1990s, we expect the results to be even better. Why? Because in the early 1990s, only 40 percent of men had organ-confined disease. But by 1998, this number had increased to 80 percent. Someday, as more men undergo regular PSA screening and diagnosis comes even earlier, we may be able to declare that virtually everyone who undergoes radical prostatectomy can be cured.

## What We Have Learned About the Probability of Cure

With the improved outcome of men diagnosed in the PSA era (1989–2006), it is possible to estimate the probability of an undetectable PSA at ten years based on the Gleason score and the pathologic stage of their radical prostatectomy specimen:

- *Group I.* Gleason score of 6 or lower. Organ-confined disease: a 99 percent chance of having an undetectable PSA level at ten years; capsular penetration and negative surgical margins: a 90 percent chance; capsular penetration and positive surgical margins: a 75 percent chance.
- *Group II.* Gleason score of 7. Organ-confined disease: an 86 percent chance of having an undetectable PSA level at ten years; capsular penetration with negative surgical margins: a 62 percent chance; capsular penetration and positive margins, a 35 percent chance.
- *Group III.* Gleason 8–10 disease or positive seminal vesicles. A 41 percent chance of having an undetectable PSA level at ten years.
- *Group IV.* Cancer in their lymph nodes. At ten years, without any treatment other than surgery, 13 percent have an undetectable PSA level.

What will be the long-term results of prostatectomy in the PSA era? These results will keep getting better. Already, in just a few years, we have seen a dramatic shift in the final pathologic stage (based on the actual removed prostate, not the educated guess made using the Partin Tables). Remember how only 30 percent of men in 1980 were diagnosed with organ-confined cancer? Even as early as 1993, after just a few years of using PSA as a screening tool, the number had increased to 55 percent, and then, by 1998, it was 80 percent.

To repeat a very important, reassuring point: *Today, because so many men are being screened with yearly PSA tests and rectal exams, early detection means that most men diagnosed with prostate cancer can be cured with effective treatment.*

---

### *ARE YOU AT HIGH RISK FOR EARLY PSA RECURRENCE?*

Some men do not fit into just one of the four groups described above; for example, a man may have a Gleason score of 3 + 4 *and* a positive surgical margin *and* positive seminal vesicles. These men have multiple risk factors that increase their risk that cancer will return. In an attempt to identify men who have a 50 percent chance of developing an elevated PSA level within three years of radical prostatectomy, investigators at Johns Hopkins Hospital and the Mayo Clinic looked at 1,800 men who underwent surgery at both institutions. This study, led by William W. Roberts, found four key factors in the men at highest risk: the presence of positive lymph nodes, positive surgical margins, positive seminal vesicles, and a high Gleason score. They gave each of these factors a certain weight (see below), and if the total score is higher than 2.84, a man's risk for developing an elevated PSA level within three years is 50 percent. This information can be helpful in identifying patients who may benefit from radiation or early adjuvant chemotherapy (see chapter 12).

| Factor | *Add* |
|---|---|
| Positive lymph nodes | 1.43 |
| Positive surgical margin | 1.15 |
| Positive seminal vesicle | 0.51 |
| Gleason score | |
| 3 + 3 | 0.71 |
| 3 + 4 | 1.42 |
| 4 + 3 | 2.13 |
| 8–10 | 2.84 |

In addition to this approach, there is currently another test (and there are bound to be others) that tries to refine the estimates of cure. It involves special stains, applied by a pathologist to the cancerous tissue, along with molecular analyses and digital imaging, and uses a computer program to quantify the results. That test is expensive (currently, it costs $2,000). Should you have it done? The Johns Hopkins pathologist Jonathan Epstein says, "Because the Gleason score and pathologic stage provide so much powerful, predictive information, it will be difficult to add to these findings to the point where it would change clinical decisions. Clearly, more information on more cases needs to be published before a final assessment is possible."

*Making Sense of Studies in Medical Journals:* There are hundreds of articles on the results of radical prostatectomy and radiation therapy in the medical journals. The results can be confusing, even contradictory. Here are a few tips to help you make sense of what you read:

- First, check the years in which the patients were studied. As the Johns Hopkins studies above illustrate, men who underwent surgery in the pre-PSA era (between 1984 and 1988) were much more likely to have advanced disease than men who underwent the same operation in the 1990s.
- Does the analysis include *all* patients, even the high-risk ones (such as the men in the Johns Hopkins study above, with a high PSA level or Gleason score and advanced pathologic stage)? Some investigators exclude their patients with positive lymph nodes and stack the deck by choosing for their studies only men with low Gleason grades, low PSA levels, and low pathologic stages. Also, because the Gleason score following a radical prostatectomy is often higher than the one estimated on the biopsy, when trying to compare the results of surgery with radiation therapy, patients need to be evaluated by the score on their original biopsy. Here the Han Tables, which use only the preoperative variables, can be useful (see chapter 6, table 6.3).
- What's the end point of the study? How do the investigators define a recurrence of cancer? Is it any detectable level of PSA, or is there a cutoff—some low-level PSA level that's considered acceptable? (In some literature, particularly studies involving radiation, it's permissible for the PSA level to go up three consecutive times, or up to 2 ng/ml from its lowest point, before the treatment is officially considered a failure. This makes it extremely difficult to compare the results of various treatments.)

## The Pathology Report Suggests My Cancer Might Return: What Happens Next?

One of the major advantages of radical prostatectomy is that it gives the patient some early, definitive answers. In contrast, when men undergo radiation therapy, there is no pathologic specimen to evaluate, and many patients find this unnerving. They ask, "You mean I just have to sit around and wait to see what happens?" Well, yes. But for men who undergo radical prostatectomy, the removed prostate is a walnut-sized crystal ball that contains a lot of infor-

## RADICAL PROSTATECTOMY IN MEN YOUNGER THAN FIFTY

In the past, very few men—only around 1 percent—diagnosed with prostate cancer were younger than fifty. However, with the widespread use of PSA testing as well as improved public awareness of prostate cancer, that number has gone up to around 4 percent. And with more men to study, we have learned something very important. We used to believe that if a younger man was diagnosed with prostate cancer, he must have a much more severe case or more advanced disease. It turns out that this was true—only because no one ever checked for prostate cancer in these men, especially in its earliest stages. This "old man's disease" wasn't on doctors' radar for younger patients. We now know that just the opposite is true—that younger men are more curable, for several reasons.

Recently, we studied 2,900 men who underwent a radical prostatectomy between April 1982 and September 2001. In this study, 341 men were younger than fifty. We found that these men had a greater chance of having organ-confined disease and that they were more likely to be cured than older men (age seventy or older). We believe that the operation is also more successful because these men have smaller prostates. There is more tissue surrounding the prostate, and the margins of resection (the surgical border between healthy tissue and cancer) are wider. Finally, in younger men, the neurovascular bundles are located farther from the prostate and are easier to preserve. This provides a win-win situation—an excellent chance for cure with improved quality of life.

mation about the future. If the cancer is organ-confined, you know there was no better way to completely eliminate the local cancer. If there is capsular penetration with negative margins, again, the surgery did the best job any form of treatment could do.

But what if the margins are positive or cancer was found in your seminal vesicles or pelvic lymph nodes? What should you do? Will any other form of treatment help right now? Let's say, for example, that you've had your first PSA test after surgery, and it was undetectable. But from studying the pathology report, you can see that the probability that your PSA level will stay undetectable is not that high. Is it possible that you can act now to get rid of any remaining cancer cells? Should you have radiation therapy to the prostate bed, the area where the prostate used to be? What about hormonal therapy?

Should you consider chemotherapy—or maybe one of the nonhormonal forms of treatment being tested at your medical center? We'll discuss all of these options in chapter 12. But let's not jump the gun. The major question we need answered right now is, if the PSA level is going to rise in the future, where are the PSA-making prostate cancer cells? Are they still in the old neighborhood—the prostate bed—and if so, is it possible to eliminate them once and for all?

There are two possibilities here. One is that some cancer cells have indeed escaped the prostate locally but are still in the prostate bed—and that radiation to this area could kill them forever. The other possibility is that these cells have escaped and are hiding, incognito, at a distant site. In this case, radiation to the prostate bed won't do a thing except cause new complications by needlessly treating an area already free of cancer. Eliminating these stray bits of cancer calls for a more systemic approach—that is, a medical treatment that affects the whole body, not just an isolated section of it.

## Micrometastatic Spread of Cancer

To determine whether cancer cells are present locally and might be killed by radiation, at Hopkins we carried out a study of the first fifty-one men who had rising PSA levels after radical prostatectomy. These men were followed until it became clear *where* these cells were located; the cancer either returned locally or showed up as distant metastases. If the cancer turned out to be in distant sites, this meant that the cancer had already flung out micrometastases—invisible flecks of cancer—into the bloodstream long before the time of surgery. We found that local recurrence was rare in men who had Gleason scores of 8 or higher, or who had cancer found in their seminal vesicles or lymph nodes during surgery; these men were more likely to have micrometastatic spread of cancer. (This study is discussed further, below.) Thus, the men who were at highest risk for developing a recurrence of cancer were those least likely to benefit from radiation to the prostate bed, and we didn't recommend postoperative radiation to these men.

So what should you do? In the past, the most common systemic help for men with a rising PSA levels after treatment for prostate cancer was hormonal therapy. However—we will cover this in detail in chapter 12—*we do not advise starting hormonal therapy early*, because we do not believe that it actually affects the cells that are most likely to cause trouble in the future; these cells are hormone-resistant. But chemotherapy is able to kill these cells. Today, there is increasing interest in the early use of chemotherapy, possibly combined with hormonal therapy, immediately after radical prostatectomy. The idea here is to go after cancer as soon as possible and to hit it hard. This approach is being used with success in women with breast cancer. Recent studies have also shown that Taxotere (docetaxel) prolonged life in men with hormone-resistant prostate cancer. Excited by this, scientists now are hopeful that using chemotherapy even earlier— way before cancer reaches the hormone-resistant stage, while the cancer is much more vulnerable—may prove much more effective (see chapter 12 ).

### What If a Positive Margin *Does* Mean that There's Still Cancer in the Area?

As we've discussed, not everyone with a positive margin has cancer left behind. However, some men do. One reason may be that the surgeon did not go quite far enough—didn't take out enough tissue— when removing the prostate. Another, more common situation is that the cancer has extended outside the prostate, beyond the point where a surgeon could remove further tissue—for example, on top of the rectum. If, indeed, cancer is still in the local area, should you undergo external-beam radiation therapy to the prostate bed?

Evidence from two recent studies may be of help here. One, carried out in the United States, involved nearly five hundred men who had cancer that extended beyond the prostate and who were randomly assigned either to radiation therapy or observation and followed for an average of ten years. The other trial, done in Europe, involved more than one thousand men, with an average follow-up of five years. The findings in both studies were very similar. Although immediate radiation therapy delayed the time to PSA failure, it did not change the risk of developing distant metastases or dying from prostate cancer. However, it is possible that over a longer follow-up period, the results could change. What does this indicate? We would expect that, if the cancer is *only* in the local area, immediate radiation therapy might help. But if there is micrometastatic spread of cancer, radiation would not be of much benefit. What these studies don't show us, however, are the results of a third option. What if these men are followed carefully, with regular PSA measurements, and they undergo radiation therapy at the time when their PSA level begins to rise? Besides putting off the side effects of undergoing two aggressive treatments within a very short span of time in many men who would never go on to have symptoms of recurrent cancer, would the results be just as good? Unfortunately, it will take many patients and many years to answer this question, and no such study is currently under way.

### What Should I Do If My Surgical Margins Are Positive?

First, talk to your surgeon and find out what his or her experience has been with radiation therapy in cases like yours. The important question of whether you should receive radiation therapy needs to be answered based on your surgeon's experience with patients like you who were in the same situation.

## What Should I Do If My PSA Comes Back After Surgery?

PSA is a very sensitive marker for the recurrence of prostate cancer. In fact, it's probably the most sensitive marker there is for any cancer. Because PSA is made only by prostate cells, when PSA levels become elevated after a radical prostatectomy, this suggests that some cancer cells are still present (although in a rare case, it is possible that some benign tissue was left behind, which is causing PSA to show up in the blood).

But before we talk about this, let's make sure you're not having it tested too soon. You should not have your PSA tested until about two or three months after surgery. Next, if your PSA is elevated more than three months after surgery, the first thing to do is have it checked again. Making PSA measurements is tricky, and some laboratories are not able to measure PSA at its lowest levels. (See PSA Anxiety: The Downside of Ultrasensitive Tests, below.) For most men, an elevated PSA level means that cancer is present. If you repeat the test and it,

## PSA ANXIETY: THE DOWNSIDE OF
## ULTRASENSITIVE TESTS

You've had the radical prostatectomy, but deep down, you're terrified that it didn't work. So here you are, a grown man, living in fear of a simple blood test, scared to death that PSA—an enzyme made only by prostate cells, but all of your prostate cells are supposed to be gone—will come back. Six months ago, your PSA level was 0.01 ng/ml. This time, it was 0.02 ng/ml. You have PSA anxiety. You are not alone.

This is the bane of the hypersensitive PSA test: *sometimes, there is such a thing as too much information.* Daniel W. Chan, PhD, is a professor of pathology, oncology, urology, and radiology and the director of Clinical Chemistry at Johns Hopkins. He is also an internationally recognized authority on biochemical tumor markers such as PSA and on immunoassay tests such as the PSA test. This is some of what he has to say on the subject of PSA anxiety.

The only thing that really matters, he says, is, "At what PSA levels does the concentration indicate that the patient has had a recurrence of cancer?" For Chan, and the scientists and physicians at Hopkins, the number to take seriously is 0.2 ng/ml. "That's something we call biochemical recurrence. But even this doesn't mean that a man has symptoms yet. People need to understand that it might take years before there is any clinical, physical evidence."

On a technical level, in the laboratory, Chan trusts the sensitivity of assays down to 0.1 ng/ml, or slightly less than that. "You cannot reliably detect such a small amount as 0.01," he explains. "From day to day, the results could vary—it could be 0.03, or maybe even 0.05"—and these "analytical" variations may not mean a thing. "It's important that we don't assume anything or take action on a very low level of PSA. In routine practice, because of these analytical variations from day to day, if it's less than 0.1, we assume it's the same as nondetectable, or zero."

Recently, investigators from the Mayo Clinic evaluated the performance of seventeen different commercial PSA assays and their accuracy at low PSA levels (lower than 0.5 ng/ml). They found that most of them were precise in measuring down to a concentration of 0.4 ng/ml. But at 0.2 ng/ml, the variation among these laboratories was great. For this reason, if your PSA level is elevated, you should have it checked with an assay that is known to be accurate at low levels. At our institution, we trust the Tosoh assay.

too, is elevated, the next question is where is the cancer? Is it still localized to the prostate area, or has it spread elsewhere? Were there some cancer cells that slipped outside the prostate—which are still hanging around the old neighborhood, the prostate bed—that were not removed at the time of surgery? Or have the cells escaped to a distant site?

### My PSA Is Elevated: Should I Get Radiation?

Could radiation therapy (this is called salvage radiation) eradicate any remaining prostate cancer cells? Or would it just cause new complications by needlessly treating an area already free of cancer? This is not an easy question to answer—in part because PSA is so very sensitive, and when so few cancer cells are present, they can't be seen by any of the usual imaging studies, such as MRI or CT. Two studies by Johns Hopkins researchers have shed much light on these troubling questions. The first, led by the urologist Alan Partin, studied rising PSA levels in fifty-one men after radical prostatectomy. In 30 percent of these men, cancer returned locally; in 70 percent, the cancer showed up as distant metastases. Based on this study, the scientists found they can estimate which course the cancer will take using the combination of Gleason score, pathologic stage (the definitive extent of a man's cancer, determined after surgery, when a pathologist looks at the actual prostate specimen and dissected lymph nodes, if any), and timing—when the PSA level starts to rise and by how much.

Men most prone to distant metastases, they found, will have one or more of these conditions: Gleason scores of 8 or higher, cancer found in their seminal vesicles and lymph nodes during surgery, or a rise in PSA within a year after their surgery. On the other hand, men with Gleason scores of 7 or lower, no cancer found in their seminal vesicles and lymph nodes, and increases in PSA several years after surgery were more likely to have a local recurrence of cancer—which means their cancer may still be cured with external-beam radiation treatment to the prostate bed, where some residual cancer cells may yet be hiding.

Another study, whose results were published in the *International Journal of Radiation Oncology * Biology * Physics* by radiation oncologists at Johns Hopkins, took these findings one step further by evaluating men who went on to receive salvage radiation therapy for an elevated PSA after surgery. Their results were similar to the findings of the Partin study—men with Gleason scores of 8 or higher or a higher PSA level (greater than 1.0 ng/ml) and men who had never achieved an undetectable PSA level after surgery had significantly lower chances of achieving success with radiation. However, even among these men, there were a few in whom the PSA level dropped—and stayed low—after radiation. Research at other institutions has produced similar findings. Given these results, is it worthwhile for some of these men to receive radiation?

The results of one of the largest studies attempting to answer this question were published in the *Journal of the American Medical Association*. Scientists studied more than five hundred men who underwent radiation therapy after radical prostatectomy at five academic hospitals. Overall, exactly half of these men had successful PSA control for at least four years after radiation. (PSA control, in this case, was defined as not having two rises in PSA level after it reached its nadir, measured after the radiation therapy. The way PSA is measured after radiation therapy is discussed later in this chapter.)

In this study, radiation therapy was less likely to be successful in men with Gleason scores of 8 or higher, a higher PSA (higher than 1.0 ng/ml ), and prostate cancer that had reached the seminal vesicles. Radiation also was not likely to help men who had negative surgical margins. "This is logical," explains the Johns Hopkins radiation oncologist Danny Y. Song, "because patients with negative margins whose PSA persists after surgery are more likely to have residual disease *outside* of the prostatic bed, as opposed to those whose margins were positive at surgery, where disease is likely to remain in the area" (and thus can be targeted with the radiation). Men with a PSA doubling time of longer than ten months had more success with radiation as well. "Patients who did not have these negative factors achieved a four-year PSA control rate of 77 percent," says Song. But there was good news for some men with higher Gleason scores as well, he adds. "Even men with Gleason 8–10 disease, if they had positive margins, a longer PSA doubling time, and received early salvage radiation, were able to attain four-year control rates of 81 percent."

In almost all studies of men receiving radiation therapy after a radical prostatectomy, one message stands out: *the lower the PSA level at the time of treatment, the better.* "Although no one has determined an absolute cutoff beyond which radiation does not work, most studies have shown differences in outcome once PSA rises beyond the 1–2 ng/ml range," Song advises. "Because of this, at Johns Hopkins, we encourage patients to seek an evaluation sooner rather than later to see if they are an appropriate candidate for salvage radiotherapy."

At the same time, there is no absolute cutoff beyond which salvage radiotherapy has *zero* chance of working (unless a man is known to have metastatic cancer). If you are in this boat, should you pursue radiation? An important point to consider, Song notes, is that right now, the only major alternative is hormonal therapy, "which is not a curative option." He adds, "Although radiation has possible side effects, with better treatment planning, using CT and three-dimensional or intensity-modulated radiation, these side effects are less than they used to be. The rates of urinary incontinence after salvage radiotherapy are similar to those in patients undergoing surgery alone." A recent study, whose results were published in the *Journal of Clinical Oncology,* reported the side effects seen in men receiving salvage radiation therapy. In this study, men who had full urinary continence before radiation had it afterward. Only about one in ten men required medication for rectal side effects (intermittent light bleeding and passing mucus or loose stools). A similar percentage of patients required treatment for a urethral stricture, but these were found in men who had already experienced a urethral stricture before radiation therapy, or they were related to a local recurrence of cancer.

Ultimately, it comes down to two things: One is the likelihood of success. The other is the possibility that your prostate cancer—even if you have a detectable PSA level—may not cause significant problems for the rest of your life. The good news is that for many men with PSA recurrence after surgery, it may take a long time—if ever—for problems to develop. (For more on this, see What Happens If PSA Comes Back Again or If I Have Distant Metastases? below.) If you can otherwise expect to live for many years and have the favorable prognostic factors mentioned above, you should strongly consider undergoing radiation therapy.

*Before You Undergo Radiation After Radical Prostatectomy*

Your doctor may want you to undergo some further tests. If there is a slight chance that the cancer may have spread beyond the local area, your doctor may suggest a bone scan, chest X-ray, and pelvic CT scan or MRI (all of these are discussed in chapter 6). The main reason for these tests is *not* because your doctor expects them to be positive, but to establish a baseline of information. (For example, if you have bone pain in years to come, your doctor can look at the bone scan and say, "Oh, that's the old football injury; see—it hasn't changed in five years.") You probably do not need a biopsy of the prostate bed. If you are going to have radiation therapy after prostatectomy, it's because all signs point to a local recurrence of cancer. It might be tiny—so tiny, in fact, that a biopsy might be falsely negative. If local recurrence is likely (based on the criteria described above), even if the biopsy were negative, radiation would still be your best course of action. So why have a biopsy you don't need? Similarly, if all evidence suggests that the PSA is coming from distant metastases, a biopsy is not necessary—because even if it were positive, radiation therapy to the prostate bed will not cure you, and it can cause side effects. Another test, called a ProstaScint scan, is often difficult for physicians to interpret, and thus may not be worth the time and money.

---

### IF YOU HAVE A RISING PSA LEVEL AFTER RADICAL PROSTATECTOMY

**M**en most likely to benefit from radiation after prostatectomy:

- Gleason score of 7 or lower, and
- Negative seminal vesicles and lymph nodes, and
- Recurrence of PSA more than four years after surgery.

**M**en least likely to benefit:

- Gleason score of 8 or higher, or
- Positive seminal vesicles or lymph nodes, or
- PSA recurrence within a year after surgery.

## What Happens If PSA Comes Back Again or If I Have Distant Metastases?

The return of PSA is a possibility that strikes terror in the heart of every radical prostatectomy patient; in fact, for many men, the dreaded PSA tests after surgery can be almost worse than having the operation itself. Although radical prostatectomy provides excellent cancer control in most men with clinically localized disease, in the past, about 20 to 30 percent of men have experienced a detectable PSA level within ten years of surgery. This number is getting better and will continue to do so as more men have their cancer detected early. But still, the worry is there: what will you do if your PSA is no longer undetectable? *The good news is that you may not need to do anything for years.*

In a landmark paper, the results of the largest, most complete study of the return of PSA after radical prostatectomy were published by Johns Hopkins doctors who have laid out guidelines to help patients and doctors know what to do if PSA comes back. They have produced a simple chart that accurately predicts a man's risk of developing metastatic cancer. It's the postoperative equivalent of the Partin Tables and, like those tables, this chart has the potential to be of great help as doctors and patients make decisions about what to do next.

As we've discussed, PSA is very sensitive in detecting any recurrence of cancer. That's because only prostate cells make PSA—so if it goes up after a radical prostatectomy, it means prostate cells are still present somewhere. For all intents and purposes, it means the cancer has come back, and that is extremely frightening. The first thing many patients want to know is, "How long am I going to live?" And the first thing many doctors want to know is, "When should we begin treatment, and how should we treat this man?" Does the man have a local recurrence of cancer that would respond to radiation, or does this represent micrometastases to lymph nodes and bone?

Until recently, there has been no way to tell. However, two studies from Johns Hopkins, whose results were both published in the *Journal of the American Medical Association,* have begun to unravel the mystery. In the first study, published in 1999, we evaluated 315 men who developed an elevated PSA level (defined as being higher than

0.2 ng/ml) after radical prostatectomy. This study included men in whom radiation therapy—given at the time PSA increased—failed to control the disease. We set out to answer some important questions: For patients who had metastases, how long would it take before these became visible on a bone scan? And, once that happened, how long would they live? The news was actually quite good: Most men did very well for a long period of time. On average, it took *eight years* from the time a man's PSA first went up until he developed metastatic disease—which suggests that there is no need to panic at the first sign of a rise in PSA level. Even better, at fifteen years after surgery, 82 percent of men were still free from metastatic disease. Even after developing metastatic cancer (detected by bone scans), men still lived an average of five years—and if the metastases showed up more than seven years after surgery, men had a 70 percent chance of being alive seven years later.

"When men see their PSA levels rise again, they think that means the cancer is back and they need to get treated right away," says the Johns Hopkins oncologist Mario Eisenberger, a coauthor of the study. "But men often live for years without having the cancer spread. This information will better equip doctors and their patients to decide what treatment—if any—is most appropriate."

## Who Needs Aggressive Treatment?

The second landmark study, published in 2005, found that not all recurrence is equal and that not all men need aggressive treatment—or any treatment right away if cancer comes back. In this study, spearheaded by Dr. Stephen Freedland, we looked at the long-term outcomes of 379 radical prostatectomy patients (out of the five thousand men who underwent this procedure at Johns Hopkins between 1982 and 2000) who, after surgery, developed an elevated PSA level. Some of these men underwent radiation therapy to the prostatic bed, but their PSA level either did not go down or continued to rise. Our goal was to see who had died from the cancer and who was alive and well, and to try to understand what made the difference in these men.

From this study, we developed reference tables for physicians and patients that help determine which men are going to be in trouble and in need of more aggressive treatment, and which men have

## IF MY PSA BEGINS TO RISE AFTER SURGERY, WILL MY BONE SCAN BE NORMAL?

This chart estimates the likelihood that a man with an elevated PSA level will remain free of metastatic prostate cancer (seen on a positive bone scan) at three, five, and seven years from the time of his initial increase in PSA after a radical prostatectomy. It is based on three factors: when his PSA first went up after radical prostatectomy (was it more or less than two years?), his Gleason score on the radical prostatectomy specimen (was it greater or less than 8?), and the time it took for his PSA level to double during the two years after the first elevation (was it more or less than ten months?).

If you have a Gleason score of 5–7 and your time to first PSA recurrence was greater than two years:

- If your PSA doubling time was greater than ten months:
  Your chance of not developing metastasis (having a positive bone scan) in:
  - Three years: 95 percent
  - Five years: 86 percent
  - Seven years: 82 percent
- If your PSA doubling time was less than ten months:
  Your chance of not developing metastasis in:
  - Three years: 82 percent
  - Five years: 69 percent
  - Seven years: 60 percent

If you have a Gleason score of 5–7and your time to first PSA recurrence was less than two years:

- If your PSA doubling time was greater than ten months:
  Your chance of not developing metastasis in:
  - Three years: 79 percent
  - Five years: 76 percent
  - Seven years: 59 percent
- If your PSA doubling time was less than ten months:
  Your chance of not developing metastasis in:
  - Three years: 81 percent
  - Five years: 35 percent
  - Seven years: 15 percent

> If you have a Gleason score of 8–10 and your time to first PSA recurrence was greater than two years:
>
> - Your chance of not developing metastasis in:
>     Three years: 77 percent
>     Five years: 60 percent
>     Seven years: 47 percent
> - And your time to first PSA recurrence was less than two years:
>     Your chance of not developing metastasis in:
>     Three years: 53 percent
>     Five years: 31 percent
>     Seven years: 21 percent

a slow-growing cancer that may not cause trouble for years—those who are relatively safe and can be carefully watched. Table 10.1 estimates the chances that a man will die from prostate cancer five, ten, and fifteen years from the time his PSA first goes up after surgery.

The difference between high- and low-risk recurrence can mean a matter of years. Some men in the low-risk group lived more than sixteen years after their cancer returned, with no sign that the cancer had spread to bone. We found that the severity of recurrence depended on three risk factors:

- *PSA doubling time.* Based only on the PSA values during the first two years after PSA reappeared, how long did it take for the PSA level in the blood to double? Less than three months, between three and nine months, from nine to fifteen months, or more than fifteen months?
- *Gleason score:* Is it 7 or lower, or Gleason 8 to 10? and
- *Time from surgery to the return of PSA.* Was it within three years or afterward?

If a man's PSA doubled in less than three months, his risk of dying from prostate cancer was much higher than that of a man whose PSA doubling time was more than a year. The same holds true for the time from surgery to the return of PSA. If PSA appears on a blood test within three years after surgery, that man is at higher risk than is a man whose PSA returns in five years.

TABLE 10.1

## IF MY PSA BEGINS TO RISE AFTER SURGERY, WHAT IS THE LIKELIHOOD THAT I WILL *NOT* DIE FROM PROSTATE CANCER?

Estimate of the risk of not dying from prostate cancer in men who have an elevation of PSA following radical prostatectomy. The numbers in parentheses are the 95 percent confidence limits (the likelihood that 95 percent of patients would be between these two numbers).

Before looking at this table, you must realize that this is the worst-case scenario. All of these men were treated more than five, ten, or fifteen years ago, at a time when prostate cancer was typically diagnosed at a more advanced stage. Also, the many new and upcoming tools for the management of advanced disease that you will receive were not available to them. Your outlook will undoubtedly be much better.

### A: FIVE-YEAR ESTIMATE

| PSA doubling time (in months) | Recurrence > 3 years after surgery | | Recurrence ≤ 3 years after surgery | |
|---|---|---|---|---|
| | Gleason sum < 8 | Gleason sum > 8 | Gleason sum < 8 | Gleason sum > 8 |
| 15 or more | 100 (98–100) | 99 (98–99) | 99 (96–100) | 98 (90–100) |
| 9.0–14.9 | 99 (70–100) | 98 (75–100) | 97 (76–100) | 94 (63–99) |
| 3.0–8.9 | 97 (81–100) | 94 (74–99) | 91 (67–98) | 81 (46–95) |
| Less than 3 | 92 (70–98) | 83 (52–96) | 74 (37–93) | 51 (19–82) |

### B: TEN-YEAR ESTIMATE

| PSA doubling time (in months) | Recurrence > 3 years after surgery | | Recurrence ≤ 3 years after surgery | |
|---|---|---|---|---|
| | Gleason sum < 8 | Gleason sum > 8 | Gleason sum < 8 | Gleason sum > 8 |
| 15 or more | 98 (96–100) | 96 (93–98) | 93 (80–98) | 86 (61–96) |
| 9.0–14.9 | 95 (75–99) | 90 (58–98) | 85 (49–97) | 69 (30–92) |
| 3.0–8.9 | 84 (62–94) | 68 (37–89) | 55 (25–82) | 26 (7–62) |
| Less than 3 | 59 (29–83) | 30 (10–63) | 15 (3–53) | 1 (< 1–55) |

### C: FIFTEEN-YEAR ESTIMATE

| PSA doubling time (in months) | Recurrence > 3 years after surgery | | Recurrence ≤ 3 years after surgery | |
|---|---|---|---|---|
| | Gleason sum < 8 | Gleason sum > 8 | Gleason sum < 8 | Gleason sum > 8 |
| 15 or more | 94 (87–100) | 87 (79–92) | 81 (57–93) | 62 (32–85) |
| 9.0–14.9 | 86 (57–97) | 72 (35–92) | 59 (24–87) | 31 (7–72) |
| 3.0–8.9 | 59 (32–81) | 30 (10–63) | 16 (4–49) | 1 (< 1–51) |
| Less than 3 | 19 (5–51) | 2 (< 1–38) | < 1 (< 1–26) | < 1 (< 1–2) |

The differences in risk turned out to be great. If you are a man who has all the low-risk features—if your PSA doubling time is greater than fifteen months, your Gleason score is below 8, and your PSA comes back after three years—your odds of being alive fifteen years later are 94 percent. Best of all, you do not need further treatment, because if you're alive and well fifteen years after surgery with no further treatment, anything we do to treat you is unlikely to improve on that and probably would only affect your quality of life.

In contrast, if you are a man at highest risk—if your PSA doubling time is less than three months, your PSA returns within three years, and your Gleason score is 8 or higher—your odds of being alive fifteen years after surgery are less than 1 percent. This means that you *do* need further treatment, including joining clinical trials and starting more aggressive therapy.

### Where Do I Go From Here?

The above information can help you and your doctor decide whether you would benefit from immediate treatment if your PSA comes back after radical prostatectomy. In chapter 12, we talk about all the options that men in this situation should consider.

## Cancer Control After Radiation Therapy

How many meters in a mile or yards in a kilometer? Comparing the cancer control results of radical prostatectomy and radiation therapy is not always as easy as you might think. For surgeons, the definition of success after radical prostatectomy is simple: A PSA level of 0.1 ng/ml or lower is considered "undetectable." A PSA level of 0.2 ng/ml or higher signals a recurrence of cancer, because there should be no remaining prostate tissue to make any PSA. But with radiation, it's more complicated for several reasons. There is no standard, definitive PSA cutoff point between success and failure, and although PSA is still useful as a marker, PSA levels require some interpretation. This is because the killing effect of radiation is directed at cancerous prostate tissue, not at normal prostate tissue. The entire prostate is not eliminated; some tissue remains behind, and PSA usually doesn't go away completely.

To understand why this happens, let's take a brief look at radio-biology—the biology of radiation therapy. As we discussed in chapter 9, radiation isn't like a machine gun, blasting indiscriminately at good and bad tissue alike and destroying everything equally. Instead, radiation's effect is different on normal tissue than it is on cancer. Low, regular doses of radiation do a better job of killing cancer cells, but normal cells are not as easily damaged by this gentle approach. At larger doses, however, the opposite is true. Normal cells are more susceptible, and cancerous cells somehow are able to hang in there and withstand the assault. "This is why we use multiple treatments of radiation instead of one single, large blast," explains the Johns Hopkins radiation oncologist Danny Song. "We learned long ago that our patients could receive curative treatment without being left with a lot of normal cells injured in the immediate area."

For many men who have completed radiation therapy, then, some normal prostate tissue survives and continues to make small amounts of PSA. This presents radiation oncologists with a difficult challenge when interpreting PSA scores after radiotherapy: is this "good" PSA, pumped out by the remaining normal tissue, or is it "bad" PSA, still being made by a few renegade cancer cells that somehow survived the radiation? Right now, there is no way to tell (although it's possible that new assays, such as those described in chapter 5, might one day be able to say, "This PSA comes from normal cells. Not to worry!" or "This PSA is being made by cancer"). Instead, the most common strategy has been to watch the *trend* of PSA—to see what it does over time, with the idea that if it's coming from benign tissue, the PSA level should remain stable, but if it's coming from cancerous tissue, the PSA will creep back up as the cancer cells multiply.

Over the last decade, the standard criteria for relapse, or bio-chemical failure, after radiation has been the consensus definition of the American Society for Therapeutic Radiology and Oncology (AS-TRO). As the name suggests, this was based on the agreement of a panel of experts, who in the 1990s met and chose to define PSA failure after radiation therapy as *three consecutive rises in PSA* (taken at least three months apart from each other) after it reaches its nadir—the lowest point PSA reaches after treatment. (PSA nadir is a key concept in radiation therapy for prostate cancer. Because radiation's effect is gradual, it may take two or three years for PSA levels to hit rock bottom. Some men reach this nadir much more quickly—within months—and some men take much longer—several years. Ideally, once PSA has reached its lowest level, it should stay put.) Although the ASTRO definition has proven useful, it has not been perfect, and not all radiation oncologists agree that this is the best way to measure success or failure.

One criticism has been that PSA increases are not always consecutive. A man's rise in PSA with one test might be followed by a transient decrease in the next, followed by another increase. Although there may be recurrent cancer, under the ASTRO definition, this man's treatment would still be considered a success—even though it's just a technicality. "Fortunately, any astute radiation oncologist will not blindly follow the consensus definition in making treatment decisions," comments Song.

A quirk of the ASTRO definition is that, over a short period of time after treatment, it really can't tell us much. This is due to the gradual nature of radiation's effects; cancer cells die, but it's a slow death. Patients who eventually turn out to fail treatment may see their PSA levels drop for months or even years after treatment, notes Song. "If the results are evaluated too soon, many patients can't know whether their cancer has been controlled."

Another potential problem: if a man has had hormonal therapy before or during radiation, this can have a profound effect on his PSA level. It causes an immediate drop due to the shutdown of testosterone (for a detailed discussion of hormonal therapy, see chapter 12). For men who have received a luteinizing hormone-releasing hormone (LHRH) agonist, it takes, on average, about six months for testosterone levels to return to normal. The time it takes to recover testosterone levels in the blood is shorter in men who have received hormonal therapy for less than four months than it is in men who have received hormonal therapy for more than two years. Thus, in men who received hormonal therapy, the low PSA level may be artificial—the result of low testosterone levels rather than the effect of radiation. Then, if a man stops taking hormonal therapy, his PSA will begin to rise. Eventually, the effect of the radiation takes over, and the PSA level will sink back down and reach its nadir, but this may happen well after the hormonal therapy has worn off. Because it can take two to even six years for a man to reach his PSA nadir after radiation, this initial "false rise" in PSA level after the hormonal therapy ends might lead to needless worry from a wrongful diagnosis of bio-chemical failure when he's actually cancer-free.

Finally, there's the phenomenon of PSA "bounce"—and this, too, can confound results under the ASTRO definition. While PSA declines after radiation, men who are ultimately headed for a healthy, low, stable PSA level may see it suddenly go up; think of it as PSA's last fling. This bounce is transient and is generally defined as a sudden rise of at least 0.5 ng/ml, quickly followed by a decrease to prebounce levels. This usually occurs around nine months after treatment and may happen in as many as a third of men after either external-beam radiation or brachytherapy. In some studies, it seems more likely to occur in younger men, and "ironically, men who de-velop a PSA bounce ultimately tend to have better disease-free sur-vival than men who did not have a bounce," notes Song. However, the ASTRO consensus definition may falsely identify some of these men as having a relapse—again, leading to unnecessary anxiety.

A study whose results were published in the *Journal of Urology* evaluated nearly five thousand patients from nine hospitals who had received external-beam radiation therapy alone and had been fol-lowed for an average of six years. The study looked at how well the ASTRO criteria and other definitions could predict actual clinical failure (the development of distant metastases or the return of can-cer in the irradiated prostate). Despite its stellar acronym, the ASTRO definition did not prove to be outstandingly superior; in fact, the re-searchers found, some of the alternate definitions of biochemical suc-cess or failure were slightly better.

In 2005, another panel of radiation oncologists met to discuss a replacement for the ASTRO definition. They decided to define treat-ment failure as a PSA level that has risen 2 ng/ml higher than a man's PSA nadir (the lowest level it reached following treatment). This definition has been correlated more accurately with long-term results in all patients, and it takes into account such factors as hor-monal therapy and the PSA "bounce." Failure is now considered to occur when the PSA level reaches the nadir + 2 value. Still, it takes time to determine this value, so this equation should not be used to gauge the success of treatment in men with less than two years' worth of PSA tests after radiation therapy. Furthermore, the consensus panel that developed this definition cautioned, "Physicians should use individualized approaches to managing young patients with slowly rising PSA levels who initially achieved a very low nadir and who might be a candidate for salvage local therapies" (see below). Called the Phoenix definition, this is the new standard measure of the success of radiation therapy. And even this isn't the one-size-fits-all, perfect definition of biochemical failure for all men who have undergone radiation. Nor is there a single best approach if a man's cancer does return after radiation. (See What Happens If My PSA Goes Up after Radiation Treatment? below). The good news is that the longer a man's PSA remains stably low after radiation, the less likely he is to have a return of cancer down the road.

Some men wonder whether any healthy prostate tissue left behind could someday turn into cancer. "There is no evidence to suggest that this occurs, and in theory it is unlikely," says Song. "In addition to its direct killing effect on cancer by destroying its DNA, radiation is also known to impede the development of the new blood vessels that cancerous tissues rely on." (This process, called angiogenesis, is discussed in chapter 12. Basically, without new blood vessels to feed them, cancers can't advance.) "This effect remains long after treatment. The main question is whether the patient is free of cancer," he continues, "not whether it's the original cancer or one that developed from benign tissue remaining after radiation. If you're comparing the results of radiation with other forms of treatment, there is no need to 'adjust' the results for new cancers. The results are reported for *any* evidence of prostate cancer, regardless of origin."

## Cancer Control After External-Beam Therapy

As we've just seen, one problem for doctors and patients wrestling with statistics and results is simply figuring out how success and failure are measured by the authors of a particular study. Another is that we probably need to reassess the longest, most mature data we have on the older, standard external-beam approach. The old picture of radiation is no longer accurate, and it's unfair and illogical to compare the results from even a decade ago with those achievable today. For one thing, it has become clear that in the past, many men didn't get

## MIXING APPLES AND ORANGES:
## USING TWO STANDARDS TO DETERMINE CURE
## WITH SURGERY AND RADIATION THERAPY

Although it is clear that the same standard to define cure cannot be used for both surgery and radiation, is it possible to compare the outcomes of the two therapies? Doctors Matthew Gretzer and Matthew Nielsen attempted to make this comparison by applying the ASTRO and nadir + 2 definitions to 2,700 men who underwent a radical prostatectomy at Johns Hopkins.

First, the ASTRO comparison. Using the surgical definition for failure (PSA less than 0.2 ng/ml) at five years after surgery, 85 percent of the men were cancer-free; at ten years, 77 percent; and at fifteen years, 68 percent. But using ASTRO criteria—requiring three consecutive rises in PSA and backdating failure to the midpoint between nadir and the first rise in PSA—90 percent of those same men were cancer-free at five, ten, and fifteen years. Thus, applying the ASTRO criteria artificially improved the patients' probability of being free from cancer at fifteen years from 68 percent to 90 percent. Many men are told that radiation therapy cures everyone—that 90 percent of men are cured, and no one fails after five years. But unfortunately, these results are based on the ASTRO guidelines, which simply overestimate the probability of cure. Thus, men must be cautious in interpreting any comparison of these therapies based on ASTRO criteria, because it may be misleading.

Next, the nadir + 2 comparison. This performed better, but there were still some problems. Using the surgical definition (PSA less than 0.2 ng/ml) at five years after surgery, 88.6 percent were cancer-free. At ten years, 81.2 percent, and at fifteen years, 78.1 percent remained cancer-free. (These results were better than those of the earlier study, because we evaluated men who underwent surgery in more recent years.) Using the nadir + 2 definition, the comparable numbers at five, ten, and fifteen years were 94.6 percent, 89.4 percent, and 84.3 percent, respectively. However, for men who developed biochemical failure, the average time to the identification of an abnormal PSA was 2.8 years using the surgical definition and eight years using nadir + 2. This was most evident in men who developed a local recurrence; at ten years, failure was identified in 80 percent of these men using the surgical definition, but in only 7 percent with nadir + 2. The reason is that the nadir + 2 definition has been optimized to identify men who are destined to develop metastatic disease. For this reason, the consensus panel that developed this definition cautions, "Physicians should use individualized approaches to managing young patients with slowly rising PSA levels who initially achieved a very low nadir and who might be a candidate for salvage local therapies."

The analysis above is helpful only if you are trying to convert the results following surgery to the same language used by radiation oncologists. However, be careful in trying to compare the results of radiation head-to-head with the results of surgery, because the surgical results are usually based on the Gleason score after a radical prostatectomy; this is often higher than the initial score on the biopsy, and this artifact makes surgery look better. Thus, if you want to try to compare the results of surgery with radiation therapy, patients in both treatment groups need to be evaluated by the Gleason score on their original biopsy. Here's where the Han tables can be of use (see chapter 6).

enough radiation to do the job of killing all the prostate cancer. For another, many men who received radiation were what doctors call adversely selected for this approach, because their cancer was too extensive for them to be cured by surgery. Unfortunately, this means that many men who received radiation in the past probably did not have curable disease to start with. Plus, the technology today is markedly better than it was a few years ago. And finally, one of our best markers for determining the extent of disease, PSA level, was not able to be measured when most of these men were treated.

The new conformal techniques have brought great promise to radiation therapy. Still, because these techniques have been in widespread use for only about a decade, there can be some uncertainty in understanding the results. The clearest short-term yardstick may be the PSA nadir (discussed above). One study of 743 patients at Memorial Sloan-Kettering Cancer Center in New York confirmed that higher-intensity radiation does a better job of achieving a rock-bottom PSA level. Of the men who received higher doses—76 to 81 Gy—90 percent achieved a PSA nadir of 1.0 ng/ml or less; 76 percent of men who received 70 Gy and 56 percent of men who received 64.8 Gy achieved those low PSA levels. But there was a trade-off—the men who received higher doses of radiation also had a significantly higher rate of gastrointestinal side effects, urinary tract complications, and impotence. To overcome these side effects at high doses, intensity-modulated radiation therapy (IMRT) has an advantage.

Another study, of patient records pooled from nine different medical centers, looked at PSA nadirs, the time it took for men to achieve PSA nadirs, and the men's risk of developing distant metastases. The researchers found that the lower the nadir PSA, the lower the risk of distant metastases. Men who had a PSA nadir of less than 0.5 ng/ml had a 3 percent risk of developing cancer at distant sites at eight years after treatment, but men with a PSA nadir higher than 2.0 ng/ml had a 27 percent risk of having distant metastases at eight years. They also found that men who received a dose of greater than or equal to 70 Gy tended to reach a lower PSA nadir and to have better cancer control.

The new, high-dose, conformally directed, external-beam techniques for radiation therapy have been in widespread use for about ten years (IMRT is more recent). At five years, in favorable patients (men with low-grade, early-stage cancer), cancer control rates of 91 percent have been reported.

### What About Proton-Beam Radiation?

Is it better than the more commonly used photon-beam (external-beam) radiation at controlling cancer? "There is little reason to believe so," comments Song. "Cancer cells respond the same way to both." In published reports detailing PSA nadirs, cancer control, and side effects, there are no significant differences seen between proton-beam radiation and other modern radiation techniques.

## Cancer Control After Brachytherapy

How effective is brachytherapy? In recent years, this has been the subject of heated debate. Radiation seeds are like little grenades inserted directly into a prostate tumor. In theory, each radioactive seed blasts a targeted area of tissue, ultimately destroying the prostate. In practice, however, it hasn't been that simple. In the 1960s and 1970s, brachytherapy was very popular, because it appeared to have fewer side effects than surgery. Back then, doctors used a freehand technique—crude by today's ultra-sophisticated standards—and placed the seeds somewhat randomly during open surgery. Basically, they eyeballed it, estimating where the seeds should go. The coverage was uneven—some of the target tissue was obliterated, but other tissue was left unscathed—and the procedure's ability to control cancer ranked a distant third behind radical prostatectomy and external-beam radiation. The procedure wasn't well suited for men with large or high-grade tumors. Also, because most implantation regimens focused only on the tissue within the prostate and ignored the seminal vesicles and tissue outside it, the seeds were unable to reach cancer that had spread locally.

Brachytherapy today is far better. Instead of the old freehand approach, doctors now use sophisticated, high-tech guidance systems, working with ultrasound or CT and crafting a custom-designed template for each patient, placing the seeds more accurately and closer together. The ideal patient for brachytherapy is someone with a moderate-sized prostate, few urinary symptoms (minimal urgency or frequency and with a strong stream), and organ-confined disease.

How do the results compare with those of external-beam radiation or surgery? According to the Johns Hopkins radiation oncologist Song, there is no straightforward answer. "This is a question that is frequently a source of spirited debate between radiation oncologists and surgeons, and like most debates, the issues involved are complex."

One problem, again, is that the definitions of success after prostatectomy and radiation are different, and the currently accepted ASTRO and Phoenix definitions are not perfect (see above). Another issue is patient selection. "Consciously or unconsciously, it has been noted that urologists often select for surgery those patients who are likely to do well regardless of treatment," comments Song, "referring the less-favorable patients for treatments such as radiation. It's akin to having the first pick of the litter." The bottom line, he adds, is that multiple studies have shown similar results for both brachytherapy and radical prostatectomy. National consensus panels such as the National Comprehensive Cancer Network, made up of experts in urology and radiation oncology, including doctors from Johns Hopkins, have stated that surgery and radiation should be considered effective therapies with somewhat different toxicity profiles.

In medical research, the gold standard for determining which treatment is better is the randomized trial in which carefully matched patients are randomly assigned to one treatment or the other. And ideally, such a study is performed not only at one center but at many, so the results are based on the practices and skills of many physicians and treatment teams, making the results broadly applicable. Large studies have the resources to make sure that patients are followed for many years. Unfortunately, a study that attempted to do this—to enroll two thousand men and randomly assign them to receive either brachytherapy or prostatectomy—failed miserably. "In the United States, patients are highly involved in making their treatment decisions and often have trouble with the idea of letting a statistical process determine which treatment they will receive, rather than being able to decide on their own," Song notes. "Previous attempts to perform similar studies between external-beam radiation and surgery have also failed for this very reason, which is partially why there is still ongoing debate after so many years."

## Combining Brachytherapy with External-Beam Radiation

Several years ago, when brachytherapy was becoming established as a treatment for localized prostate cancer, some radiation oncologists worried that the seeds alone would not prevent cancer at the capsule of the prostate from spreading outside it. For this reason, they decided to hedge their cancer-killing bets, adding low-dose (45 to 50 Gy) external-beam radiation to brachytherapy. This practice continues in many centers. Some physicians prefer to start with external-beam radiation; others put the seeds in first. To minimize side effects, the two treatments are often separated by a three- to five-week break.

Support for this double-barreled approach emerged from research published by doctors at the Pacific Northwest Cancer Foundation, a hospital in Seattle, who used this technique in patients with higher risk factors, such as a Gleason score of 7 or higher. At ten years, this group of men had better PSA control than the men who had received brachytherapy alone for lower-risk disease. Another study, published in the *Journal of the American Medical Association*, compared results of external-beam radiation, radical prostatectomy, brachytherapy with hormonal therapy, and brachytherapy alone for men with low-, intermediate-, and high-risk prostate cancer. The study found that brachytherapy alone was not as successful in men with intermediate- to high-risk prostate cancer as compared with the other treatments. These results suggested that men with a Gleason score higher than 6 or a PSA level greater than 10 ng/ml should receive additional therapy. In other studies as well, combination treatment was found to be superior to brachytherapy alone.

However, critics of these studies have noted that the differences in the Seattle treatment groups could be because the external-beam radiation made up for "cold spots" among the seeds, which were implanted early in the brachytherapists' experience. The second paper was hampered by the fact that there were relatively few patients who received brachytherapy alone, limiting the statistical power of the study. Other radiation oncologists have argued that if cancer does extend beyond the prostate, it does so only at a magnitude of 1 to 3 millimeters—well within reach of the seeds' therapeutic range. Retrospective comparisons have been published showing no differences between men treated with brachytherapy alone versus those treated with brachytherapy combined with external-beam radiation. In some studies, Gleason scores and PSA levels appear to be similar in both groups. "If this is the case," asks Song, "why did the physicians chose to give some patients both treatments and other patients brachytherapy alone?"

There is less controversy regarding the side effects associated with the two options. Results from several studies show that the combination treatment carries a higher incidence of erectile dysfunction and rectal and urinary side effects. Currently at Johns Hopkins, only men with one or more unfavorable characteristics are treated with both brachytherapy and external-beam radiation; men with Gleason scores of 6 or lower and other low-risk factors are offered brachytherapy alone. There is little justification for performing combination treatment in favorable, low-risk patients, since the results with brachytherapy alone are quite good. Fortunately, the Radiation Therapy Oncology Group is currently performing a randomized trial to address the issue of the role of external-beam radiation in patients receiving brachytherapy. In this study, men with intermediate-risk prostate cancer receive either brachytherapy alone or brachytherapy combined with external-beam radiation.

A recent study led by Michael J. Zelefsky, a radiation oncologist at Memorial Sloan-Kettering Cancer Center, involved more than 2,600 patients who underwent brachytherapy at eleven different centers. These men were treated between 1988 and 1998. (Remember, in looking at any study involving men treated in the pre-PSA era, the results will undoubtedly be worse than those in men undergoing treatment today.) No patients received hormonal therapy; men were treated with either iodine-125 or palladium-103. At eight years, 82 percent of favorable-risk patients were cancer-free using the ASTRO definition (this number was 74 percent using the nadir + 2 definition). The same statistics for intermediate-risk patients were 70 percent and 61 percent, respectively. Not surprisingly, the long-term results were significantly affected by the quality of the implant. When the study focused on men who had received a dose higher than 140 Gy to 90 percent of the prostate, between 90 and 92 percent of these men were cancer-free at eight years. This emphasizes the importance of finding the right doctor who can reliably deliver these results. The nadir PSA level achieved after treatment was also important. Patients who reached a PSA nadir of less than 0.5 ng/ml had eight-year PSA relapse–free survival outcomes of 92 percent and 86 percent (depending on the use of iodine-125 or palladium-103, respectively). Although there were some slight differences in outcome based on the isotope used, these differences were not statistically significant.

### What About High-Dose-Rate (HDR) Brachytherapy?

High-dose-rate (HDR) brachytherapy, which uses high-powered, temporary seeds (described in chapter 9), is still a relatively new option. It has been used mostly on men with intermediate- or high-risk disease. So far, there have not been head-to-head comparisons between these two forms of brachytherapy. Some studies have shown that HDR brachytherapy plus external-beam therapy has better cancer control rates than external-beam radiation alone. However, the doses used in the patients receiving external-beam radiation alone were low (approximately 66 Gy) compared to recent standards.

### Which Form of Radiation Therapy Is Best?

This is the $64,000 question. And the answer is . . . we don't know. Again, no long-term studies are long-term *enough* yet to tell us how men fare with brachytherapy, conformal external-beam radiation therapy, or a combination of the two, with or without the addition of hormonal therapy.

What will the results of these radiation treatments be after ten or fifteen years? This is a crucial question for healthy men under age seventy-five who can expect to live long enough to really need to know the answer. But nobody knows. And in an era of constantly refining techniques and technology, the downside is that when the treatment changes, the results achieved with the outmoded therapy lose their meaning. As you look at the results of a certain form of radiation treatment or a particular hospital's success rate, you have the right to know such criteria as:

- What was the preoperative PSA level, clinical stage, and Gleason score of the patients they treated? (If all the patients were in the elite, low-risk group, then the five-year success rate *ought* to be good.)
- What are the researchers using as an end point? Is it the nadir + 2, or the ASTRO definition—or some other standard?
- In what era were their patients treated? Before or after PSA testing came into widespread use?
- Are they comparing apples to apples—men treated during the same era?

## What Happens If My PSA Goes Up After Radiation Treatment?

The purpose of radiation treatment is to disable the prostate, to stop cancer there from continuing to grow. Because the prostate is the source of PSA, if PSA continues to be made and its level begins to rise, there are two possibilities. Either the cancer has reactivated locally, within the prostate or surrounding tissue, or a distant metastasis—a tiny bit of cancer that probably escaped the prostate before treatment began—has started causing trouble.

It is sometimes difficult after radiation therapy for a man to know where he stands, because cancer often takes its time in announcing itself; it usually takes several PSA measurements before a man and his doctor can figure out whether treatment has failed. Some men worry that this period of uncertainty is a window of opportunity for curing prostate cancer. If the initial decision to perform radiation therapy was made because of the presence of advanced disease or older age, then most studies on salvage treatments after radiation therapy has failed have found no difference in cancer control, as long as men received extra treatment before their PSA levels reached 10 ng/ml. If you are being closely followed by your doctor and it turns out that the radiation alone has not killed the cancer, this should be clear long before your PSA level reaches this point. However, it's worth repeating that the consensus panel that developed the nadir + 2 definition advises, "Physicians should used individualized approaches to managing young patients with slowly rising PSA levels who initially achieved a very low nadir and who might be a candidate for salvage local therapies."

If your PSA level continues to rise, what should you do? To determine whether you are a candidate for surgery after radiation, you will need to have a prostate biopsy to confirm that the cancer recurrence is local; you will also need a bone scan and CT scan or MRI of the abdomen and pelvis to rule out the possibility that cancer has spread to distant sites. The guidelines above (see "What Should I Do If My PSA Comes Back After Surgery?") may one day be adapted for men who have failed radiation treatment, but the overriding principles can be useful here in identifying the probability of metastases. If you have a high Gleason score (8 or greater), or if the PSA level begins to rise early after radiation therapy, or if the PSA level has a rapid doubling time, it is more likely that you have metastases than a local recurrence, and in this case, you should seek systemic therapy (see chapter 12).

### Salvage Therapy

If the cancer appears to have stayed put—to be still localized to the prostate bed—what are the options? Salvage radical prostatectomy, salvage brachytherapy, and cryoablation.

In the past, with standard radiation therapy and with less sophisticated brachytherapy, performing a radical prostatectomy on a man who had undergone radiation treatment was a surgeon's nightmare. The prostate was adherent to everything around it and very difficult to remove cleanly; in fact, it was often necessary to remove the bladder as well. The side effects were high, particularly the risk of incontinence and rectal injury. With the advent of 3-D conformal

external-beam therapy, it may be easier to perform surgery as a salvage procedure. There is too little information yet available about salvage surgery after brachytherapy to make a judgment. Under the best
circumstances, in men who appear to have no evidence of distant
metastases, the likelihood of being cancer-free following a salvage radical prostatectomy at five and ten years is about 50 percent and 30 percent, respectively. The price for this in quality of life, however, is high.

One of the largest studies to look at radical prostatectomy after radiation comes from the Mayo Clinic. At an average of forty
months after radiation, 199 men underwent either prostatectomy
or cystoprostatectomy (removal of prostate and bladder). Urinary
extravasation (leakage of urine into tissues) occurred in 15 percent
of men, and 22 percent had bladder neck contracture. Urinary incontinence (defined as a need to wear pads) developed in 44 percent,
and 4 percent had rectal injury during surgery. The percentage of
men who had erectile dysfunction was not recorded, but this is almost inevitable with salvage prostatectomy. At five years after surgery, 58 percent of men remained free of cancer. Other studies of
salvage prostatectomy have reported that between 55 and 69 percent
of men remained cancer-free.

## Salvage Cryoablation

Recently cryoablation—freezing the prostate, discussed in chapter 9—
has been considered as a plan B for radiation patients with rising PSA
levels. Although there is little long-term information available on how
this affects the tumor, the complications are high, as with any salvage
procedure. Early studies found that complications were much worse
if the urethra was not warmed during the procedure (in an attempt
to kill the entire prostate). In one study, this resulted in "urinary incontinence, impotence, tissue sloughing (during urination), prob-
lematic voiding symptoms and/or perineal pain (pain between the
rectum and scrotum) in a substantial number of patients." Urethral
warming has resulted in fewer of these complications, although incontinence, pelvic pain, impotence, and urinary retention still remain
substantial risks.

More recent results of salvage cryoablation are based on biopsies
of prostate tissue taken several months after treatment. In one study,

106 men underwent cryoablation for biopsy-proven, clinically local-ized cancer after radiation therapy. It was encouraging that three to twenty-four months after treatment, only 14 percent of these men had a positive biopsy, but 42 percent of the men had viable prostate glands, and 27 percent had viable stroma—in other words, working prostate tissue and structural support, which means that the prostate was not destroyed. These results are more troubling than reassuring, especially since only four cores of tissue were removed for the biop-sies. Thus, it is fairly certain that the biopsies could not completely es-timate the actual incidence of residual cancer. We do not yet have any long-term results on salvage cryoablation using the newest, third-generation equipment.

How does salvage cryoablation after radiation compare to salvage radical prostatectomy? Although salvage radical prostatectomy has more complications, it actually may control the disease better. In a ret-rospective study of men treated with either salvage radical prosta-tectomy or salvage cryoablation, in which the men were matched for their pretreatment PSA level and Gleason score, PSA levels continued to increase in 67 percent of the men treated with salvage cryoablation, compared with only 30 percent of the men who underwent salvage radical prostatectomy. This suggests that salvage cryoablation may provide inferior cancer control.

### What About Additional Radiation?

This is a third option—either additional external-beam radiation or brachytherapy. There are a few reports describing the use of brachytherapy as a salvage procedure after external-beam radiation. These reports have included a variety of patients, some with disease that had a low likelihood of being controlled with treatment limited to the prostate alone. However, preliminary results suggest that sal-vage brachytherapy may be effective for some men, especially those who have PSA levels of less than 10 ng/ml. The risk of incontinence has been reported to be as high as 25 percent, although this was with the older, uniform loading technique (see chapter 9), which has been associated with higher incontinence for brachytherapy in general. In-creased rates of pelvic or penile pain, proctitis, and impotence have also been noted. Note: *If you are considering this option, it is essential that the procedure be performed by someone who is skillful in delivering further radiation to an already irradiated area.*

Your doctor may want you to start long-term hormonal therapy. If you are otherwise feeling fine and have no evidence of metastatic disease, this may or may not be a good idea. There is some evidence suggesting that beginning hormonal therapy soon after radiation failure may improve metastasis-free and overall survival, but this is an area of much controversy and debate. A PSA doubling time of less than three months has been associated with a high risk of clinically significant cancer progression; in this situation, you and your doctor should strongly consider starting hormonal therapy or looking at other options, such as participation in clinical trials. Otherwise, hormonal therapy, discussed in detail in chapter 12, is nothing to enter into lightly. Many men have very slow, gradual elevations in their PSA levels for years and have no symptoms of cancer. If you're not on hormonal therapy, you can enjoy a normal life (including a normal sex life) and simply be followed closely with watchful waiting. Then—only if or when you develop symptoms from local recurrence or metastatic disease— you can consider further treatment. The field of treating advanced disease is constantly changing, and there are many new, exciting, and hopeful advances. These are discussed in chapter 12.

## How Well Do Cryoablation and Thermal Ablation Work?

Again, there is a downside to evolving technology: there are no long-term studies to help us evaluate the success of third-generation cryoablation in controlling cancer. Whenever any technology is improved, the clock starts all over again for scientists who are evaluating its success. As we've discussed earlier in this book, even if a miracle cure comes along tomorrow, it won't be proven to eradicate prostate cancer until the men who have been treated with it have been cancer-free for at least a decade. The earliest way to determine success is by looking for a local recurrence of cancer, based on biopsies, but there isn't much information available yet. It is somewhat encouraging that 81 percent of the patients in one study did achieve a low PSA level (0.4 ng/ml or less) at three months of follow-up, and 78 percent of low-risk patients remained free from a biochemical recurrence of cancer at twelve months. However, how do we define biochemical recurrence? Many investigators use the ASTRO definition, which we discussed above, and which probably is not appropriate for evaluating cryoablation. Ideally, in the long run, we would hope that the yardstick used for success here would be a persistent, long-term PSA level of 0.4 ng/ml or lower.

Is cryoablation effective? To answer this question, we need thoughtful studies that not only determine the risks of late complications but that demonstrate cryoablation's long-term success in controlling cancer. Unfortunately, because the third-generation technique is so new, long-term results on cancer control are not yet available. Even the pioneers of this treatment do not recommend it for the young, otherwise healthy man who most likely has organ-confined disease. However, as reported by two researchers from Allegheny University of Health Sciences in Pittsburgh in the journal *Contemporary Urology*, there is a role for cryoablation. It is a "very viable option for patients with bulky lesions, high-grade lesions, clinically localized legions with high PSA, radiation failures, and for those patients whose age or comorbidity [other health problems] make them a suboptimal candidate for conventional surgery." For example, the researchers stated, cryoablation may benefit a man with stage T2b, Gleason 8 cancer who has a PSA of 20 ng/ml. "Even if biochemical 'cure' is not obtained, one can achieve very effective local control with low morbidity," or side effects.

What if cancer comes back after cryoablation? There is no question that cryoablation can be repeated—it can and is. But if it fails again, what's next? One study suggests that radiation therapy after cryoablation may be useful. In this study of fifty patients, salvage radiation therapy reduced PSA levels to less than 1.0 ng/ml in most men while causing few side effects. However, we do not have long-term results on the success of salvage radiation after cryoablation.

**What About Thermal Ablation?**

This is the new kid on the block, and it's so new that the only available results are from short-term studies. In one study of sixty-three men, only one-third of them developed a PSA level of less than 0.2 ng/ml four to eight weeks after treatment. The lowest PSA achieved—

the PSA nadir—was less than 0.2 ng/ml in one-third of the men, 0.2–1.0 ng/ml in another third, and greater than 1.0 ng/ml in the other third. A man's likelihood of developing a low PSA level immediately after treatment correlated well with his likelihood of remaining disease-free at three years. This was 100 percent in the men who had a PSA nadir less than 0.2 ng/ml, 74 percent in the middle group, and only 21 percent in the men with a PSA nadir greater than 1.0 ng/ml. However, these disease-free survival results use the ASTRO criteria, which are notoriously unreliable in providing the short-term follow-up picture. We do not yet have enough information to state how well thermal ablation will control prostate cancer over the long term.

## Final Thoughts on Treatment for Localized Prostate Cancer

What's the best form of treatment for localized disease? This is a major dilemma for men and their doctors, because it's a moving target. There are multiple options with varying definitions of success. Study results can vary widely, depending on the stage of disease at which a patient is treated, making comparisons even more difficult, because men undergoing different treatments may not have had exactly the same characteristics before treatment.

Surgeons will sometimes tell you that in the past, when radiation therapy was used to treat localized prostate cancer, even with improved treatments, the failure rates were higher than everyone had hoped. Obviously, with all forms of treatment, radiation, and surgery, more patients experience a recurrence of their cancer than anyone would like. Essentially, every incremental advance in radiation therapy has brought better results for patients. With state-of-the-art imaging and high-dose delivery techniques, it is much more likely than it was in the past that all prostate cancer cells will be killed. Indeed, we now have more long-term follow-up studies to show that this is the case.

In addition to this uncertainty about outcomes, you must take into consideration some of the external factors that can sway someone's decision about treatment type. The news media are constantly reporting what's new. That's their job; but it's not always clear from the newspapers and TV that "new" doesn't always equal "best." Prostate cancer is a well-publicized disease these days (unlike the bad old days, when men didn't speak of the disease and either didn't know to get tested for it or were afraid of what they'd find out). At least once a month, we hear about some celebrity or political figure who is diagnosed with prostate cancer and what form of treatment he has chosen. It's easy to think, "That guy is a multimillionaire; he must have the best doctors in the world, and if this is what he's chosen, it must be the best treatment there is." Well, sometimes it is, sometimes it isn't. Also, in today's world of instantaneous everything, many patients have the idea that they should be able to receive effective treatment without any complications—that they should be cured today and be able to play golf tomorrow.

There are more subtle factors at work here, too. In today's health-care economy, many physicians are being strongly affected by reimbursement patterns. Insurance companies and HMOs are paying less for traditional surgery. Frankly, many urologists have found that they can make more money during the same period of time it would take to perform one very difficult operation by performing two outpatient procedures that require no postoperative care. Finally, the companies that make devices and the pharmaceutical companies that make drugs are in a high-stakes business, where marketing their wares to patients and physicians (through advertisements, Internet Web sites, and carefully placed stories in the media) can bring in astronomical profits. So when you sit down and talk to your doctor about what you should do, take into consideration these outside influences. Ideally, you should be seen by both an experienced urologist and radiation oncologist in a single center that offers care in multiple methods of treatment where you can be assured that you are not being persuaded into one type of treatment just because that's its specialty.

What's the best form of treatment? The traditional way to determine this, for any disease, is randomized clinical trials, in which men are randomly assigned to undergo one form of treatment or another, and the long-term results are eventually collected. If this route is taken in prostate cancer, it will take many years for results to become available. While this would be a very good thing to do, we are fortunate that all information to date suggests that surgery and contemporary radiation therapy are effective forms of treatment. Until such a definitive trial takes place, what do we do in the meantime? One problem is that men choose specific medical centers for a reason—namely, that center's expertise in a particular form of treatment. It is unlikely that a man who goes to a center known for its strength in one particular treatment would choose another form of treatment in the interests of impartiality and the betterment of science.

I believe the quickest, most reliable results will come from non-randomized comparisons of treatment by a blue-ribbon registry. Experts in all the fields here—urology, radiation oncology, and medical oncology—should name their most respected, impartial colleagues to a registry that can compare treatments performed at different centers. This registry should agree on the characteristics of the candidates for treatment—their age and any other illnesses they may have—and should develop a stratification of risk to determine, in groups, who is curable and needs to be cured using standard, easily available criteria such as PSA level, Gleason score, and clinical stage. These thoughtful experts should also agree on ways to evaluate the quality of life of men before and after treatment. When all of this is in place, they should enlist medical centers of excellence—centers where the side effects are the lowest and cure rates highest—to participate so that comparable patients given different forms of treatment at separate institutions can be compared. With a powerful resource such as this, over the next decade, we can learn with confidence which form of treatment is truly better.

# 11

# ERECTILE DYSFUNCTION AFTER TREATMENT FOR LOCALIZED PROSTATE CANCER

## ▶▶▶ READ THIS FIRST

Men who have trouble with erections after surgery or radiation therapy have normal sensation and normal sex drive and can achieve a normal orgasm. Their only trouble may be in achieving or maintaining an erection. That's the bad news. The good news is that this problem, called erectile dysfunction (ED), can always be treated.

Why does ED occur? There are many reasons in addition to the fact that a man has had prostate treatment. Aging is one reason for ED. But ED can also result from medical conditions such as atherosclerosis, diabetes, or hypertension; from certain medications; from the overuse of alcohol, cigarettes, or other drugs; and even from emotional or psychological problems.

The bottom line is that for most men, ED does not have to be a permanent situation. If there's a will, there's generally a way.

The important message here is that after treatment for prostate disease (except for men treated with hormonal therapy), recovery of sexual function is almost certain. Take heart! You will get through this.

## What Is Erectile Dysfunction?

As its name suggests, erectile dysfunction (ED) is trouble having or maintaining an erection. There's no minimum age requirement for ED; it can happen to any man at any time. It's especially common after treatment for prostate cancer with radical prostatectomy or radiation therapy. Having ED does not mean your sex life is over—far from it. In fact, a man with ED has *normal sensation and normal sex drive and can achieve a normal orgasm.* He may just need a little help with erections. And this is a problem that can be fixed.

The purpose of this chapter is to let you know two things: First, that you're not alone. By age sixty-five, about 25 percent of all men—those who have been treated for prostate cancer as well as men who have never had it—experience at least some trouble with ED. In the United States alone, ED affects an estimated ten to thirty million men. (Note: ED is different from the loss of libido, or sex drive, that results from hormonal therapy—discussed in chapter 12.) A report from the Massachusetts Male Aging Study suggests that the incidence of ED triples from 5 to 15 percent between ages forty and seventy. Aging (and the general nerve loss that goes along with it; see below) is one reason for ED. But ED also can result from medical conditions such as atherosclerosis, diabetes, hypertension, or multiple sclerosis; from certain medications; from the overuse of alcohol, cigarettes, or other drugs; and even from emotional or psychological problems.

The second point here is that help is available. For most men, ED does not have to be a life sentence. If there's a will, there's generally a way.

## AFTER RADICAL PROSTATECTOMY, TESTOSTERONE GOES UP

Some men experience a loss of libido—sex drive—after radical prostatectomy. This is different from impotence, or difficulty with erections. It's not about having trouble with sex—it's about not wanting to have it at all. Some scientists have theorized that perhaps after surgery, there is a decrease in male hormones (particularly testosterone), and perhaps this accounts for the diminished libido in some men.

But a Johns Hopkins study has found that this is not the case; in fact, it's the opposite of what we suspected. Before we go any further, let's take a quick look at testosterone. The story begins in the brain—in the pituitary gland, which makes a hormone called luteinizing hormone (LH). In the chemical chain of events involved in the production of testosterone, the pituitary is the thermostat, the regulator that controls the testes—the furnace, in effect. The furnace cranks out heat—testosterone—which, in turn, stimulates the prostate. The level of testosterone in the blood is constantly monitored by the brain, which regulates how much LH is needed.

This study showed that when the prostate is removed, LH goes up— and so, then, does testosterone—suggesting that the prostate somehow produces a substance that controls LH secretion. The investigators were studying the effect of radical prostatectomy on these hormones in sixty-three men, wondering whether some change in hormonal makeup might explain the loss of libido experienced by some men after surgery. In normal men, the major factors that influence sexual function are blood flow, nerve supply, and hormones. A great deal of attention has been placed on studying how to avoid disrupting the nerve supply and blood supply during surgery—but up to this point, there has been little attention paid to what happens to the hormones.

The newly discovered information, that the pituitary gland makes more LH after radical prostatectomy, suggests that the prostate is also making an inhibitor that regulates the release of LH from the pituitary, raising the fascinating idea that the prostate itself may influence hormone levels in an effort to modulate its own growth.

The increase in testosterone is not noticeable, but it certainly dispels the theory that a loss of male hormones contributes to a loss of sex drive. Instead, a more likely cause of this diminished libido after surgery is the lack of psychogenic erections. This occurs early on after surgery (see What Can Go Wrong? below). Another cause may be depression, and fortunately, treatment can restore the sex drive.

## What Happens in Normal Sexual Function?

Normal erection in men can be reduced in medical terms to a vascular event. But this seems too simple a description for the delicate, complex interplay between blood vessels (veins and arteries) and nerves. The penis itself is a remarkable structure, made up of nerves, smooth muscle tissue, and blood vessels. It has three cylindrical, spongy chambers that are essential to erection; one of these is called the corpus spongiosum, and the other two are called the corpora cavernosa.

When sexual function is normal, this is what happens. A man becomes sexually aroused. A substance called nitric oxide is released by the nerve endings, and the smooth muscle tissue in the penis begins to relax. The spongy chambers (also called sinusoids) within this smooth muscle tissue begin to dilate. Meanwhile, arteries continue to pump blood, as usual, into these spongy chambers of the penis. As the penis elongates, the veins are stretched; they clamp down against the thick tissue that surrounds the corpora cavernosa—shutting themselves off so the blood can't leave the penis. The chambers become engorged, and this keeps the penis inflated during sexual activity. An erection is born.

After ejaculation, nitric oxide stops being released; the smooth muscle tissue contracts, and the blood flow to the penis is reduced—the veins ease their viselike grip. Once again, blood is allowed to leave the penis, and the erection goes away.

## What Can Go Wrong?

There are four components to normal sexual function in men—libido (sex drive), erection, emission of fluid (ejaculation), and orgasm. All of these elements are regulated separately; there is no centralized sex control center.

### Libido

The sex drive is controlled by two things—male hormones and psychological and environmental factors. The main male hormone that affects libido, testosterone, is made in the testicles. When this hormone supply is shut off—as it is in hormonal therapy (actually, hormone-deprivation therapy) for advanced prostate cancer—testosterone levels fall considerably, to extremely low levels. When this happens, most men on hormonal therapy lose all interest in sexual activity. Men who have undergone a radical prostatectomy or radiation therapy may also experience a loss of libido, but it's not caused by the loss of testosterone, and it's not usually as severe. There is some evidence that radiation therapy may cause a slight decrease in the production of male hormones, although this is unlikely to be significant enough to reduce sexual function. Surprisingly, after radical prostatectomy, testosterone levels actually go *up* (see above). The most likely cause of diminished libido after surgery is the early loss of erections that are brought on by visual and mental stimulation; these are called psychogenic erections. As we'll discuss later, most men rely on these signals to increase their libido, and when they are absent, they sense that they've lost interest in sexual activity. (It's like thinking, "The lights aren't on; therefore, nobody is home"—without even knocking on the door to find out!) Other causes may be stress, performance anxiety, or depression. Many men find that if they take a vacation and get their mind off their work and other problems, they lose an overlay of stress they may not even have realized they've been carrying around, and their sex drive returns. It's also common for men to become distracted by fretting about the mechanics of sexual relations rather than the pleasure of intimacy. When a man sits around and broods about whether he's going to have an erection—when he agonizes over the thought of disappointing his partner or even starts to obsess about various blood vessels doing or not doing their jobs right—it probably isn't going to happen. This is known as performance anxiety. And finally, after any major treatment or trauma to the body (this is common in men after a heart attack, for example), depression can occur. Paradoxically, it may be even more acute when the treatment is successful. Depression is one of the body's natural responses to stress, and in many men, treating the depression restores the sex drive to normal. For all of these reasons, many men may perceive a decrease in their sex drive, which usually returns over time, as these problems correct themselves one by one.

## Erection

Probably the most common sexual problem for men after prostate treatment is the inability to have an erection sufficient for sexual intercourse. The nerves that lead to and from the penis are extremely important to erection. Particularly essential are nerves in the two bundles that sit on either side of the prostate (see the illustrations in chapter 8). Even if these nerve bundles are not removed during radical prostatectomy, they can still be damaged by the surgery. They also can be injured during radiation treatment and other procedures, including cryoablation. But remember, *these nerves are necessary only for erection—not for sensation, and not for orgasm.* The nerves that are responsible for sensation travel outside the pelvis for a long distance. These nerves are not close to the prostate and should not be damaged. Loss of erection after radical prostatectomy or radiation is what doctors call multifactorial—in other words, it's probably not caused by one single problem.

In the most skilled surgeon's hands, if both neurovascular bundles are preserved during a radical prostatectomy, potency should return in at least 80 percent of men in their forties and fifties and in 60 percent of men in their sixties. However, only about 25 percent of men over age seventy are potent after surgery. Why are the numbers so much lower? We think a large part of the problem is something that comes with the territory of aging in general—a gradual loss of all nerves, including those involved in erection. When a younger man undergoes a nerve-sparing radical prostatectomy, it's likely that about 20 percent of the nerves involved in erection are damaged, 60 percent are preserved normally, and 20 percent are temporarily disabled but eventually recover. This explains why for most men, sexual potency doesn't just snap back like a coiled spring.

So at best, a younger man after prostatectomy has about 80 percent of these nerves left for erection. But as we age, we constantly lose nerves. By age sixty, a man has only about 60 percent of the nerves he was born with—which means that if 20 percent of them are damaged by treatment for prostate cancer, only about 40 percent remain. This explains why ED is more common in older men after surgery and in men in whom it is necessary to remove one neurovascular bundle.

Erection problems also can result from vascular injury—damage to the blood vessels in the penis. For a normal erection to occur, the arteries that supply blood to the penis must be intact. This blood supply can suffer after radiation treatment; in fact, damage to these arteries is believed to be the main cause of ED after radiation treatment, although recent studies suggest that radiation may also injure the neurovascular bundles. In a few men, this blood supply can also be reduced by radical prostatectomy—even though the major arteries that supply the penis do not normally travel next to the prostate. In these men, for some reason, the major blood supply to the penis runs *inside* the pelvis—instead of outside, as it does in most men, and so these arteries can be damaged inadvertently during radical prostatectomy. At Johns Hopkins, once we recognized this, we modified our surgical technique, and now any major arteries that run on top of the prostate can be saved.

Another major problem with erections in men after radical prostatectomy or radiation therapy results from a problem called venous leak. Remember, as blood flows into the penis and it elongates, veins stretch and clamp down against the thick tissue that surrounds the corpora cavernosa, shutting them off so the blood can't leave the penis. However, early on after radical prostatectomy, the blood flow into the penis may not be rapid enough to cause these veins to go into their "stretch and automatically close" mode. Imagine a bucket with a hole in it, with water running in and then running out (except in this case, it's blood flowing in but draining back out, because the veins can't dam it up properly). For these veins to clamp down, the penis must be fully engorged. If a man never gets a full erection, there's a constant leak. Also—yet another consequence of aging—as men get older, the fibrous tissues that surround the penis weaken, and this, too, undermines the ability of the veins to hold in the blood.

## Emission

In normal ejaculation, several events must take place. Sperm, which are made in the testicles, travel to the epididymis, a "greenhouse" in which they mature. During orgasm, sperm are rocketed from the epididymis through the vas deferens during a series of powerful muscle contractions. They shoot through the ejaculatory ducts and mix with fluid produced by the prostate and seminal vesicles. Simultaneously, a muscular valve in the bladder neck slams shut, forcing this fluid out the only possible exit—through the urethra and penis to the outside world, rather than backward into the bladder.

After radical prostatectomy, there is usually no emission of fluid because the prostate and seminal vesicles, which produce the vast majority of this fluid, are gone, and the vas deferens has been shut off. (Thus the term "dry ejaculation." A few men, however, do continue to produce a small amount of ejaculate. This fluid comes from the nearby Cowper's glands; like the prostate and seminal vesicles, these are known as sex accessory tissues.)

After radiation therapy, many men also have a loss of ejaculate fluid because the glands responsible for making this fluid are dried up. In any event—no matter what causes dry ejaculation—the lack of fluid should not interfere with orgasm. This is because orgasm doesn't really have much to do with the prostate. Think about it—women don't have prostates, yet they do have orgasms. Here's why.

**Orgasm**

Orgasm happens primarily in the brain. For orgasm to take place, there must be sensation and stimulation. In men who are impotent after radical prostatectomy or radiation therapy, sensation is not interrupted; therefore, orgasm should always be possible and it should be no different from the way it was before treatment. Many men don't realize that they can have an orgasm without an erection, and they're surprised to hear that half of the people in the world have orgasms without an erection—women. (Again, it's different for men receiving hormonal therapy for prostate cancer; orgasm is not an issue because—although a few can still have erections—the treatment causes a loss of interest in sexual activity.)

Note: A recent study suggested that some men, up to 14 percent, feel pain during orgasm after radical prostatectomy. For most of my patients who experience this problem, it gradually diminishes over time. It may be that there is a spasm of the sphincter at the time of orgasm. For this reason, treatment with an alpha-blocking drug such as Flomax (tamsulosin) can improve the problem or cause it to resolve completely.

## What Can You Do About ED?

Talk to your doctor. The first thing you can expect is to have a detailed history taken and a physical exam performed. The doctor is going to try to pinpoint the exact problem and figure out what's causing it. Is it trouble with libido, erection, ejaculation, or orgasm? Even though it may seem pretty obvious—your erections were just fine before prostate cancer treatment and inadequate or nonexistent afterward—the doctor needs to rule out the possibility that any other medical or psychological problem is causing this.

You may be asked to fill out a questionnaire so you don't have to discuss details face-to-face, or your doctor may ask you some very specific questions. You'll probably be embarrassed; most men would rather be almost anywhere else, discussing almost any other topic, than in a doctor's office talking about ED. But you shouldn't be embarrassed. This is private, sensitive, confidential information. Everything you discuss in the doctor's office will remain there. Remember: This certainly won't be the first time your doctor has heard about such difficulties, and it won't be the last. There are millions of other men in the United States alone with this same trouble. And finally, remind yourself that having this discussion is the first step toward solving the problem.

Probably one of the first questions your doctor will ask is whether you ever wake up at night with an erection. Most men have several erections while they're asleep; these are usually associated with dreaming, and they happen during a particular phase of sleep called REM, the abbreviation for rapid eye movement sleep. (Because men tend to wake up in the morning with these erections, they often connect them with having a full bladder; this is just coincidence.) The idea behind this question is to make sure there's no mental or emotional problem causing the ED. In other words, if a man can't produce an erection during sexual activity but has several a night while he sleeps, this is a clue that the nature of the problem is not physiological, but psychological. This type of erection problem is called psychogenic, as we discussed above, and it's often treated successfully with counseling. After a radical prostatectomy, things are different. Many men who are potent do not report having nocturnal erections, and some men who are not potent do have them.

How can this be? We don't know yet. However, we do know that the stimuli following surgery are different, and most men who are not potent but have nocturnal erections will eventually be able to have intercourse.

Your doctor will also ask whether you have a history of cardio-vascular disease. Men who have had a heart attack; who have coronary artery disease, hypertension, or elevated blood lipids; or who smoke have a greater chance of having vascular problems. Aside from the obvious health risks, smoking causes arteries to contract. Smoking is an easily reversible cause of ED; if you quit smoking, you could greatly improve your ability to have an erection. One of the first steps in erection is for the arteries to dilate; they fill up the penis with blood. If they're contracted, they won't be able to dilate very well. The arteries in the penis are the same size as the arteries in the heart. If you have heart disease, hypertension, atherosclerosis (hardening of the arteries), or high cholesterol (which can contribute to heart disease), it is very likely that the arteries in the penis are already narrowed.

Neurological diseases—diabetes, for example—can cause ED. Also, certain drugs may contribute to sexual problems, and combined with prostate treatment, they may result in ED. Cimetidine (Tagamet), for example, is a drug used to treat ulcers; but it's also an antiandrogen; it blocks the action of testosterone. Other medications that can cause ED include drugs that treat high blood pressure, such as beta-blockers and thiazides; medications that treat depression, such as monoamine oxidase inhibitors and tricyclic antidepressants; antipsychotic drugs; sedatives; drugs that treat anxiety; and drugs of abuse, such as opiates. (And don't forget alcohol and cigarettes—they're drugs, too.) Basically, it's a good idea if you're on any medication—even herbal or dietary supplements—to check with your doctor to make sure the side effects don't include ED. Switching from one drug to another may make a big difference.

### Diagnostic Tests

Your doctor may want you to undergo further evaluation, which may include something called a nocturnal penile tumescence test. This sounds like a form of torture, but all the name means is that it's a test to see whether you have erections during your sleep. If your doctor suspects a problem with penile blood flow, you may need to undergo pulsed Doppler evaluation. This test uses high-resolution ultrasound to evaluate the arteries' blood supply to the penis. Another test involves the injection of smooth muscle relaxants through a small needle directly into the penis; the idea here is to see whether an erection can be produced. If this shot doesn't cause an erection, this is a good hint that there's a vascular problem—trouble with arterial blood flow. Sometimes during this test a man develops an erection but gradually loses it; this usually signifies that there's a problem with the veins—they're not shutting off the blood supply, so the blood is escaping from the penis, and thus the erection is failing. Note: Surprisingly, psychological factors can prevent the penis from becoming erect in spite of this powerful pharmacological stimulation. This shows the true influence of mind over matter, and here again, counseling may provide significant help.

## Recovery of Potency After Radical Prostatectomy

You've had a radical prostatectomy, and one or both bundles were preserved, which means that the potential for erection is there. So what's the problem? Why isn't it happening?

The first bit of advice your doctor will probably give you here is "Be patient. Erections return gradually." Maybe better advice is "Be very patient. It can take up to four years for some men to experience full recovery of potency. Your body has been through a trauma; it needs time to recover." Now, this doesn't mean you should give up on sexual relations until the day you wake up with a full erection or until four years go by—whichever happens first. By no means. Also, know that the erection you have two months after surgery is not the same one you'll have two years from now. *Most patients experience an improvement in their erections over time; the quality improves month by month.*

Before surgery, men became sexually aroused, had an erection, and then pursued sexual activity. But after radical prostatectomy, the stimuli that cause an erection are different; visual and mental stimulation are not nearly as important as tactile sensation—what the penis can feel directly. Usually, shortly after surgery, the only way a man

## PEYRONIE'S DISEASE AND RADICAL PROSTATECTOMY: IS THERE A LINK?

Peyronie's disease is a disorder of the connective tissue within the penis that can cause curvature during erection. It's fairly rare—diagnosed in only 26 out of 100,000 men each year, most of them in their fifties and sixties. But Johns Hopkins urologists have spotted what they believe may be a small yet significant trend: Peyronie's disease seems to be more common in men who have had a radical prostatectomy. Is this just coincidence? The age group is roughly the same. Or does the procedure itself—or a man's recovery from it—somehow contribute to development of the disease?

"Peyronie's disease is like arthritis of the penis," says the urologist Jonathan P. Jarow, who specializes in the treatment of erectile disorders. "When you get scar tissue deposited in the connective tissue of your joints, you get arthritis. It's a similar problem in the penis." Sometimes this buildup of scar tissue causes a telltale bend, or curvature, in the penis (which appears only during erection). It may also manifest itself as palpable or painful lumps—which may be terrifying for a man to discover. "Many men worry that they have penile cancer," says Jarow, "but we can tell just by examining them exactly what it is." He hastens to reassure his patients that although the disorder may be annoying, it is not life-threatening: "Men aren't going to live any longer or shorter because of it."

Although nobody knows what causes Peyronie's disease, scientists believe that it's related to a series of minor injuries—or, as Jarow explains, "wear and tear." One theory "is that it's due to repetitive, minimal trauma to the penis from buckling that occurs when you're attempting sexual relations with an incomplete erection, and that this repetitive trauma leads to buildup of scar tissue." Peyronie's disease appears to be more common among men who have ED, notes Jarow. "It's not clear whether it's secondary to some of the treatments, such as vacuum erection devices or injection therapy, or whether it's due to having erection problems to begin with and is independent of the treatment."

In a study of sixty-four radical prostatectomy patients, three men developed "rapid appearance of new-onset Peyronie's disease" after surgery, says Jarow. "This sounds very low. But if you compare that to the incidence of Peyronie's disease in the general population, it's one-thousand-fold greater."

In some men, there may be an inherited component to Peyronie's disease (as there is with other connective tissue disorders). Jarow is seeking men with a family history of the disease in hopes of finding genetic proof. "If we can understand the mechanism behind Peyronie's disease, we may be able to prevent it in men undergoing radical prostatectomy in the future, as well as in other men."

The good news is that Peyronie's disease does not progress forever. "In some men [fewer than 20 percent], it goes away completely by itself," says Jarow. "For most people, it eventually stabilizes. The pain goes away. The lump becomes less prominent, and the curvature lessens. In just about everybody, the disease process, the deposition of scar tissue, stops with time."

Men who were fully potent when the disease began generally remain so, Jarow notes. "In other words, erection problems—specifically, problems with rigidity—are a rare result of Peyronie's disease in general." But most men who have had a radical prostatectomy have at least some temporary trouble with erection; thus, treatment depends on a man's specific symptoms.

"If a man's problem is curvature—if the penis is bent so he cannot engage in sexual activity or it's uncomfortable to his partner—then we can do an outpatient surgical procedure to straighten the penis," says Jarow. "If, however, he has significant curvature that prevents sexual relations and problems with rigidity, then he's treated with insertion of a penile prosthesis combined with penile straightening," also an outpatient procedure. If a man simply has erection problems but no serious curvature, he is "treated like anyone else with an erection problem, starting with pills, then shots, then the vacuum device, then, if necessary, a penile prosthesis."

can achieve an erection is with direct sexual stimulation. This changes the sequence of events. Before surgery, visual or psychogenic stimuli would bring on an erection, which led to interest in sexual activity. Now, men need sexual stimulation to produce an erection sufficient for intercourse. Over time, psychogenic erections almost always return. For now, you will need to be proactive. In other words, you and your partner need to bypass the brain as an instigator or even a middleman and speak directly to the penis. Thus, don't be afraid to experiment with sexual activity.

If you have a partial erection, go ahead and attempt intercourse— vaginal stimulation is the best stimulation to improve your erection. So don't wait until you have the perfect erection. (If you do, you could be waiting a long time and missing out on this important aspect of your life.) Use whatever erection you have to attempt vaginal penetration; you will probably find that the erection soon becomes much firmer. The use of lubricants such as Astroglide (available at most drugstores) also will help tremendously. Remember, you can have an orgasm even without an erection (and don't be surprised that it is dry—see above).

Early on, however, erections are often not sufficient for traditional vaginal penetration. One common reason for this is the venous leakage described above. Even though the arteries are doing their job and filling the penis with blood, producing a partial erection, the veins aren't keeping the blood trapped inside the penis. To improve this situation, many men find that if they attempt sexual activity standing up, they'll be able to achieve a much firmer erection. (The escaping blood has to travel all the way back up to the heart, and this takes longer if a man is standing up than if he's lying down.) Sexual activity can continue either while a man remains standing or while he's kneeling. Also, it may help to attempt entry from behind; the vagina opens more easily if a woman is bending forward.

Another way to combat venous leakage is for men to place a soft tourniquet at the base of the penis before they begin foreplay or sexual stimulation. The purpose of the tourniquet is to keep blood in the penis once the stimulation causes the arteries to dilate and penile blood flow to increase. The tourniquet doesn't impede blood flow into the penis; it just keeps it from going back out. You can achieve the same effect with a rubber band, a ponytail holder, an O-ring that you can buy in a hardware store, or—if you're brave enough to venture into a novelty store—a device called an erection ring.

## To Sum Up

The return of sexual potency is different in every man. For some men, it can take as long as four years for full potency to return. For others, intercourse is possible just a few weeks after surgery. In any case, you don't have to wait for the penis to become erect on its own.

It's worth repeating that almost all men who can't obtain an erection after radical prostatectomy still have normal penile sensation and are able to achieve a normal orgasm. Therefore, even if you are not having erections—and even if you need some extra help—your recovery of sexual function is almost certain. Take heart. As for the extra help you may need, there are five basic approaches, discussed below.

## Loss of Potency After Radiation Therapy

Radiation's effect on potency is much more gradual than surgery's immediate impact. Sexual function may be fine immediately after radiation therapy. However, ED may develop gradually over the next one or two years. The slow, late progression of ED has been blamed on radiation damage to the arteries that provide blood to the penis. However, there is some recent evidence that radiation also may damage the neurovascular bundles, especially after brachytherapy. In an effort to protect these delicate nerves and reduce the chances of impotence, radiotherapists are developing new ways to estimate the amount of radiation delivered to this area.

## Solutions to the Problem of ED

Before we go any further, let's just say right here that some men have very little sexual activity before treatment for prostate cancer and frankly aren't that interested afterward. That's very common, particularly in older men, and there is absolutely nothing wrong with a man who is not concerned about having an erection.

However, many men who were very sexually active before treatment want this part of their lives to continue. What's next? The first thing that needs to happen is that you need to involve your partner. The worst thing you can do—take it from a doctor who has seen the unnecessarily devastating effect ED can have on patients' relationships—is to clam up; wrap yourself up in shame, self-pity, failure, anger, or any other negative emotion you can think of; retreat to a distant corner of the bed; sulk; agonize; and not talk to your partner about this. Your partner should understand what's going on and should be part of the solution.

Second, as mentioned above, experiment early (as soon as four weeks after surgery, sooner after radiation treatment). Anything you can do to bring new blood into the penis will speed up your recovery of spontaneous erections. Many men don't understand this. They don't want to use a crutch because they think it will slow down the body's own efforts to recover potency. This is hogwash. Think of it, if you will, as recovering from any other injury—a broken leg, for example. At first, crutches are necessary. Two of them. Then, as you get stronger, maybe you taper down to one crutch, then a cane. Then you walk, run, and join a marathon, if you wish. The same is true for sexual activity. Experiment early—with a tourniquet, O-ring, or elastic band, if necessary—and if you need more help, we suggest the following crutches, in this order:

- ED drugs—phosphodiesterase inhibitors, such as Viagra, Cialis, and Levitra
- Intraurethral therapy
- Penile injection therapy
- Vacuum erection devices
- Penile prostheses (implants)

We suggest you begin with a pharmacological approach—ED drugs, such as Viagra (sildenafil), Cialis (tadalafil), and Levitra (vardenafil); intraurethral therapy; or an injection—because these truly bring new blood flow into the penis and are most likely to jump-start the spontaneous recovery of erections. Some men worry that if they start using some of these approaches, they will always need them— they'll become dependent on them, and spontaneous sexual activity will never return. *This couldn't be farther from the truth. These approaches will actually speed up recovery by bringing in blood flow to the penis.* Think of them as a crutch. Once spontaneous activity begins to recover, you can throw them away.

### ED Drugs

Phosphodiesterase inhibitors—including Viagra, Cialis, and Levitra— are a remarkable breakthrough. (Note: Although they are similar, these drugs are not all the same, and one of them may turn out to be more effective for you than another.) They work very well in many men after radiation therapy and in men after radical prostatectomy, too— but *only if the neurovascular bundles have been spared.* (Investigators who report that ED drugs aren't terribly effective after radical prostatectomy are probably working with men who did not undergo an effective nerve-sparing operation.)

ED drugs have been called wonder drugs. What does this mean? Will they put a spring in your step, revitalize your relationship, pay your bills, and generally solve all your problems? No. Are they instant erection pills? No. Contrary to the plots of some recent TV sitcoms, and despite many a comedian's monologue, taking one of these drugs is not followed by a hearty "boing!" Instead, to understand what happens, we need to take a brief look at the biochemistry of erection.

Several years ago, researchers discovered that the chemical messenger, or neurotransmitter, nitric oxide plays a crucial role in erection. We discussed this briefly above, but here are some of the nitty-gritty details. When a man is sexually stimulated, tiny nerve endings in the penis release nitric oxide, which causes the smooth muscle tissue in the penis to relax and the blood vessels to dilate. If an erection, like every chemical process in the body, is a domino effect, or cascade of events, then nitric oxide is roughly step one. For the next link in the chain, nitric oxide activates another chemical switch, called cyclic GMP—known in scientific terms as the second messenger; this is the active agent within the blood vessels and smooth muscles that causes the dilation and relaxation. Here, we might consider cyclic GMP to be the gasoline running the engine. How much cyclic GMP you have determines how strong your erection is and how long it lasts. Obviously, erections aren't meant to last forever, so there is also an off switch—another chemical, an enzyme called phosphodiesterase. Now, cyclic GMP is active in many organs of the body, and the off switch phosphodiesterase comes in many forms, each specifically targeted to various tissues. In the penis, the particular type of phosphodiesterase that's active is called type 5. ED drugs act by blocking the action of type 5 phosphodiesterase (which is why you may also see them referred to as "PDE-5 inhibitors"). In this way, they amplify the action of whatever cyclic GMP is present.

## Side Effects

Most ED drugs have little effect on other tissues in the body—except for Viagra, which temporarily causes minor vision disturbances (a blue color is seen by 3 percent of men who take it). This is because Viagra also affects type 6 phosphodiesterase, which is in the cones of the retina. The other major problem with these drugs affects men who are taking a form of nitrate—nitroglycerin, for instance—for heart disease. Both ED drugs and nitroglycerin can lower your blood pressure; together, they can lower it to a dangerous level.

Otherwise, the list of side effects for these drugs is relatively modest. Most common are headaches (in 16 percent), flushing (in 10 percent) and an upset stomach (in 7 percent); men also may experience muscle aches, back pain, and a runny nose. (Flushing is more common with Viagra and Levitra; muscle aches and back pain are more common with Cialis.)

How well do ED drugs work after radical prostatectomy? At Johns Hopkins, in the experience of men who are unable to have intercourse more than one year after an operation in which both neurovascular bundles were spared, 80 percent are able to have successful intercourse after treatment with an ED drug. But again, not only are these not instant erection pills, they may not even work very well in the first few months or even the first year after surgery. We think this is because the nerves are temporarily paralyzed. However, as these nerves recover, ED drugs work better and better. Thus, if you take an ED drug six weeks after surgery and it doesn't work, you should try again every month until it does.

Also, be sure you're taking it right. All of these drugs begin to work within about twenty minutes. But if you take an ED drug with food, especially fatty food, this can delay stomach emptying so that the drug just trickles in small amounts into the small intestine and never reaches the high blood levels necessary to facilitate an erection. This problem is most evident with Viagra, less so with Levitra, and not a problem with Cialis. The reason for this relates to each drug's length of action. The effect of Cialis can be felt for as long as thirty-six hours; thus, it lingers in the bloodstream for a long time. Levitra can last as long as eight hours. The most fleeting drug here is Viagra, which only lasts about two hours, at most. Thus, for Viagra to work, it needs to reach a high level in the blood fairly quickly, and if there's fatty food in the stomach (or a big meal of any kind or one rich in dairy products), this just won't happen. If you're going to take Viagra on a full stomach, you might as well not take it at all; it's a waste. Viagra works best on an empty stomach. Then, it takes about an hour to reach its peak strength in the blood. At this point, a man needs to have sexual stimulation. (Remember, immediately after surgery, just thinking about sex isn't going to be enough. Here, sexual stimulation needs to be tactile.) Soaking in hot water increases blood flow in the pelvis; this might be a good way to spend the hour between the time you take Viagra and you attempt intercourse. (This has also been reported to improve the effectiveness of MUSE—see below.) Remember, Viagra does not create an erection; it only facilitates one.

### What Dose Should I Take, and When Should I Begin Taking It After Surgery?

As long as you have no contraindication (medical reason not to use a drug), it makes sense to start out with the maximum dose. For Viagra, that's 100 mg, and for Levitra and Cialis, it's 20 mg. If the drug works at that dose but there are side effects, you can always try taking less. The most cost-effective way to do this is to get a pill cutter (available at drugstores and at many online health stores) and just split the pills in half. The next question is, how often should you take it? Some doctors believe that you should take one of these every night or every other night, for the first year after surgery. I encouraged my patients to do this for a while and did not see any dramatic effect; I've been told by a respected colleague in Europe that he had a similar finding. Thus, I think that it's probably best to take an ED drug as needed for sexual activity. However, there is no question that by bringing blood flow into the penis, it does help rehabilitate and encourage recovery of erectile function. Whether you decide to take one every day, every other night, or as needed, I strongly encourage you to begin taking an ED drug about four weeks after surgery.

### Who Should Not Take ED Drugs?

If you have any history of cardiovascular disease, retinitis pigmentosa, or significant liver or kidney disease, talk to your doctor before you take ED drugs. Despite the fact that they're mainly targeted at the penis, ED drugs are not safe for men with certain medical conditions.

*Do not take Viagra if:*

- You are taking any form of nitrate, such as nitroglycerin.
- You have had an irregular heartbeat or heart attack in the last six months.

- You have low blood pressure (lower than 90/50 mm Hg).
- You have high blood pressure (greater than 170/110 mm Hg).
- You have congestive heart failure or chest pain.
- You have retinitis pigmentosa.

ED drugs are broken down by an enzyme in the liver. If you have severe liver dysfunction, the action of these drugs may be prolonged severely. Also, the breakdown of ED drugs can be delayed significantly by eating grapefruit or drinking grapefruit-containing juices or by taking drugs such as cimetidine (Tagamet), ketoconazole (Nizoral), erythromycin, or protease inhibitors (for the treatment of HIV). If you fall into one of these categories, you must discuss the risks of taking an ED drug with your internist first.

Some men who have used ED drugs to have intercourse have had heart attacks and died. This is probably not a direct effect of the drug, but was probably related to the exercise associated with intercourse. Many men who have heart disease do not exercise or don't exercise regularly. These are the weekend warriors who have heart attacks after exertion they're not accustomed to—playing pickup basketball, perhaps, or shoveling snow or moving heavy furniture. If these men have ED, they may rarely experience intercourse and the sexual excitement that goes with it. However, if ED drugs make them able to have intercourse and this causes them to exercise to a point where they shouldn't, this is probably the reason for the heart attacks. The safest bet for you is to talk to your doctor first. If you can't exercise or you have any other limitations on your physical activity, do not take an ED drug.

## Which ED Drug Works Best?

There have been no good comparisons of all three drugs done in a single study. It's safe to say that all of them are effective and that one drug may work better for one man and another for a different man. Indeed, it may be that there are genetic variations in the phosphodiesterase type 5 enzyme that may influence the way each man responds to and tolerates these drugs. Because Cialis has a window of thirty-six hours, it is associated with less planning and pressure on the partner. Some doctors believe that Levitra may have fewer side effects. Which one

## WILL IT MAKE ME GO BLIND?

In 2005, a scary story made the news—a published study of about thirty men who developed blindness soon after taking Viagra. This frightened many men (and activated several personal-injury law firms, who advertise class-action lawsuits against Pfizer, the maker of Viagra, on the Internet). But this blindness occurred in thirty men out of about *twenty million* who had taken the drug. The study's investigators identified that this problem occurred *only* in men who had NAION (nonarteritic anterior ischemic optic neuropathy), which is the most common acute optic nerve disease in adults over age fifty. Its typical victims are people with other health complications—such as diabetes, hypertension, coronary artery disease, or hyperlipidimia—and people who smoke.

Fortunately, if you are a smoker or if you have one of these conditions and are worried that you might be at risk for NAION, you don't have to wait for it to happen. You should go to an ophthalmologist and be examined for the anatomical abnormality that leads to this problem; it's called low cup-to-disc ratio, or crowded disc. It is not known for certain whether taking Viagra absolutely caused the blindness in these thirty men or whether they would have developed it eventually because they had this abnormality and were at high risk. But if you turn out to have this predisposing factor, which may affect one or both eyes, you should seek your opthalmologist's advice before you take an ED drug.

should you get? The best way to find out is to get samples of all three from your urologist. Try each one to see which works best for you—and give each more than one chance. Just because it doesn't work the first time, you may find that in a different setting—possibly with a more empty stomach, for instance—one may work better than another. We are fortunate to have three effective drugs to choose from.

### How Long Will I Have to Stay on an ED Drug?

In a study of men after radical prostatectomy who were taking Viagra, at three years, 71 percent were still responding to the drug. Of the remaining patients, half of the men stopped taking it because of the return of normal erections, and the other half stopped because the drug didn't seem to help anymore. These results suggest that the vast majority of men with erectile dysfunction after radical prostatectomy who initially respond to ED drugs continue to do so at three years and are satisfied with the effect.

## Other Pharmacological Approaches

New medications not yet commercially available may join the market within a few years. One is an oral form of phentolamine (Regitine). Another is apomorphine (Apokyn), a drug that acts centrally in the brain as a dopamine agonist. Apomorphine has been reported to induce erections in as many as 60 percent of men with ED. However, it has undesirable side effects that are not conducive to romance—mainly, the fact that many men who take it become nauseated or vomit. Also, it appears that a drug called a melanocyte-stimulating hormone (MSH) may have a powerful effect on libido. As we mentioned earlier, many men, for reasons that are unclear, state that their libido is reduced after treatment for prostate cancer. One reason for this is depression, and antidepressants can be of great help here. There is a new superpotent MSH analog that has been effective in inducing erections in early studies, even in men with psychogenic ED.

### In the Future

We've talked about why injury to the nerves that control erection can cause ED. A number of experimental studies currently under way are aimed at preserving these nerves. In animals, several studies have shown that growth factors may enhance the recovery of nerve function more rapidly. There is also some exciting evidence that gene therapy may one day be used to transfer growth factors directly into the penis and boost nerve stimulation.

New methods of application are also under study. Scientists are working on a topical approach—salves or gels that contain vasodilators (drugs that cause blood vessels to open up) such as prostaglandin (Alprostadil), papaverine (Pavabid, a calcium channel–blocker derived from the opium poppy), or nitroglycerin.

## Intraurethral Therapy

Another type of pharmacologic treatment is the use of agents that can be placed directly into the urethra. One of these is called

MUSE (medicated urethral system for erection), a tiny suppository that contains a vasodilator called prostaglandin E1 (Alprostadil). The best thing about MUSE is that it's easy to administer. First, urinate (to empty and moisten the urethra). Then, place a suppository into the end of the urethra while you are standing. Then, massage the penis for fifteen minutes while the drug is absorbed; it may help to use a tourniquet at the base of the penis as well. MUSE works in about 40 percent of patients. However—and this is a big "however"—MUSE probably won't be ideal for many men after radical prostatectomy. For some reason, prostaglandin E1 often causes severe pain in men who have undergone a radical prostatectomy. But men who have ED for other reasons (including ED after radiation therapy) do not experience such pain, and for these men, it can be a valuable resource.

## Penile Injection Therapy

Injection therapy is one of the best ways to bring new blood flow into the penis and encourage the recovery of sexual function. Again, the ideal situation is that you won't need this forever—consider it a crutch or a jump-start, as described above, until your body recovers enough to handle erection on its own.

How does it work? The keys to a normal erection are for the arteries to open and fill the penis with blood and for the veins to close, so the blood can't escape the penis. The smooth muscle tissue also needs to relax. Several drugs can produce erections by making these events happen; most of these are in a class of drugs called alphablockers, which are used to treat some forms of hypertension and also to treat benign prostatic hyperplasia (BPH). They are vasodilators; they open up blood vessels, making a wider channel for blood to go through. They also cause the smooth muscle tissue to relax and the veins to close. The main advantage here is that these drugs produce an absolutely normal erection. Some of these erection-producing drugs include papaverine (Pavabid), phentolamine (Regitine), and prostaglandin E1 (Alprostadil).

It usually takes less than five minutes for one of these drugs to work, and the erection can last as long as a couple of hours. It will be important for your doctor to determine the lowest possible dose you need to achieve an erection; this will help reduce the risk of side effects. Other ways to help lessen side effects include limiting injections to no more than once a day and using an insulin syringe (which has a smaller needle than many syringes) to minimize pain and bleeding from the injection site. Also, you should compress the site where the needle went in for three minutes after the injection; this also helps reduce bleeding and tissue damage.

Again, a common side effect for men after radical prostatectomy is that prostaglandin E1 treatment is often very painful. These men should ask their physician to prescribe a different blend of injection, called Tri-Mix, which contains papavarine, phentolamine, and smaller amounts of prostaglandin E1. This may reduce the pain considerably.

Penile injection is not for everybody. These erection-producing agents may not help men with vascular problems. However, they do work in most patients. Because of the nature of this therapy—giving the penis a shot—it obviously is not ideal for men who can't see well, men with poor hand-eye coordination, or men who are very overweight. Also, because many erection-producing drugs reduce blood pressure, this therapy can cause problems for some men with heart disease.

One side effect is that if the injection is too strong, it can produce a prolonged erection that may require medical therapy to be relieved. Some doctors ask patients who opt for penile injections to sign a consent form because of some other side effects—some of them long-term—associated with the injections. These can include tiny blood clots, burning pain after injection, damage to the urethra, or minor infection. But the worst is that in some men, over time, painless, fibrous knots of tissue build up in the corpora cavernosa, which can cause the penis to become curved. (For more on this condition, also called Peyronie's disease, see above.) Doctors aren't entirely sure why this happens; it may be related to the frequency of injection, the strength or dosage of the drug used, and the amount of bleeding resulting from the shots. Some doctors believe compressing the site at the time of injection may be critical to minimizing this risk; also, keeping the dosage to a minimum or using a blend of several drugs may help.

## Vacuum Erection Devices

The idea here is to create suction using an airtight tube that is placed temporarily around the penis. An attached pump withdraws air, creating reduced atmospheric pressure—a vacuum—around the penis, causing it to become engorged with blood. The penis becomes erect. Then a constricting ring, like a rubber band around the neck of a balloon, keeps the blood trapped in the penis so the erection can be sustained. (This imitates the clamping action of the veins in normal erection.) It usually takes about five minutes to produce the erection, and it generally lasts for about half an hour. (The erection probably shouldn't last much longer than that; leaving the constricting band on too long can cause distention or swelling due to fluid retention in the penis.)

This erection is not quite the same as a normal erection—it begins only above the constricting band. But it is sufficient for successful intercourse. However, the penis is usually cold and sometimes numb, and from the man's standpoint, the erection is often less than desirable. Also, because this approach does not bring new blood flow into the penis, it may not do much to facilitate the recovery process. Vacuum devices have few complications; these can include trouble with ejaculation, pain in the penis, and tiny, pinpoint-sized bruises. (Men taking aspirin or other blood-thinning medications may be more likely to experience such complications.) Some men are highly satisfied with the result of vacuum devices; others are not.

## Penile Prostheses (Implants)

Penile implants, or prostheses, are available in several varieties; the simplest are bendable, and the more complicated ones are inflatable or mechanical. The implants are not a new idea, but they have improved considerably since they were first introduced about thirty years ago. The bendable prostheses, for example, were exactly the same size all the time—whether or not the penis was in the erect position—which, as you can imagine, often proved awkward in social settings. Earlier models of the inflatable prostheses that did allow for a nonerect size sometimes failed to work and needed to be replaced.

If these relatively clumsy but functional early designs were the prosthetic equivalent of the typewriter, then the latest models are more like a Macintosh—sleek, sophisticated, and user-friendly. They are more reliable, easier for surgeons to implant, and designed to look more natural in the nonerect phase—even the bendable prostheses, which are more malleable than before. And they can restore sexual function entirely to normal.

Now, most prostheses are implanted into the penis through an incision in the scrotum. Some of the more complicated devices involve a pump and a reservoir for fluid, housed in the abdomen or scrotum, and inflatable chambers, which are placed in the corpora cavernosa. (Fluid is pumped into the penis to create an erection and is held there by a valve. Afterward, the valve is released, and the fluid returns to the reservoir.)

Penile prostheses used to be offered routinely to most impotent men. Now, with other good treatments available, many urologists have come to regard penile prostheses as a last resort because they do involve surgery—and thus they carry the risk of complications. These can include infection, scarring, damage within the corpora cavernosa, or a problem with any part of the prosthesis. However, these side effects are relatively rare. Most men who have penile prostheses are satisfied with the result and have a normal sex life.

Prostate cancer is tough on everybody. Wives, partners, and family members feel the stress of prostate cancer and treatment, too. You're all sharing the burden of this disease. Your priorities change, your focus shifts, and your usual best lifeline—each other—may temporarily flag from the physical and emotional stress. The worst thing you can do during this recovery process is try to go it alone. The best thing you can do is talk about it with each other, your doctor, other patients and their partners, a counselor, or a member of the clergy. And go back and read this chapter over again, as many times as you need to, because it is full of hope. Be patient. You *will* get your life back.

# 12

# HELP FOR ADVANCED PROSTATE CANCER

## ▶▶▶ READ THIS FIRST

As you are reading this, scientists are working on the cure for advanced prostate cancer. Research on advanced prostate cancer has exploded with whole new classes of innovative, cancer-fighting drugs and treatments targeted at various stages of the disease. Perhaps even more exciting, scientists are rethinking their strategies for giving these drugs—going after prostate cancer when it is still relatively young and vulnerable, hitting it hard, and hoping to change the course of the disease. The bottom line: even when cancer has escaped the prostate, there is still much hope—more now than ever before.

### HORMONAL THERAPY

The mainstay for the management of advanced disease is hormonal therapy—shutting down the hormones that feed the prostate and nourish the cancer. Unfortunately, some prostate cancer cells aren't affected by hormonal therapy at all. These are called hormone-resistant (or androgen-independent) cells.

When a man starts hormonal therapy, the early results are successful and highly encouraging: the tumor shrinks, prostate-specific antigen (PSA) levels drop in the blood, and the patient feels better. When this happens, many men rejoice, believing the cancer cells to be utterly defeated. But only the hormone-dependent cancer cells have been affected, and the drop in PSA level may be misleading. So when PSA falls, it signals that the cancer is responding to treatment—which is good, but it's no guarantee that the cancer is completely gone. The cancer cells that have nothing to do with hormones are unaffected by them.

There are several forms of hormonal therapy, which can be used individually or in combination. They are all designed to accomplish the same goal: to lower testosterone levels in the blood. The most direct and least expensive way to control testosterone is to surgically remove a man's testicles; this is called an orchiectomy, or surgical castration. The same effect can be accomplished medically with drugs called LHRH (luteinizing hormone-releasing hormone) agonists, LHRH antagonists, or antiandrogens. For obvious reasons, this is the most popular approach today.

## WHEN SHOULD YOU BEGIN HORMONAL THERAPY?

First, if you have metastases to bone, bone pain, or a large mass of cancer that is obstructing your kidneys or bladder, you need to start hormonal therapy now. In this situation, hormonal therapy is the right course of action—one that can make a huge difference in your quality of life and can protect your body from the ravages of cancer.

But what if you have no cancer in your bones and no sign that anything is wrong, except a rising PSA level after surgery or radiation or the presence of cancer in your lymph nodes, and you feel fine? Many doctors would advise you to start hormonal therapy as soon as possible. Others—and I'm in this group—believe that there is no evidence that starting hormonal therapy immediately, as opposed to later, will prolong life. But doesn't early hormonal therapy delay the progression of cancer? The answer is yes and no. It delays your *knowledge* of progression. Hormonal therapy does two things. It stops cells from making PSA, and it shrinks the hormone-sensitive cell population; a man's PSA falls, and it takes longer for his bone scan to become positive for metastases. But it doesn't stop the clock; the hormone-insensitive cells continue to grow silently.

## WHAT ELSE IS THERE BESIDES HORMONES?

Many new drugs—and these are a far cry from the old chemotherapy drugs with their buckshot approach—killing everything, good and bad, in range while having a limited effect on prostate cancer. These new treatments work like high-powered rifles with only one target in their sights: prostate cancer cells. They're specifically designed to target the biological mechanisms involved in cancer progression and metastasis. They can be grouped based on their mode of attack. The most exciting strategies are immunotherapy, gene therapy, drugs that put roadblocks in the way of cancer's progress and keep it from invading other tissues, drugs that slow down the cancer growth rate, and drugs that interfere with the way cancer cells communicate. As these new treatments become available, scientists and clinical doctors are figuring out the smartest ways to use them. For example, vaccines are more likely to work when the tumor burden is very low; angiogenesis inhibitors are more effective before metastases are evident. We are rapidly approaching an entirely new era of cancer treatments.

### COMPLEMENTARY MEDICINE

Can changing your diet help slow down the progression of prostate cancer? We don't know. It is not reasonable to assume that diet can reverse cancer after the fact—that it can "unring the bell." However, it may help. If you want to change your diet to reduce your intake of fat and increase your intake of soy, you should do it. But be careful not to lose too much weight too quickly. A rapid 10 percent drop in your weight can compromise your immune system, which may be the main self-defense mechanism holding your cancer in check.

A final word for caregivers: take care of yourself, too. You need your strength—emotional as well as physical—now more than ever. We have some advice for you in this chapter, too.

## Revolution in Treating Advanced Prostate Cancer

As you are reading this, scientists are working on finding the cure for advanced prostate cancer. There have never been so many promising drugs being developed for prostate cancer, and never before have doctors been so hopeful about their ability to help men with advanced disease—cancer that either has spread beyond the prostate or cancer that has returned after surgery or radiation.

Research on advanced prostate cancer has expanded with whole new classes of innovative, cancer-fighting drugs and treatments targeted at various stages of the disease. Perhaps even more exciting, scientists are rethinking their strategies for giving these drugs. Armed with the guidelines (discussed in chapter 10) that, for the first time, allow doctors and patients to predict what will happen if a man's PSA returns after treatment, oncologists, radiation oncologists, and urologists are working together to go after prostate cancer when it is still relatively young and vulnerable, hitting it hard and hoping to change the course of the disease.

What a difference in hope this is from even a few years ago! Traditionally, oncologists began chemotherapy in men with advanced prostate cancer only after other treatment—surgery or radiation followed (sometimes even years afterward, when men developed symptoms of advanced cancer) by hormonal therapy—failed to control the cancer. But over the last few years—in breast and colon cancer, as well as prostate cancer—there has been a sea change in scientific thinking. As the Johns Hopkins oncologist Mario Eisenberger puts it, "Why should we wait until it's a last-ditch effort? Why not go all out first? This is the main principle behind most clinical trials."

In the past, oncologists have been unwilling to take a man who is, for all practical purposes, healthy—who has steadily increasing PSA levels, but no other symptoms of disease—and make him sick. Chemotherapy drugs have been notorious for their side effects, which often include vomiting, hair loss, and debilitating fatigue.

But the newest generations of drugs have fewer side effects. They're smarter and more specific, and many of them are aimed at containing prostate cancer rather than eradicating it. Most are less toxic than conventional chemotherapy and can be taken orally, with no need for hospitalization. There are many new treatment approaches, but the basic ideas are to stabilize the disease and inhibit growth. "So ideally, in men with minimal disease, they may delay further progression of cancer and thus the development of symptoms. And if they're used in men with more advanced disease who are well, these men may *stay well for a longer period of time*," says the Johns Hopkins oncologist Michael Carducci.

Carducci and Eisenberger, a pioneer in developing and refining drugs to treat prostate cancer, have identified key groups of men with advanced prostate cancer, all of whom have different needs and who probably respond best to different drugs.

- Men who have undergone surgery who have been identified as having a high risk of cancer recurrence.
- Men who have undergone surgery and/or radiation who have a detectable PSA level, but no other evidence that the cancer has spread.

- Men with metastatic disease in whom hormonal therapy has lost its effectiveness (this is also called hormone-refractory cancer).

"Most of the drugs have traditionally been developed and tested in this last group of men," says Carducci. "But increasingly, the drugs are showing few or limited side effects, and laboratory models suggest that they work best in patients who have hardly any disease."

The bottom line, to paraphrase a popular saying, is that it's not your father's prostate cancer anymore—at every step of the way. Even when cancer has escaped the prostate, there is still much hope—more now than ever before. We will cover these and other new approaches in this chapter.

## Treatment of Advanced Prostate Cancer: An Overview

As we will discuss in depth, the mainstay for the management of advanced disease today is hormonal therapy. But before we begin to talk about it, let us add that all of us who treat prostate cancer hope that this will not be the case forever—or even for very many more years. Obviously, the best thing would be to prevent prostate cancer from ever developing. We're not there yet, either, but we're closer. The next best thing would be to catch it in every man while it's still confined to the prostate and to cure it with surgery or radiation. And the next best thing after that would be to find a way to stop the cancer, to stop whatever feeds it, to stop it from spreading—or, if it has spread, to kill it where it lies. One thought is that we might control prostate cancer—as we do diabetes and heart disease—with some form of daily medication to keep it in check. Another thought is that we might be able to treat it for a time with a medical version of the weed killer Roundup—kill the cancer by preventing it from getting nourishment—and then not even need to use further medication. (We will talk about some promising drugs that work along both of these lines, along with many others, later in this chapter.) With these scenarios, men would not need long-term hormonal therapy. And doctors would rejoice right alongside their patients, because we hate it, too.

*Nobody* likes hormonal therapy. But we prescribe it because it works. For some men, it can work for many years. Hormonal therapy

## WHAT IS METASTASIS?

We've used this word a lot in the book, along with its plural form, metastases—another pair of words doctors use interchangeably. When a person develops a metastasis, we say the cancer metastasizes.) And you probably know that it means cancer that has spread to a distant site, using the body's own transportation routes—the bloodstream or lymph nodes. But what does this mean for you?

First, having advanced prostate cancer doesn't necessarily mean that you have *any* obvious metastases. In fact, you may have no symptoms associated with advanced cancer for years. The only indication that you still have prostate cancer hiding somewhere in your body may be that you have an elevated or rising PSA level, and *by itself, this is nothing to be afraid of.* Crazy PSA numbers can't kill you. "It's not like blood sugar, or potassium, or poisonous chemicals," notes the Johns Hopkins oncologist Mario Eisenberger. "It will not, by itself, make you feel sick." It's just something we measure.

Metastasis is a process, and in prostate cancer, as compared to other forms of cancer, it usually happens slowly. For example, in lung or colon cancer, cancer cells that are on the move can reach other organs in weeks or months. But in prostate cancer, this same process can take years. The good news is that, for most men, even if your PSA level is on the rise, "there is ample opportunity to try standard and experimental treatments," says Eisenberger, "and still allow our patients to spend many productive years in their work and with their loved ones." (See If My PSA Begins to Rise After Surgery, Will My Bone Scan Be Normal? and Table 10.1 in chapter 10.)

But when prostate cancer does metastasize, it seems to make a beeline for bone. Some men wonder if this means they then have bone cancer; it does not. The cancer in the bone is still prostate cancer; if you were to have it biopsied, a pathologist would see prostate cancer cells in there. This cancer still makes PSA, and it would have a Gleason score, except we don't assign a Gleason score when a biopsy is done outside of the prostate gland. When metastasis does happen, a man's PSA level can skyrocket—over 25 ng/ml is common, and some men have PSA levels in the hundreds or even thousands. And yet—here's a paradox—some men with the most aggressive tumors can have low PSA levels. This is because these tumors are working so hard to cause trouble that they have little energy left over to make PSA.

Prostate cancer also may spread to the liver or lung. A man's symptoms usually tell us where the metastasis is; for example, if it's in the bones, the patient can usually feel it. But not always; some men who have bone involvement may have other problems instead or in addition.

If the bone marrow is affected, a man may become anemic (develop a low red blood cell count), which can cause fatigue, weakness, and shortness of breath. If it's in the liver, a man may feel nothing but may experience unexplained weight loss, a decrease in appetite, and nausea. If it's in the lungs, he may feel shortness of breath or chest pain, or develop a cough.

But most prostate cancer metastases are in the bone and bone marrow. In 90 percent of men with metastases, the bone is the main site; 20 percent of men have lymph node involvement, and only about 5 to 10 percent have metastases in vital organs such as the liver or lung. Why is this? There's something about the bone and bone marrow that prostate cancer cells are drawn to, says Eisenberger. "Prostate cancer cells establish a direct line of communication with the bone and bone marrow, telling them—sometimes in advance—what they would like to have in place in order to grow and spread further. The bone, in turn, will see that this is done very early and will do everything it can to create and maintain optimal conditions."

But now that we know this, we can use it as a weapon. "In fact," Eisenberger continues, "one major strategy to treat prostate cancer today is to target the bone to prevent the growth of the cancer, simply by changing the environment. Studies are now being conducted to test bone-targeted approaches even before the cancer cells reach it. This is very important, because one of our major tools to treat advanced prostate cancer, hormonal therapy, can eventually weaken the bone and create a favorable environment for the cancer cells to grow." (Bone-targeted strategies are discussed later in the chapter.)

means shutting down the hormones that feed the prostate and sustain the cancer. (Note: Androgens are male hormones, and many doctors use these two words interchangeably. This may be confusing; hormonal therapy is also called hormone or androgen deprivation, or hormonal or androgen ablation.) Prostate cells need male hormones to grow and develop—think of a houseplant that flourishes because it receives a steady supply of fertilizer. If the supply of hormones is shut off, the normal prostate shrinks but does not disappear. If a houseplant doesn't get fertilizer, it doesn't die, either. It might struggle along on nothing but sunlight and water, but it still hangs in there. Normal prostate cells can survive without hormones, and so can cancerous prostate cells. Not having the hormones is a setback—one from which it can take years for prostate cancer to recover—but it's not a lethal blow. In fact, some prostate cancer cells aren't affected by hormonal therapy at all.

Why doesn't hormonal therapy serve as a knockout punch for prostate cancer? Because prostate cancer is heterogeneous, which means it's a cellular melting pot. It's a bunch of different cell types mixed together. When all of these cells are confined within the prostate, the fact that they're not all alike is not much of an issue. No matter how many different kinds of cells there may be, if they're all in the prostate, *bang*—they're all equally dead when the prostate is surgically removed or effectively irradiated. But when some cancer cells have escaped to distant sites, this diversity becomes a major challenge. A drug or hormone treatment that targets only one kind of cell won't have any effect against another variety; the "one-size-fits-all" approach doesn't work here. Plus, some of these cells have learned to be resistant—to grow in the absence of male hormones. These are called androgen-independent or androgen-insensitive cells. (And cancer that seems to defy hormonal therapy is called hormone-refractory disease.)

When a man starts hormonal therapy, the early results are successful and highly encouraging: the tumor shrinks, PSA level drops in the blood, and the patient feels better. When this happens, many men rejoice, because the cancer cells seem to be utterly defeated. But in the prostate, *only the hormone-dependent cancer cells have been affected*, so the drop in PSA may be misleading. Guess what controls the production of PSA? Hormones. When male hormones are shut off, the PSA-making process may indeed stop, but this doesn't necessarily mean that the cancer cells are dead or that they've stopped growing. In animal models, scientists have shown that cancer cells can continue to grow even when PSA is no longer made. One process has little do to with another; in fact, the nastiest, most malignant cells don't make much PSA anyway. So, when the PSA level falls, it signals that the cancer is responding to treatment—which is good, but it's no guarantee that the cancer is completely gone.

The cancer cells that have nothing to do with hormones just go on about their merry, proliferative business, oblivious to the hormonal war being fought just cells away. Say you had a weed problem in your garden, and instead of spraying Roundup, you sprayed Raid. What effect would this have on the weeds? Not a lot.

Scientists believe that these androgen-independent cells probably inhabit the prostate for years; they don't suddenly appear one day after the cancer is diagnosed. Ultimately, the androgen-independent cells manage to dominate through two different means. One of these is genetic drift. In this case, each time the cancer cells reproduce, or divide, they accumulate more mutations and become increasingly malignant. In the process, cells that used to depend on hormones manage to wean themselves; they learn to survive without them. The other mechanism is called clonal selection. Here, the most malignant cells (which originally may have been in the minority) grow faster than the better-differentiated, more sedate cells. Over time, they overtake these more normal cells. This may actually be aided, inadvertently, by hormonal therapy: the androgen-dependent cells shrink back, and the androgen-independent cells take their place.

## Hormonal Therapy

### *Specific Ways to Control Hormones*

Doctors have long known that hormones play a major role in the life of the prostate. In 1786, an English surgeon named John Hunter became the first to demonstrate in animals that a radical operation—castration—caused the sex accessory tissues, including the prostate, to shrink. But it wasn't until the 1930s that anyone discovered *why* this happened. At the University of Chicago, Charles Huggins discovered that removing the testes shut down production of testosterone. And when shots of testosterone were injected into castrated animals, shrunken sex accessory tissues were restored to normal size and function. This Nobel Prize–winning research resulted in another valuable finding—that castration also could shrink prostate cancer.

Huggins also was able to achieve the same effect chemically; he found he could shut down testosterone with doses of female hormones called estrogens. Estrogens blocked a signal transmitted in the brain by the pituitary gland called luteinizing hormone (LH), which stimulates testosterone. The oral estrogen, called DES (diethylstilbestrol), produces what's known as chemical castration; it lowers testosterone levels, just as removal of the testicles does.

For now, hormonal therapy means one of two main choices: surgical castration, a one-shot treatment; or chemical castration, a lifetime of medication. Loss of sexual function is likely with almost every kind of hormonal therapy; 90 percent of men on hormonal therapy lose sexual drive and the ability to have an erection.

What's the best method of stopping these male hormones? Think of a car going through a series of checkpoints—points A, B, C, and D—to cross over a border into another country. You want to stop this car from reaching the other side. At what point do you stop it? Do you set up a roadblock at point A, the first stop? Or do you wall off the border at point D, so the car can never cross over? Or do you divert the car at some point along the way? The androgens that affect the prostate reach their destination through a multistep process that begins in the brain. Medical roadblocks are now available to stop or detour this process at point A (the brain), point D (the prostate), or several spots in between.

### How Hormonal Therapy Works

Each therapy targets a different link in the chain of hormonal interactions that affect the prostate. Some of them work better than others, and some are more expensive. The chain of hormonal actions is long and complicated; put down on paper, it's a confusing jumble of letters, mostly consonants, that looks like alphabet soup. And if you're like most men, just thinking about this muddle will make your eyes glaze over. But, stripped down to its essential steps, this code is not so tough to crack—you can do it! (And you need to master this information so you can not only understand what your doctor's talking about but help choose the treatment option that's best for you. See fig. 12.1.)

To understand this hormonal chain, let's start at the beginning— the brain, where the hypothalamus makes, among other things, a substance called LHRH (luteinizing hormone–releasing hormone), which acts as a chemical signal. It's dispatched in pulses, like Morse code or flashes of light, to the nearby pituitary gland. Its message? "Make LH and FSH," it tells the pituitary.

LH (luteinizing hormone) and FSH (follicle-stimulating hormone) are other chemical signals, and they bring us to the testicles, or testes, where LH motivates certain cells (called testicular Leydig cells) to make testosterone. (FSH has its major effect on sperm production.)

And testosterone brings us to the prostate. Testosterone circulates

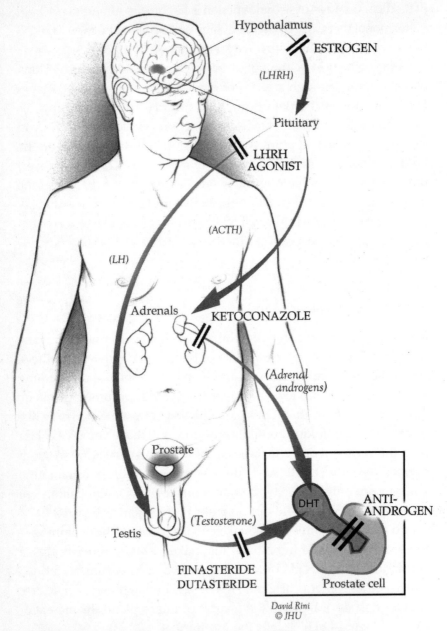

**FIGURE 12.1   Where Men Make Hormones and Where Hormonal Therapies Actually Work**

There are drugs that block either the effect of testosterone and other androgens (anti-androgens dutasteride and finasteride) or the production of testosterone itself (LHRH agonists, estrogens, and ketoconazole).

in the blood and enters the prostate by diffusion, like water through a tea bag. Soon it undergoes a metamorphosis: testosterone is transformed by an enzyme called 5-alpha reductase into a hormone called DHT (dihydrotestosterone)—which is more than twice as powerful as testosterone. Several studies have shown that the prostate contains less 5-alpha reductase when it is cancerous; therefore, DHT is not believed to be as important in prostate cancer as it is in the normal prostate or in benign enlargement of the prostate (BPH). Both testosterone and DHT can bind to the same receptor in the prostate cell, like two different keys fitting the same lock. (DHT *really* binds to it with great affinity; testosterone does not cling as strongly to the receptor.) When DHT or testosterone hooks up to the receptor, this complex attaches to DNA, which then activates certain genes.

Testosterone in the blood circulates back to point A, the hypothalamus, which acts as a thermostat. It measures the level of testosterone and decides whether to boost or cut back on its LHRH production, and the cycle begins all over again (scientists call this a feedback loop).

Also, the adrenal glands, which sit on top of the kidneys, make weak male hormones called adrenal androgens, including androstenedione, dehydroepiandrosterone (DHEA), and dehydroepiandrosterone sulfate (DHEAS), plus small amounts of testosterone. These are minor players, believed to make up only 5 percent or less of the total androgen stimulation to the prostate. Their total effect on the prostate has been a controversial issue (see below).

So there are several potential checkpoints in this chain of events. Currently, hormonal therapy agents can target the hypothalamus (LHRH), the pituitary (LH, FSH), the adrenal gland (adrenal androgens), the testes (testosterone), and the prostate (DHT). They can be used individually or in combination.

## Surgical Castration

The surgical removal of a man's testicles (also called an orchiectomy) is the most direct and least expensive way to control testosterone. As surgical procedures go, it's simple. The operation can be performed under spinal anesthesia (for a description of spinal anesthesia, see chapter 8) or, if the patient is not strong enough to tolerate this, even a local anesthetic. A surgeon makes a small incision in the scrotum and brings out each testicle individually through this opening. Then the surgeon cuts the vas deferens and blood vessels that supply each testicle, and the testicles are removed. Some surgeons perform what's called subcapsular orchiectomy. In this operation, the surgeon opens the lining of the testicles and empties the contents of each one. The lining is closed again, and this empty shell is placed back inside the scrotum—so nothing looks different; in other words, no one can tell from outward appearance that there's nothing inside the scrotum. The basic differences here are cosmetic—and therefore psychological—and for some men, this makes the thought of castration easier to accept.

After surgery, patients usually can go home from the hospital the same day—or, at the very latest, the next day. The only major complication to worry about with surgical castration is bleeding. However, this shouldn't be a problem if the surgeon makes a point of checking that all bleeding is stopped before the scrotum is closed and that a compression dressing is left in place to control the smaller, harder-to-see blood vessels.

Castration works fast; it reduces the body's amount of testosterone by 95 percent almost immediately and permanently. *Boom*; within about three hours of surgery, testosterone levels begin to plummet to a level called the castrate range. This is considered the gold standard, an important point of comparison in monitoring the success of hormonal therapy, as certain drugs are judged by their ability to reduce testosterone to this range.

Some doctors used to believe that several months after castration, the body began producing more testosterone at other sites—and that this was the reason prostate cancer continued to grow. This is not true. There is no delayed increase in testosterone and, anyway, that's not why prostate tumors keep growing. They continue to spread because of the cancer cells that are *not* affected by hormonal therapy.

What happens to the prostate tumor? It begins to shrink, and men with symptoms of obstruction or pain caused by the cancer begin to feel better right away.

Castration's advantages are that it is effective almost immediately and its results are permanent—there's no need to take daily medication. And, because it is a one-shot treatment, it's relatively inexpensive.

*Specific Side Effects*

Its disadvantages are certainly psychological (this can vary, depending on a man's age and stage of illness) and cosmetic. To help alleviate the stigma of castration, some surgeons perform what's called a subcapsular technique—see above—in which only the testosterone-producing parts of the testicles are removed, and the outer shell remains. (Also, testicular implants—which make the testicles appear normal—are available for some men.) However, castration is irreversible, and for many men this is too final a treatment. (For a discussion of the general side effects of hormonal therapy, see below.)

## Medical Castration

Medical castration can be accomplished in three ways: by shutting down the hypothalamic-pituitary connection (see above), by directly blocking the ability of the testicles to make testosterone, or by blocking the effects of testosterone at the target organ—the prostate. (See fig. 12.1.)

*Drugs That Shut Down the Hypothalamic-Pituitary Connection*

*Estrogens*
Many men, for many reasons, don't want to undergo surgical castration, so they opt for chemical castration—taking drugs that accomplish the same result.

DES, the main oral estrogen, targets a different checkpoint—the hypothalamus. It works by blocking the release of LHRH. In turn, the pituitary stops making LH, and this virtually shuts down the Leydig cells, the testicles' testosterone-making factories. So testosterone drops to the castrate range.

The effect is not as speedy as with surgical castration; it generally takes ten to fourteen days for testosterone to fall to the castrate range. And it's not permanent—in most cases, the testicles start making testosterone again soon after a man stops taking DES.

We talk about DES here because it's the most widely used oral estrogen, and it's the gold standard of estrogen therapy (but no longer the mainstay of hormonal therapy) for prostate cancer. Other compounds, such as Premarin (conjugated estrogens) and ethinyl estradiol (both used for estrogen replacement by women during menopause) have been used, although they are not considered as effective as DES. A drug called polyestradiol phosphate (Estradurin), used mainly in Europe, is injected once a month and may be easier to tolerate for men with gastrointestinal problems. Another drug, called chlorotrianisene (Tace), is a synthetic estrogen that lowers testosterone but doesn't completely shut down its production; it also permits the body to make a little bit of LH. Because its estrogenic activity is weak, it requires large doses to be effective. For this and other reasons, we no longer use Tace as a treatment for prostate cancer.

Twenty years ago, oral estrogens—easy to administer and much cheaper than other forms of treatment—were the foundation of medical treatment for advanced prostate cancer. They aren't today, mainly because of their major, potentially fatal side effect—they raise your risk of having a heart attack or developing a blood clot. European physicians use Estradurin in hopes of lowering these risks. Some physicians believe that the clotting complications of oral estrogens happen because the hormones are absorbed by the intestine and metabolized in the liver. This can be avoided when the injectable form of the drug is used, because the body processes it differently. However, the efficacy and safety of Estradurin compared with DES were never well established, and the drug was never widely used. Even efforts to make estrogen easier to tolerate—delivering it in a skin patch, for instance, to minimize nausea and vomiting—have not proven worthwhile (see below).

Decades ago, doctors gave high-powered doses of DES—10 to 20 mg a day—thinking that it would not only eliminate testosterone but also possibly kill cancer cells. This didn't happen; testosterone was lowered, but that was it. Then, studies by the Veterans Administration showed that lower doses could achieve the same results. But even 5 mg a day proved to be too much. One study found that over time, men on 5 mg of DES a day died from heart disease caused by the estrogen, not from prostate cancer! Then doctors tried 3 mg and then 1 mg a day. *And 1 mg of DES a day proved sufficient to suppress testosterone with fewer cardiovascular side effects.* A large study in Europe found that men on 1 mg of DES a day showed no signs of irreversible damage to the cardiovascular system.

Other studies have proven that there is no statistical difference in the life span of men who were castrated and men who took 1 mg of DES a day. Some doctors argue that it takes 3 mg of DES a day to lower testosterone to the castrate range. This is true. However, if there's no difference in the length of survival, and the heart-related side effects are fewer with 1 mg than with 3 mg, what's to be gained by taking the higher dose? The very interesting aspect of this finding is that men can live just as long by taking the lower dose—and not even lowering testosterone to the castrate range. This adds more fuel to the fire that combined androgen blockade (discussed below)—eradicating every last iota of male hormone—is not important or necessary. Still, because even with 1 mg a day, DES can cause cardiovascular problems, many doctors believe even this slim risk is not worth the benefits and prefer other forms of hormonal therapy.

### Other Specific Side Effects

Estrogens cause painful enlargement of the breasts, a condition called gynecomastia. This problem can be minimized, however, with one to three low-dose treatments of radiation given directly to the breast before estrogens are started. Edema (water retention, which causes swelling in the ankles and legs) is also common and may complicate problems in men with heart disease and high blood pressure; however, this swelling can be reduced significantly with diuretics. Some physicians also recommend that their patients on DES take an aspirin every day to help them avoid other cardiovascular side effects, such as thrombophlebitis (blood clots in the legs), and to lower the risk of this clot migrating to the lungs (this is called a pulmonary embolism) or heart. Because of the risk of cardiovascular problems, men with a history of heart disease or thrombophlebitis should not use estrogens as their main form of treatment. Also, older men (over age seventy-five) do not tolerate them well. (For a discussion of the general side effects of hormonal therapy, see below.) Estrogens can also cause thinning of the skin and the loss of body hair, including facial hair.

### Conclusion

One mg of DES a day is just as effective as higher doses, and 1 mg of DES is just as effective as surgical castration in prolonging life. However, because even this very low dose can cause cardiovascular side effects, most doctors believe that it's just not worth the extra risk. Men with a history of heart disease or stroke, men who have had a blood clot, and men over age seventy-five should not take any form of estrogen.

---

## ARE "NATURE'S REMEDIES" BETTER?

Several years ago, the next big thing to come along was a "natural" preparation called PC-SPES. There were hyped-up headlines and fervent patient testimonials, and the word "breakthrough" was bandied about with great frequency. What caused all the ruckus? A combination of eight herbs, most of them used in Chinese medicine, including saw palmetto. This herb was once believed to improve urinary symptoms in men with BPH; however, a recent randomized trial, whose results were published in the *New England Journal of Medicine,* showed that it was no better than a placebo. PC-SPES also had several potent phyto-estrogens ("phyto" means that they come from plants). It acted like any other estrogen: it suppressed testosterone and caused PSA to plummet in virtually all men. It was also very expensive, costing from $200 to $500 a month.

And yet men swore by it. So great was the hype surrounding this drug that some men with localized disease started taking it—in effect, hitching their wagon to this unproven star. Men with curable cancer and no symptoms subjected themselves to great quality-of-life changes—loss of libido, erectile dysfunction, breast enlargement and tenderness, a reduction in overall body hair, edema, and a significant drop in lipoprotein levels—all of which they could have achieved with a low dose of DES bought for $5 to $15 a month. Many of these men seriously compromised their odds of being cured of cancer by making this effort to delay the disease. (Again, hormonal therapy does not put prostate cancer on a block of ice, because the hormone-insensitive cells keep on growing.)

Wow, that drug was really something else, you might say. Actually, you really could say this, because it turned out that PC-SPES really *was* something else. Scientists studying a batch of the drug found out something startling: the drug was spiked! It was laced not only with DES but with a blood thinner called warfarin (Coumadin), and with an addictive tranquilizer, alprazolam (Xanax). The Food and Drug Administration (FDA) acted quickly to pull the drug off the market, and the company that made it was fined.

What have we learned from this? Did it just confirm scientists' bias against unconventional, alternative medications? Not at all. Can natural, herbal remedies—those not spiked with anything else, that is—really be that powerful and effective? Certainly. One of the most effective herbal medicines in the world is used to treat heart disease. It's digitalis, and it comes from the leaf of a plant. Doctors are very interested in herbal compounds. In fact, Mario Eisenberger and other Johns Hopkins scientists are currently studying one mixture of botanical extracts called Prostasol (previously known as PC-PLUS). It has virtually no side effects and some effectiveness against cancer.

Now, the argument from proponents of herbal medicine is, "Doctors just don't trust herbals on principle, no matter how effective they are." Not true. Doctors just don't trust *anything* until it has been proven to be safe and effective. (Remember, the first rule of medicine is "Do no harm.") And as this PC-SPES episode has demonstrated, this is the right thing to do. In a letter to the editor of the *New England Journal of Medicine*, the physician Michael Katz, of the March of Dimes Birth Defects Foundation, wrote, "what the proponents of alternative [complementary] medicine are demanding is alternative epidemiology that would accept anecdotes as proof." Another physician, writing in the same issue of the journal, commented, "While attending a conference on alternative medicine, which was organized by one of the most respected medical schools in New York City, I realized why this conference was so popular. During the coffee breaks and lunch hour, I discovered that a large number of participants were driven to learn the new "science" in order to build an "herbalist" practice, which is outside the control of and not currently reimbursed by managed care. Many were also interested in the profitable sale of these untested products to their patients."

Ouch. The message from both of these doctors—and my own advice to you—is to use the proverbial grain of salt in digesting information about any "breakthrough" product. Keep an open mind, but do your best to look past the hype.

## LHRH Agonists

Like oral estrogens, LHRH agonists shut down the production of LH and FSH. Here's how they work: LHRH is a small protein, built of ten blocks of amino acid. A synthetic substance called an LHRH analog, or agonist, made by changing one of the ten blocks, works by blocking LH (the hormone that tells the testicles to make testosterone). The hypothalamus acts like a lighthouse, sending out LHRH in signal pulses—like Morse code in flashes of light—to the pituitary gland. LHRH agonists work by providing prolonged signals—by turning on the light and keeping it on instead of just sending flashes. So these drugs trick the pituitary; because the pituitary receives no flashes, or pulses, it thinks no signal is being sent, and it doesn't make LH. In turn, the testicles do not produce testosterone.

These drugs don't work right away. In fact, for about a week after a man begins taking an LHRH agonist, his testosterone level kicks into overdrive. This is called a flare, and it happens because the constant LHRH signal initially stimulates LH production. But after about ten days, testosterone falls into the castrate range. For the first few weeks, doctors often prescribe an antiandrogen, bicalutamide (Casodex), to block this surge. A new class of compounds known as LHRH antagonists do not produce this brief testosterone flare and cause a faster reduction in testosterone than the LHRH agonists. (However, if an antiandrogen is given along with an LHRH agonist, the net effect is the same.) One such drug, called abarelix (Plenaxis), has been approved by the FDA. However, because it produced severe allergic reactions in some patients, its use is highly restricted to men with metastatic disease who really need some extra help. Men who can receive this drug are those at risk of neurological compromise from metastases, men with ureteral or bladder outlet obstruction, or men with severe bone pain that defies even narcotic painkillers. If you are given this drug, you must always wait in your doctor's office for *at least thirty minutes* after getting each shot. If a serious or life-threatening allergic reaction happens, it is usually soon after getting an injection. *Tell your doctor right away if you feel warm, faint, or light-headed, or if you have chest tightness, shortness of breath, redness of your skin, or swelling of your face, eyelids, tongue, or throat.* These could be signs of an allergic reaction.

The most commonly prescribed LHRH agonists are leuprolide (Lupron) and goserelin (Zoladex). In large studies, researchers have found that these LHRH agonists are equivalent to treatment with DES or surgical castration in their ability to lengthen the time until the cancer progresses and to prolong survival.

### To Sum Up

LHRH agonists are basically equivalent to DES in testosterone-lowering and life span–lengthening results, and both are basically equivalent to surgical castration. The chief advantages of LHRH agonists are that they negate the need for surgery and they don't carry the risk of cardiovascular complications that can accompany estrogen treatment. Also, they don't cause breast swelling as often as treatment with estrogens.

### Specific Side Effects

LHRH analogs require an injection. Long-acting agents need to be injected either monthly or every three or four months, and new pumps have been developed that dispense medication for a whole year. However, they must be implanted, and this requires a small incision to be made, under local anesthesia. Other disadvantages include the tremendous expense—LHRH agonists cost thousands of dollars a year. (For a discussion of the general side effects of hormonal therapy, see below.)

## Drugs That Block the Effects of Hormones at the Prostate

### Antiandrogens

These drugs don't care how much LHRH, LH, testosterone, or DHT you make; it doesn't matter to them. (Actually, antiandrogens cause testosterone levels to go *up* because of an increase in LH.) All they do is make sure testosterone and DHT don't reach their targets—the receptors. In other words, antiandrogens act as dummy keys in the "locks," or receptors. When testosterone and DHT reach the receptors, there's already a key sitting in the lock, so they can't enter the lock and activate the receptors. Therefore, the tumor doesn't get the hormones it needs to nourish its androgen-dependent cells.

Bicalutamide (Casodex), flutamide (Eulexin), and nilutamide (Nilandron) are the most widely used antiandrogens. Casodex and Nilandron are given once a day, while Eulexin requires two tablets, three times a day. Because of this (and also because it has more side effects, including diarrhea and liver abnormalities), Eulexin is rarely used today. In Europe, cyproterone acetate (Androcur, Procur) is also common. (This drug, however, acts like estrogen, and rather than stimulating testosterone, it actually suppresses the hypothalamic-pituitary connection, so it lowers LH, thus reducing testosterone.)

Originally, antiandrogens were used for specific reasons in combination with other treatments. For example, their most common use, even today, is to block the surge, or flare, of testosterone that occurs during the first week or ten days after treatment with an LHRH agonist. (To stop this surge, antiandrogens are usually given for the first month of treatment with an LHRH agnoist.) Antiandrogens also have been given to men who needed more urgent treatment—men who came to the doctor with severe bone pain, for example, or who had large, local cancers that were obstructing urinary flow. Treatment with an antiandrogen immediately blocks the effect of testosterone and brings relief to men who are awaiting either surgical castration or for an LHRH agonist to achieve its full effect. They also have been administered chronically in combination with castration or an LHRH agonist—the form of treatment called combined androgen blockade (see below).

More recently, however, doctors have become interested in using antiandrogens, especially bicalutamide, as monotherapy—that is, as a single agent, without any other form of treatment. The main goal here is to attempt to preserve sexual function. When bicalutamide is given in doses of 50 mg, three times a day, sexual interest is maintained in many men; however, beyond one year, only about 20 percent of men remain potent. This 150-mg daily dose of bicalutamide has been used in men with various stages of prostate cancer. For men with metastatic disease, it is less effective than an LHRH agonist. In men who don't have metastatic disease, there is a major red flag. Although bicalutamide at this dose was never approved for use in the United States, it was in other countries. However, in England and Canada, the license for this use was withdrawn. This was based on the findings of a study in which men with localized disease were randomly assigned either to receive a placebo or to receive 150 mg of bicalutamide a day. More men in the bicalutamide group died—25 percent versus 20 percent of the men taking the placebo. The reason for this is unclear, but (as we will discuss later), this study's results are similar to the long-term findings of the Medical Research Council study. In this study, of men who received early hormonal therapy, the improvements in overall survival disappeared. Over time, because it is so tough on the rest of the body, prolonged hormonal therapy may do more harm than good.

Thus, men with metastatic disease should not be treated with antiandrogen monotherapy. However, for men who start taking antiandrogens when they have locally advanced disease, the survival rate appears to be about the same. Thus, there is great interest in using these drugs in men with advanced cancer that has not yet metastasized to bone. Note: As we will discuss below, no form of early hormonal therapy really prevents prostate cancer from progressing. The only thing it delays is your knowledge of this progression.

### Specific Side Effects
In addition to allowing men to maintain sexual interest, antiandrogens appear to have a lower risk of osteoporosis than surgical castration or treatment with LHRH agonists, most likely because testosterone levels are maintained. Both bicalutamide and flutamide cause breast enlargement in about 75 percent of the men who take them. Flutamide's major side effect is diarrhea. Also, it can cause significant liver damage in some men; therefore, it's a good idea for men taking flutamide to have their liver function checked after the first few months of treatment.

### Conclusion
The fact that men can retain sexual interest makes antiandrogens the focus of intense research—particularly, scientists are investigating combining these drugs with others in hopes of improving quality of life in men undergoing hormonal therapy. However, the use of high-dose antiandrogens as the only form of hormonal therapy for prostate cancer has not yet been approved in the United States. We need to understand the reason for the higher risk of death in men who receive 150 mg a day of bicalutamide before patients can safely consider this option.

### 5-Alpha Reductase Inhibitors
In prostate cells, testosterone is converted by an enzyme called 5-alpha reductase into a more potent hormone, DHT. Five-alpha reductase inhibitors—drugs such as finasteride (Proscar) and dutasteride (Avodart)—block this enzyme. Their big advantage is that they preserve potency, because testosterone levels in the blood remain unchanged.

These drugs work well in shrinking BPH, in which DHT plays a major role. But in prostate cancer, testosterone is more of a villain than DHT, and finasteride and dutasteride do little to stop it. So by themselves, 5-alpha reductase inhibitors are not enough. Some scientists are investigating whether these drugs may prove more effective when combined with an antiandrogen (see above).

### Drugs That Inhibit the Production of Testosterone

The best known drug in this class, ketoconazole (Nizoral), got its start as an antifungal agent. Then doctors noticed that men taking it developed breast enlargement—clearly, more than fungal problems were being treated here! Doctors learned that ketoconazole blocks the production of testosterone by the testicles as well as androgens by the adrenal glands. It works quickly; taking 400 mg of ketoconazole every eight hours reduces testosterone to the castrate range within twenty-four hours. Because ketoconazole also blocks the production of steroid hormones made by the adrenal glands, low doses of cortisone are administered with it. Another drug in this group, aminoglutethimide (Cytadren), has a similar effect. Neither drug is used very commonly today. Before antiandrogens were available, these drugs were the only way to suppress testosterone quickly. However, when antiandrogens were approved, these drugs became more or less obsolete.

### Combined Androgen Blockade

This idea is not new. Investigators have been pursuing this concept since the 1930s, when scientists first began to understand the ramifications of shutting down every single hormone that could possibly affect the prostate. Some approaches have been more drastic than others—surgical removal of the adrenal glands or the pituitary, for instance.

The theory here is that even low levels of testosterone and DHT—engendered by the adrenal androgens—can stimulate cancer in the prostate, and they must be stopped. This can be accomplished by combining whatever achieves a castrate level of testosterone—surgical castration, estrogens, or an LHRH agonist—with an antiandrogen.

Combined androgen blockade became a hot topic in the medical community in the 1980s, due largely to the work of one scientist. This scientist reported that combining an LHRH agonist with an antiandrogen was far more successful than using either approach alone. But there are a few things you should know about this research: one is that *no other scientist has ever reproduced this man's original spectacular results.* In his study, 97 percent of men with advanced cancers who were treated with an LHRH agonist plus flutamide were still alive eighteen months later.

The sad truth is that in nearly every other doctor's experience, only half of patients diagnosed with metastatic prostate cancer are alive two or three years later, and no treatment, so far, has made a real difference in those numbers.

Most studies since then have shown either no difference in survival or an overall survival time lengthened by only a few months. (For more on these studies, see The Flutamide Disappointment: An Oncologist's View, below.)

Unfortunately, the idea that combined therapy can somehow stretch out the time that hormones work—lengthening by several months the time to progression of cancer—just hasn't borne fruit. These findings confirm those of another study of men on the combined treatment: in a huge analysis of about five thousand prostate cancer patients in Europe and the United States, doctors studied overall survival and found, at five years after treatment, *virtually no difference* between the men on combined androgen blockade and the men who underwent castration or took LHRH agonists alone. Again, unfortunately, this is not a stunning display of the success of combined androgen blockade.

And, after a certain point, some patients actually benefit from *stopping* antiandrogens. For example, if a man taking an antiandrogen in combined therapy begins to relapse—if his prostate cancer begins growing again and his PSA level goes up—one step his doctors should take right away is to *stop* the antiandrogen. In 20 to 25 percent of these men, PSA levels drop when the antiandrogen is stopped (see "What Happens If Hormonal Therapy Doesn't Seem to Be Working? below.).

Paradoxically, antiandrogens can make some patients who initially were helped by them worse. Exactly why this happens is not clear. In certain prostate cancers, over time, the androgen receptors (the part of the cell responsive to hormones) undergo a mutation—and all of a sudden, the antiandrogen *stimulates* the cancer. Remember, antiandrogens normally act like a dummy key in the "lock" (the receptor) whose purpose is to block testosterone and DHT from activating the receptor. With this mutation, however, the antiandrogen key actually works—it turns in the lock and activates the receptor. Because of this odd twist, some doctors have questioned the long-term value of taking these drugs and believe they should be used only for a month by men taking LHRH agonists.

### What About Quality of Life?

If the addition of an antiandrogen to castration (surgical or chemical) doesn't make life longer, does it make it *better*? In one study, scientists compared the quality of life of men given castration and a placebo with that of men given castration plus flutamide. Although most patients reported improved quality of life over time, the men in the flutamide group tended to show less improvement in most areas, particularly in the area of emotional functioning. (For more on depression and prostate cancer, see below.) Men in the flutamide group also had more trouble with diarrhea.

There is one crucial concept here that you need to understand: *ultimately—although it may take years—combined androgen blockade is going to stop working, just as every other kind of hormonal therapy does.* Anyone who leads you to believe otherwise is not doing you a favor. And if hormone treatment stops working, it's not because of the tiny amounts of testosterone and DHT being made by the adrenal androgens—in other words, it's not the fault of some renegade hormones that are sneaking through the hormonal blockade. It's because of the hormonally *independent* portion of the cancer—the cells that couldn't care less what hormones its host is taking, because *hormones have no effect on this portion of the tumor.* Using hormones to fight these cells is (going back to our bug spray analogy) like trying to kill a cockroach with weed killer instead of insecticide. The problem is, we're still looking for the right "Raid," as well.

As the Johns Hopkins scientist John Isaacs explains, "Cancer cells are very efficient. And as they keep dividing, they jettison some deadweight. One of the first pieces of unnecessary baggage to go may be the system of controls—the part of the cell that takes orders from hormones. Over time, the deadliest cancer cells survive because they become pure, stripped-down growing machines."

If blocking adrenal androgens really were the key to fighting prostate cancer, antiandrogens should produce a dramatic improvement in men who were castrated, took estrogens or an LHRH agonist, and then had a relapse. This just isn't the case. Sadly, what happens for these men is that beginning combined androgen blockade has little effect—again, suggesting that this approach is not the answer.

Finally, other studies have demonstrated that adrenal androgens have little effect on the prostate. In one investigation at Johns Hopkins, researchers studied the autopsy records of four men who had their pituitary glands removed before they reached puberty—which means that not only did their bodies fail to make LH, they failed to make a hormone that stimulates the adrenal gland, so it was virtually shut down; in other words, they had combined androgen blockade. They also studied three men who had a genetic disorder called Kallmann's syndrome (in which the hypothalamus doesn't make LHRH, and therefore the pituitary glands don't make LH or FSH) and one unfortunate man who had been castrated at age seven, when a dog bit off his testicles. None of these men ever received treatment with testosterone; at autopsy, their average age was about sixty-five. Using age-matched control (normal) patients for comparison, the investigators showed that at autopsy, there was *no disparity in prostate size* in men with both testosterone and the adrenal hormones out of commission and in men with only testosterone missing. (In all of these men, the prostate was tiny. In all but the castrated man, there were no Leydig cells, the tiny testosterone-making factories in the testicles.) In other words, *combined androgen blockade made no difference.*

## General Side Effects of Androgen Deprivation

Testosterone is the hormone that makes men feel "manly." When it is missing, some of the characteristics associated with being male vanish along with it. Side effects of castration—surgical or medical—can include a loss of muscle mass (because male hormones are involved in making men muscular) and osteoporosis ("thinning" of the bones), which eventually can lead to fractures (one study has found that the long-term bone loss is worse for men who undergo surgical castration than medical castration). The loss of bone density—because testos-

## THE FLUTAMIDE DISAPPOINTMENT:
## AN ONCOLOGIST'S VIEW

Destroy all androgens! Don't stop at shutting down the testes, the body's main testosterone-making factory. Eliminate every single one, even weak male hormones produced in tiny amounts by the adrenal glands—anything that could possibly affect the prostate. This is the concept behind combined androgen blockade, combining surgical or medical castration plus LHRH agonist drugs (castration deprives the prostate of its chief hormone, testosterone, causing the prostate cancer cells that are hormone-dependent to die) with an antiandrogen.

The idea was that this one-two punch would be far more successful than either approach alone, and it became a huge issue in prostate cancer treatment in the 1980s. Scientists around the world conducted trials of flutamide; the Johns Hopkins oncologist Mario Eisenberger conducted two of them, with about two thousand patients in total. "The first trial we did was marginally positive, a six-month difference in survival" in favor of the group of men randomly assigned to receive combined androgen blockade (versus the men who took LHRH agonists alone). Eisenberger's results were good enough for the FDA to approve the drug in 1989.

"The problem," Eisenberger says, "is that the issue continued to be controversial. There were two more positive trials, and everybody focused on those three trials" despite the fact that in one of them, the difference in survival was only about three months. "There were twenty-four other trials, all negative. This included my second trial—the largest ever done, with close to 1,400 patients. In the end, close to eight thousand patients were entered in twenty-seven clinical trials, and only three of the trials were marginally positive." Eisenberger estimates that more than $1 billion has been spent in clinical research on combined androgen blockade. The sum could be justified, he adds, "if it generated something that would consistently be shown to improve the survival of our patients." But that didn't happen. The twenty-four negative trials didn't receive nearly as much attention as the three marginally positive ones. Combining LHRH agonists or surgical castration with antiandrogens "became a standard treatment, and added substantially to the cost of prostate cancer treatment." Antiandrogens cost about $300 a month. The negative result of Eisenberger's second trial, reported in the *New England Journal of Medicine*, confirmed what he had suspected: "Men with prostate cancer don't really need an antiandrogen. Antiandrogens provide what we consider a clinically insignificant advantage." Worse, in another trial designed to look at patients' quality of life, Eisenberger found that flutamide caused men to have more hot flashes (a side effect of hormonal therapy in general), cramps, diarrhea, nausea, vomiting, and depression.

These results, Eisenberger concludes, show that men with advanced prostate cancer "don't need an antiandrogen together with castration. By not taking it, they're saving money, not affecting their quality of life, and not losing anything." Antiandrogens are best used as a backup to surgical or medical castration, he adds. "For patients treated with any form of castration who demonstrate a rising level of PSA in the blood, or if their PSA levels do not go down very much, antiandrogens represent an option. About 20 percent of patients will get a second response."

terone helps strengthen bones—may be as much as 7 to 10 percent in the first year; men who smoke may be more susceptible. Men can help prevent this bone loss by taking vitamin D supplements (400 IU daily) and boosting their calcium intake to 1,200 mg a day. There is strong evidence that drugs called bisphosphonates help increase bone density. Studies have shown that the drug alendronate (Fosamax), taken by women during menopause to treat osteoporosis and osteopenia (decreased bone mass), can help maintain bone mass during hormonal therapy. A newer and stronger drug in this class, called zoledronic acid (Zometa), has been shown to do this even more effectively. Zometa—which is thought to be twenty times stronger than Fosamax and also stronger than another bisphosphonate called pamidronate (Aredia)—also seems to help prevent bone pain and other bone complications of hormonal therapy. It is given intravenously for fifteen minutes, every three months. (Note: Specific risks are discussed with each form of hormonal therapy.)

*Protect Your Bones*

If you are starting or already receiving hormonal therapy, you should be evaluated for osteoporosis. Your risk is higher if osteoporosis runs in your family. You may also be at higher risk if you have a low body weight, if you have already broken one or more bones, if you drink a lot of alcohol, if you smoke, if you have low levels of vitamin D in your blood, or if you have taken prednisone or other steroids. (Note: If you smoke or consume excessive alcohol, here's an excellent reason to stop.

Do it for your bones.) Even if you aren't at particularly high risk for osteoporosis, you should start taking calcium and vitamin D supplements. Do you need bisphosphanates? Not particularly, according to an excellent review article written by scientists at the National Institutes of Health, published in the *Journal of the American Medical Association*, unless you have osteoporosis (or are at high risk for it) or if your cancer defies hormonal therapy and spreads to the bone.

Other general risks of hormonal therapy include anemia (because male hormones act on the bone marrow to encourage the formation of red blood cells in men), loss of sex drive, and decreased mental acuity. According to a study from Australia, whose results were published in the *British Journal of Urology International*, the loss of male hormones can mean temporary changes in verbal fluency, visual recognition, and visual memory. In older men, scientists have learned that testosterone levels are strongly linked to cognitive function—particularly verbal memory (for example, naming the months of the year backward) and mental control (for example, the ability to recall a name and address after a ten-minute delay). Impotence is not an absolute certainty; 10 percent of men do remain potent. However, they are rare exceptions to the rule. (Impotence here, unlike impotence in other situations, means the loss of libido as well as the ability to achieve an erection.) Some men also experience tenderness, pain, or swelling of the breasts (gynecomastia). This is not common after castration or treatment with an LHRH agonist, but it occurs in 50 to 70 percent of men treated with antiandrogen monotherapy and in all men on estrogens. It can be prevented by receiving low-dose radiation to the breasts *before* treatment begins or by treatment with an antiestrogen, which adds further to the cost of an already expensive regimen.

## Hot Flashes

The other major side effect is hot flashes similar to the hot flashes experienced by women during menopause—a sudden rush of warmth in the face, neck, upper chest, and back lasting from a few seconds to an hour. Although they aren't harmful to a man's health, they can be bothersome. They probably occur because the change in hormones affects the hypothalamus, the brain's thermostat for regulating body temperature. The brain's response to changes in the hypothalamus makes the body feel out of kilter. The blast of heat happens because blood vessels underneath the skin are dilating; this causes sweating, which helps bring the body back to normal temperature.

Hot flashes are unpredictable; no one knows what sets them off or what makes them go away. Some men don't have any; other men are plagued by them. There is some evidence that outside triggers such as being near radiant heaters, eating hot food, drinking alcohol, or taking certain medications can bring them on. Hot flashes can be treated with progestational drugs such as medroxyprogesterone (Provera) and megestrol acetate (Megace). It is possible that one shot can put an end to, or severely diminish, hot flashes for six months or more. For some men with an active public life and speaking engagements, taking a single oral dose of Megace before an engagement may be effective in preventing the embarrassment of hot flashes. Eisenberger cautions, "I only suggest this approach on rare occasions, and try to avoid treating hot flashes, because megestrol acetate is very similar to the androgens that we are trying to suppress—and because of this, PSA levels have been reported to rise in men who take it." If you decide to have this treatment for hot flashes, you need to have your PSA level monitored closely.

### Other Changes

Finally, many men on hormonal therapy report that they don't feel "normal." In addition, they may feel irritable and less aggressive. Subtle changes in physical appearance—differences in skin tone and hair growth—also are common. However, contrary to popular belief, there is no change in the pitch of the voice; nor, unfortunately, do balding men regrow a full head of hair. Weight gain, along with an increase in cholesterol, may be a problem as well. When the male hormones are taken away, men lose muscle mass and have an increase in body fat. There is an increase in cholesterol and triglycerides, and some men may develop glucose intolerance. All of these can raise a man's risk of developing cardiovascular problems. This should be strongly considered if you're thinking about starting hormonal therapy early, before you have any symptoms of metastatic disease, especially if you're an older man.

Note: It is important for you to know that you're not alone, and many men undergoing this same treatment are experiencing the same feelings. Ask your doctor about a local support group. (For more information, see Where to Get Help at the end of this book.)

TABLE 12.1

### TYPES OF HORMONAL THERAPY AND SIDE EFFECTS

| Treatments That Suppress Testosterone | All Side Effects |
| --- | --- |
| Bilateral orchiectomy (surgical castration) | Chronic fatigue |
| LHRH analogs (medical castration) | Osteopenia/Osteoporosis |
| | Weight gain |
| LHRH antagonists (medical castration) | Decreased muscle mass; |
| | Higher body fat |
| Estrogens | Anemia |
| High-dose ketoconazole | Hot flashes |
| | Decrease in body hair |
| | Decreased libido and impotence |
| | Metabolic problems |
| | (glucose intolerance, |
| | lipid abnormalities) |
| | Breast enlargement |
| | Depression; Reduction |
| | in cognitive function |

### How Long Do Hormones Work?

This varies from man to man, and we expect these numbers to change with the explosion of new strategies for attacking hormone-resistant cancer. Ten percent of men who are started on hormonal therapy when they have metastases to bone live less than six months. Ten percent live longer than ten years. The other 80 percent fall somewhere in the middle. Statistics have shown that half of these men live three years or fewer, and 25 percent are alive after five years.

What accounts for the extreme disparity in these numbers? It all has to do with the ratio of hormone-sensitive cells to hormone-insensitive cells in the cancer and how fast the cancer grows. In some men, nearly every cell is responsive to hormones; in other men, very

## LOSS OF SEXUAL FUNCTION:
## WHAT'S REALLY IMPORTANT HERE?

L oss of sexual function is an awful thought, one that makes most men shudder. This loss of identity is not a pleasant concept; it can be even worse when combined with the fear and uncertainty that are part of having cancer. This is a scary time, but you are not alone. It might help to talk to your doctor or family, or to men and their partners who are going through this, too (see the Where to Get Help section at the end of this book).

For many men with prostate cancer, when it comes down to choosing between sexual potency and holding off cancer, the sex life takes a backseat to survival. If hormonal therapy can truly mean the difference between life and death and you're preoccupied with sexual potency, you're missing the bigger point. (On the other hand, *if you have no symptoms of advanced cancer, this is one of the best reasons to delay hormonal therapy until you do—which may be a long time*. The long-term benefits are the same, but the difference in quality of life can be tremendous—see below.) But if you have cancer in the bones or other symptoms of advanced disease, the message is clear: taking hormones now can prolong your life, ease your pain, and make you feel better in countless ways.

One of the greatest challenges with any illness is to find a way past the physical limitations imposed on your body. Even if your sex life has moved to the back burner, you can still be intimate. In fact, intimacy—physical and mental closeness and sharing—is more important now than ever. It's easy, and very tempting, to let yourself become angry at what you *can't* do, and many people fall into this trap as they struggle to come to terms with a serious illness. This kind of frustration ultimately boils down to a control issue—it's human nature; we want to be in charge of our lives. But most of us, throughout our lives, have the point made—repeatedly—that there's remarkably little over which we have direct control. We are at the mercy of—well, God, if you believe in God; infinite other factors, if you don't.

One of the most difficult pieces of advice doctors can give to patients—but one of the best things we can do for them—is to tell them to take the hard road: Make it your daily mission to avoid bitterness, which is not only unproductive and time-wasting, it consumes your vital energy and strength like the plague. Don't just ignore negativity; go a step further, and substitute positive thoughts and actions in its place. A rabbi once told his congregation, "We all have the same amount of time—today." With this in mind, treasure every extra, precious moment you get to spend with your loved ones. Now is the perfect time to do some things you've always wanted to do—take that trip you've always dreamed of, for instance. Take your partner out dancing. Learn to sail. Teach your grand-child how to fish. Investigate your family tree, and look up long-lost rel-atives. Realize that there is so much more to living than sexual potency.

Finally, remember that *it's tough on your partner, too.* Of all the things nobody wants to talk about, this is right up there—the impact of sexual dysfunction on the partner. Karen Boyle, a urologist at Johns Hopkins and an expert in the management of sexual dysfunction, says many women in this situation describe feeling a surreal sense of loss—that there's a "stranger in my bed." For couples who have shared an active, loving relationship, the loss of intimacy can present a great hardship for the patient's partner. For example, all of a sudden, a woman's husband of thirty years isn't interested, but more devastating than any of the phys-ical aspects is that he doesn't seem to care. He has changed. As de-lighted and grateful as she is that her husband is feeling better, she is also conflicted; she is in mourning—grieving over this change in her best friend. *But this can be worked on*, says Boyle. The challenge is getting the man first to recognize the problem, to realize and understand the feelings of the woman he loves and perceive the changes in himself, and then to agree to participate in a treatment plan geared not to optimizing sexual intercourse but to optimizing sexual intimacy. Erections are not a requirement. Instead, the ultimate goal is for a dedicated, committed man to understand the needs of his partner.

few cells are hormone-sensitive. Some cancers take hundreds of days to double in size; others double every few weeks.

There is a mathematical model of how these cancer cells grow called tumor kinetics. A tumor must double in size thirty times be-fore a doctor can even feel it, before there's a centimeter of cancer. This growth is exponential—two cells, then four, then eight, and so on. Say a tumor is at its tenth doubling; it has 1,024 cells. And say that three-fourths of these cells are responsive to hormones. The patient is castrated, and all the hormone-responsive cells drop out of the pic-ture, leaving only 256 cells. What happens? These cells aren't affected by the hormones; they continue to grow. The now smaller tumor doubles. There are 512 cells. It doubles again—1,024 cells. It's back to where it started. And when it doubles again, there will be twice as many cells as before.

Now say only 1 percent of this cancer is not responsive to hor-mones. It's going to take many more doublings before this tumor be-comes dangerous. So how long hormones work depends on two things: the ratio of hormone-resistant cells to hormone-dependent cells and how long it takes for the cancer to double in size. Relapse will come a lot sooner in a man whose cancer doubles every thirty days, for example, than in a man whose cancer takes one hundred days to double. Unfortunately, today we have no way to predict these two important numbers.

## When Should You Begin Hormonal Therapy?
## Some Factors to Consider

Of all the issues in the field of prostate cancer treatment, this remains one of the most controversial. In fact, many well-informed, thoughtful individuals have reached diametrically opposed conclusions, often based on information from the same studies. One group says, "Start hormones right now. Time's wasting, and if you start hormones today, you can delay the progression of the androgen-insensitive cell population and add years to your life." The naysayers believe there is no evidence that hormonal therapy cures prostate cancer, nor does it have any effect on the androgen-insensitive cell population, which for so many men is the factor that eventually determines life and death. They say that starting hormonal therapy early will only add side effects and will actually take life out of the years a man has to live, without adding any years to that life. Still another group says, "Let's use hormones intermittently. We'll start and stop them, maintain the quality of life, and have the best of both worlds." And finally, there's a new group using what's called step-up treatment. Here, men start with innocuous therapies that have little effect and hardly any side effects and then increase the intensity of treatment (and the potential for side effects) as the cancer progresses. We will discuss all of these approaches in detail.

Finally, there's something that might fit in the category of "worldly issues." You should be aware that the medical debate in this area is strongly influenced by factors that often don't get talked about openly. The pharmaceutical industry makes at least $1 billion a year on hormonal agents for the treatment of prostate cancer. There is no question that they look after their financial interests by stoking the furnace to keep sales (prescriptions) up. This happens in many ways—through direct advertising; cleverly disguised Web sites; distribution of multicolored "scientific summaries" that endorse the widespread use of their products; or surreptitious support for medical meetings at fancy spas, at which "experts" (who receive generous honoraria, frequent-flier miles, and a free trip) promote the company cause. The massive financial and political clout—and largesse—of the pharmaceutical companies is widespread and well known among physicians of every specialty, not just urology. Not all physicians are swayed by it; many aren't. But it's out there, it's yet another element in this complicated mix, and it's something for you to take into consideration. Now, all that said, let's discuss the timing of hormonal therapy.

First things first: We need to get one thing straight right away: *If you have metastases to bone, bone pain, or a large mass of cancer that is obstructing your kidneys or bladder, you need to start hormonal therapy now.* In this situation, hormonal therapy is the right course of action—one that can make a huge, vital difference in your quality of life and can protect your body from the ravages of cancer. Also, you should select some form of treatment that will drive your blood testosterone to the lowest level—either an LHRH agonist (accompanied for the first month by an antiandrogen to block any possible flare reaction—described above) or the surgical removal of both testes. This is not the time for treatment with an antiandrogen alone—you need effective, immediate action. Also, if your bone scan is positive for metastatic disease—even if you don't notice any symptoms—you should start hormonal therapy now. (Note: If you start hormonal therapy, do not have another bone scan right away. When the hormonal therapy begins working, the cancer in the bone goes away, and normal bone cells begin to rebuild the bone. These cells soak up the dye used in the bone scans and may give the false impression that the bone is "hotter" than before. To avoid confusion and needless anxiety, you do not need a bone scan unless your PSA level begins to rise or you develop bone pain.)

But what if you have no cancer in your bones and no sign that anything is wrong—except a rising PSA level after surgery or radiation or the presence of cancer in your lymph nodes—and you feel fine? Many doctors would advise you to start hormonal therapy as soon as possible. The rationale here, as one oncologist puts it, is to "treat the tumor while a greater percentage of cells are responsive to hormones, and the patient should do better." Advocates of this approach also believe that it preserves quality of life, because it delays the onset of symptoms.

Others—and I'm in this group—believe that there is no evidence that starting hormonal therapy now, as opposed to later, will prolong life. (This is discussed in detail below.) However, if a man adopts this philosophy, he must be followed very closely so that hormonal therapy can be started before any symptoms develop. This means a man should go back to the doctor every six months or fewer. At each visit, he should be questioned closely about any signs or symptoms that could be bone pain, undergo a physical exam to check for any increase in the size of a local tumor, have a bone scan every six or twelve months or any time a new pain develops, and have blood tests—a PSA test and a serum creatinine test to measure kidney function. (An elevated creatinine level in the blood may signal that the cancer has silently obstructed the kidneys.) Other blood chemistries such as alkaline phosphatase should be measured at least once a year.

## Does Early Treatment Prolong Life?

The real issue in debating when to start hormonal therapy does not relate to symptoms and quality of life, because if you choose delayed hormonal therapy and are followed carefully, you will be started on active hormonal therapy at the earliest signs of progression (such as a positive bone scan), before you have any symptoms. This will delay the adverse side effects of hormonal therapy as long as possible. Instead, the simple question is: Does early hormonal therapy prolong life? The best evidence to date is based on a study done by the Veterans Administration Cooperative Urological Research Group. (See fig. 12.2.) When prostate cancer began to progress in the men on the placebos—this eventually happened to 65 percent of the men with locally advanced disease and all of the men with metastases to distant sites—they began hormonal therapy, too. The study, though not originally intended for this purpose, turned into a comparison of early hormonal therapy versus delayed treatment. *There was no difference in survival between the men who started hormonal therapy late and the men who had been on it all along.*

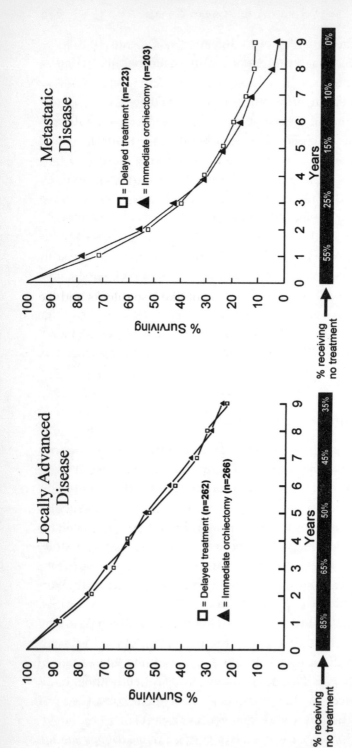

**FIGURE 12.2  Does Early Hormonal Therapy Prolong Life?**

These two graphs show the results from the Veterans Administration Cooperative Urologic Research Study 1, of 954 men with prostate cancer. The men were randomly assigned either to immediate surgical castration or were given placebo therapy and followed closely until their cancer progressed, at which point they underwent definitive hormonal therapy. The percentage of men left untreated is shown in the dark band below the x-axis. With follow-up intervals up to nine years, there is no difference in survival in the men who received early versus later treatment. This study must be addressed by anyone who tries to argue that early hormonal therapy prolongs life—because if it does, then what's wrong with this carefully executed, long-term study of almost one thousand men? [Modified from Blackard, C.E., D.P. Byar, W.P. Jordan, *Urology* 1:553-560, 1972; reproduced with permission.]

This study, as your doctor will probably tell you, took place more than thirty years ago. Why are we quoting something that clearly is old news? Because its results are rock solid and still hold up today—because, unfortunately, there have been no breakthroughs or improvements in hormonal therapy over the last fifty years. Because, ultimately, hormones aren't the answer for the long haul. Hormonal therapy never cures; at best, it palliates cancer, often for many years. What is the alternative? A new plan of attack—many different strategies are being tested today—designed to kill the cancer cells that don't respond to hormones (see below).

But what about the studies that have shown a benefit from early hormonal therapy? One of the most quoted is another study by the Veterans Administration, originally designed to determine the ideal dose of estrogen. What happened was a lot like "Goldilocks and the Three Bears": some men were randomly assigned to receive a very low dose of estrogen—too low, actually, to be effective. Some received a very high dose—so high that it caused cardiovascular toxicity. And some men got an intermediate dose that turned out to be "just right." These three groups of men were then compared with men treated with a placebo. The men treated with the intermediate dose did better; they lived longer. But about half of the men on a placebo and the men who might as well have been on a placebo (those in the "too low" dosage group) never received hormonal therapy—so this study didn't really turn out to be a comparison of early versus late treatment with hormones. Instead, it compared early treatment versus no treatment. This happened because many investigators in this study misinterpreted the first Veterans Administration study. They believed that first study showed that hormonal therapy did not prolong life; they missed the fact that the men in the placebo-treated group eventually did receive hormones.

More recently, scientists in Great Britain, in an investigation similar to the first Veterans Administration study, looked at the influence of early versus late hormonal therapy in men with locally advanced and metastatic disease. However, this study was not terribly uniform (for example, bone scans were available for some men, but not all), and there was no defined interval for follow-up. When the scientists first looked at the results, they concluded that men with locally advanced cancer who received early hormonal therapy lived longer.

However, the comparison wasn't that fair. For men assigned to the delayed treatment group, treatment was *really* delayed—often until men had irreversible damage from the cancer. For example, some men didn't receive hormones until they had developed a pathologic fracture or spinal cord compression (when the bones had become riddled with cancer). There were fifty-four more deaths in the delayed treatment group than in the patients who received hormonal therapy up front—but of these fifty-four men, twenty-nine *never* received hormonal therapy before they died of prostate cancer. These men were, in effect, hung out to dry—and so this study is not a true comparison of early versus late hormonal therapy. Instead, it's a comparison of early treatment versus *no* treatment or treatment that comes too late to do any good. And several years later, when they looked at the results again, they concluded that there was no overall survival difference in the early and late treatment groups.

A study from the Eastern Cooperative Oncology Group (ECOG), published in the *New England Journal of Medicine,* has received a lot of attention. This study looked at radical prostatectomy patients who turned out to have cancer in the lymph nodes. These men were randomly assigned either to receive hormonal therapy right away or to delayed treatment—hormonal therapy given only when these men developed signs or symptoms of metastatic disease. After a relatively short follow-up interval of seven years, the authors found that the men who received early hormonal therapy lived longer. However, these findings have proven somewhat surprising—at least to scientists heading similar studies. One of these is a European study in which 304 men with cancer in the lymph nodes who did not undergo radical prostatectomy were randomly assigned to early or delayed hormone therapy. In this much larger study, in which patients have been followed for an equal length of time, no significant difference in survival has been reported yet. Another study led by the Mayo Clinic retrospectively reviewed data from a large group of men with cancer in the lymph nodes, many of whom were treated with hormonal therapy. At seven years after treatment, the Mayo scientists found no overall survival benefit for men receiving early hormonal therapy. Beyond ten years, however, they identified a small subset of men (12 out of 790) with diploid tumors (which have the normal number of chromosomes—an indication that they are slower-growing) whom they felt did benefit from early hormonal treatment.

Why haven't other scientists been able to achieve the same success? One possible reason is that there weren't enough men in the ECOG study. When scientists carry out a randomized study, they need to have comparable patients in each group. This study was designed to evaluate 240 patients; however, the scientists had trouble recruiting men for the study and ended up with only 98 men. This left a smaller number in each group, and it's possible that unintentional bias might have been introduced.

More recently, there have been two informative studies conducted in Europe. One study from Switzerland involved 197 men treated with either immediate or deferred surgical castration for locally advanced prostate cancer. The Swiss scientists found that there was no significant difference in these two groups in overall survival or in the time it took for metastases to reach bone and cause painful symptoms. Another important point is that many men in this study required no treatment at all; it took so long for their cancer to progress that they died of other causes. The second study, carried out by the European Organization for Research in the Treatment of Cancer, was larger—involving 985 men with locally advanced cancer. Once again, there was no evidence that early hormonal therapy reduced a man's likelihood of dying from prostate cancer. Thus, of all the trials in which early hormonal therapy was used alone, without radiation therapy, there is only one that showed a survival benefit—the small ECOG study, in which hormonal therapy was started early in men who were found to have positive lymph nodes at the time of surgery.

## Big Difference

Now, hormonal therapy by itself is one thing, and beginning it early (and staying on it for years) is highly overrated. But hormonal therapy in conjunction with radiation therapy is something else altogether. In chapter 9, we reported that in some men, hormones plus radiation therapy can be better than radiation therapy alone. Why is this? Because *hormonal therapy makes the radiation work better*. This was most dramatically demonstrated in a study conducted at Harvard, which looked at the use of short-term (six months) hormonal therapy plus radiation in men with Gleason scores of 7 or higher and PSA levels greater than 10 ng/ml. The investigators found that after five years, there was not only an improvement in disease control but also a 10 percent improvement in overall survival. There's a big difference between these two kinds of hormonal therapy, and if your doctor is talking to you about early hormonal therapy, you need to know exactly what's being proposed: hormonal therapy alone for an indefinite time period or hormonal therapy for a finite period along with radiation therapy.

But doesn't receiving early hormonal therapy delay the progression of cancer? The answer is yes and no. It delays your *knowledge* of progression, but it doesn't stop the clock. Another way to look at it is "pay me now, or pay me later." Eventually, the result is the same. Hormonal therapy does two things: it stops cells from making PSA and shrinks the hormone-sensitive cell population. Say a man begins hormonal therapy when his PSA level is elevated, but his bone scan is negative. His PSA level will drop dramatically, and he may feel that his cancer is gone. But it's not; it has just slipped below the radar screen. Those hormone-insensitive cells continue to grow silently. There is a euphemism for this called a delay in progression. What it really is, unfortunately, is a silent progression. Over time (and this may take years), these hormone-insensitive cells will reappear on the medical radar— the PSA level will begin to rise again, the bone scan will become positive, and the tumor will begin to attack bone, producing the signs and symptoms of advanced, hormone-refractory disease.

Actually, this delay is just a time shift. Say the man waited to start hormonal therapy until his bone scan was positive. Right away, his tumor would shrink, his PSA level would fall, and the man would experience a remission of indefinite duration—until, just as in the first scenario, his hormone-insensitive cells reached a critical mass. Eventually—whether the man started hormonal therapy early or late—the result would be the same. If the man had begun hormonal therapy early, his cancer would have progressed, but he wouldn't have been aware of it. The trade-off is that he would have endured the side effects of hormonal therapy for a much longer time. If the man had begun hormonal treatment later, he would have had fewer side effects. What about peace of mind? Well, in both cases, the cancer is growing. The man who begins treatment early has a false peace of mind based on the idea that what he can't see won't hurt him. Unfortunately, as we've discussed at length, hormones are not the long-term answer to controlling prostate cancer. The best hope is in the nonhormonal approaches, which we're going to discuss a bit later.

## What I Believe

So far, there has been no convincing scientific evidence to prove that early hormonal therapy prolongs life. In chapter 10, we talked about the Johns Hopkins study that followed men who had an elevated PSA level after radical prostatectomy. We found that, on average, it took *eight years* for these men to develop metastases in the bones. We also developed a means of predicting when metastases may show up, using the Gleason score on the radical prostatectomy specimen (whether it was more or less than 8), the time after radical prostatectomy when the PSA level first increased (whether it was more or less than two years), and how long it took for the PSA level to double (whether it was more or less than ten months). Using this information, a man can quickly determine his risk of developing metastatic disease. In one of the most common scenarios, a man with Gleason 7 disease who developed a PSA level elevation more than two years after surgery who had a PSA doubling time longer than ten months had an 82 percent likelihood of being metastasis-free at seven years. On the other hand, if the PSA had gone up within the first two years and the PSA doubling time was less than ten months, then the likelihood of freedom from metastatic disease at seven years would be only 15 percent. This information can tell men how long it will be before they actually need hormones—*if they ever do*. Why should they subject themselves to these serious side effects if they don't have to, and if there is no convincing scientific reason to do so?

Whether a man is treated with hormonal therapy immediately, as soon as the diagnosis of advanced disease is made, or his doctor waits until the man has signs of progression and *then* begins treatment, we believe—and study after study proves—that *survival is exactly the same*. There is no compelling evidence that any kind of hormonal therapy works better earlier than later, when a man begins experiencing symptoms such as urinary obstruction or has a positive bone scan. And yet, it's highly unlikely that a man who is symptom-free (also called asymptomatic) is going to feel any better once he has been deprived of his normal hormones. Again, the cancer cells that ultimately prove fatal in prostate cancer are the hormone-insensitive cells. They keep right on growing, unaffected by hormonal therapy. To these cells, whether hormonal therapy comes earlier or later *does not matter*.

For an asymptomatic man, early hormonal therapy means going from feeling fine and normal to experiencing hot flashes; loss of libido and the ability to have an erection; weight gain; changes in muscle mass, skin, and hair growth; and the subtle changes in personality that accompany the loss of male hormones. As we discussed earlier, the long-term effects of hormonal therapy can include osteoporosis—loss of bone density, leaving bones more brittle and easy to break—and decreases in mental acuity. What's the point of going through this early when, ultimately, you could achieve exactly the same benefit if you wait to start hormonal therapy until there is evidence of disease progression?

The idea of early hormonal therapy appeals to many men because it's doing something rather than nothing. Many doctors, too, promote a proactive approach, telling their patients that this will delay progression of the disease. Actually, it takes a lot of time for a doctor to convince a man *not* to start early hormonal therapy—and unfortunately, many doctors don't have very much time to spend with their patients. *If you want to attack the cancer aggressively, don't pin all your hopes on hormones.* Instead, read the section below on nonhormonal approaches, and consider enrolling yourself in a clinical trial—there are many—aimed at killing the cancer cells that hormonal therapy can't touch.

## Intermittent Hormonal Therapy (Intermittent Androgen Suppression)

In searching for some kind of compromise between early and late hormonal therapy, many doctors have embraced the idea of the happy medium—intermittent hormonal therapy.

Basically, it works like this: Men start taking hormones early—after an elevated PSA score following a radical prostatectomy, for example—before signs or symptoms of advanced cancer begin. Then, when their PSA levels drop, they stop taking them and get a little "vacation" from treatment. The men are monitored closely, and at the first sign that the tumor is growing, they start taking the hormones again.

The major benefits of all this, advocates say, include better quality of life—recovery of sexual function and a greater sense of well-being during the downtime between treatments. Advocates of this approach believe prostate cancer can be cycled, like a rubber band that stretches and then—*boing!*—snaps back to a smaller state, then stretches again. And that in this way, they can stave off the emergence of the androgen-insensitive cells that ultimately prove fatal in men with metastatic prostate cancer.

There are a few problems here. The first, as we've already discussed, is that *there's no evidence that any form of hormonal therapy prolongs anyone's life when it's begun earlier than a man absolutely needs it.* So why would interrupted therapy work better? All the benefits of intermittent hormonal therapy—mainly, the better quality of life—can be had simply by *delaying* therapy until a man has signs of progression, without the serious roller-coaster effect of starting and stopping these powerful drugs. An intermittent hormonal therapy program requires disciplined and careful monitoring of PSA and testosterone levels, especially after the treatment is stopped.

## Speaking of Quality of Life

Many of the men beginning the treatment are asymptomatic, with early-stage disease—men who wouldn't be considered, by many physicians, appropriate candidates for hormonal therapy in the first place. (However, these men might be excellent candidates for a trial of one of the new therapies discussed below.) For these men—many of whom have an excellent long-term outlook without any further treatment—it's hard to justify the intensive monitoring, the expense, and most of all, the life-changing repercussions of hormonal therapy without substantial proof that this on-again, off-again approach even works.

Which brings us to the second problem: *the evidence showing that intermittent hormonal therapy is successful is largely theoretical.* Advocates cite experimental studies, not solid data from randomized clinical trials in humans—mainly because there haven't been any results published yet. In one of these experimental investigations, mice were castrated when their tumors reached a certain size. When a tumor shrank to 30 percent of its original weight, scientists transplanted it into another mouse. The tumor shrank, began to grow again, and that mouse was castrated. Then, when the tumor shrank again, it was transplanted into still another mouse, and so on. The investigators inferred from this that cycling androgens can delay the time to tumor progression—the time before the androgen-independent cells take over and hormonal therapy no longer works.

They didn't take into consideration one very basic issue: any time a tumor is removed and transplanted into another animal, it shrinks, because many of its cells simply don't survive the move. So the scientists were killing cells just by transplanting them, and the big benefits they cited were almost certainly from the transplantation, not from the hormone manipulation. The researchers could have avoided scientific criticism simply by giving the animals cycles of reversible hormone suppression. After all, this is what would be done in human patients. Investigators in another study actually did this. Their findings showed that animals that were castrated or treated continuously with DES (in other words, animals given constant, *not interrupted,* therapy) survived 50 percent longer than animals on intermittent hormone suppression.

Currently, there are several studies comparing continuous and intermittent hormonal therapy. Although none of these has been completed yet, the European Randomized Trial issued an interim report. In this study of men with a rise in PSA level after radical prostatectomy, so far there has been no difference in progression-free survival—and most importantly, no evidence that intermittent hormonal therapy delayed the development of hormonal-intensive cancer cells. At present, the American Society of Clinical Oncology considers intermittent androgen suppression to be experimental.

### Step-Up Hormonal Therapy

This is a gradual approach to hormonal therapy, and it has great appeal to many men with micrometastases, who have no signs or symptoms of cancer progression but want to "do something" now. The idea here is to start modulating the male hormones with agents that have the fewest side effects and then to escalate as needed, if the

## SHOULD YOU BE IN A STUDY?

It depends on the study and the medical institution that's conducting it. Make sure, before you enroll, that you know exactly what's being tested, how the study works—whether some patients (and perhaps yourself) will be receiving placebo treatment, for example—and whether there are any potential side effects. Generally, there are many advantages to participating in a study. Medical studies are strictly controlled, with well-defined rules (participants can stop being in the study whenever they want) and review boards that include doctors, nurses, lawyers, scientists, clergy members, and laypeople. Often, people who take part in medical studies are followed more closely, and thus probably receive better medical care, than the general public—and usually at little or no cost. (Sometimes, if a medication proves helpful, participants are even given a free supply as a reward for their help.)

Participating in a study often means gaining access to new drugs that aren't yet available to others; you may get first crack at a new breakthrough. And many people who volunteer for a medical study say that they feel they are doing something important—that their contribution will advance medical science and ultimately help other people.

"If they're motivated and feel well, patients should always explore this option," says the Johns Hopkins oncologist Mario Eisenberger. "They shouldn't give up. For many patients, being in a study gives them a new outlook and new hope."

disease progresses. For example, as we mentioned earlier, prostate cancers don't make a lot of DHT; thus, we would not expect a drug that blocks the production of DHT (a 5-alpha reductase inhibitor) to be very effective in controlling prostate cancer. And it isn't. However, it doesn't have many side effects—and so men on step-up hormonal therapy start with the most benign option, a 5-alpha reductase inhibitor. If the PSA level continues to rise or starts rising again, they move to the next level—an antiandrogen as monotherapy. If that begins to lose its effectiveness, they then add a different 5-alpha reductase inhibitor, and if that doesn't work, they then add an LHRH agonist. Although there is no scientific evidence to tell us whether this step-up therapy—in effect, a candy-coated approach to hormonal therapy—is any more or less effective than any other form of treatment, it's safe to say that it's probably a lot more expensive. But it's attractive, too. Many men feel better when their PSA level falls, especially when the treatment has few side effects. It's hard to convince these men that there is no evidence that this works—nor that any form of hormonal therapy is better than delaying treatment until there are signs of cancer progression, as discussed above. And if this is what you want to do, then you should do it.

However, there are two drawbacks, besides the expense. One is that the men who choose step-up hormonal therapy are also excellent candidates for a trial of one of the new nonhormonal therapies—and in the long run, these have a much better chance of killing the prostate cancer cells that don't give a hoot about how much, or how little, male hormone you have. Two is that it will be hard for medical science to make progress in finding ways to kill these androgen-insensitive cancer cells if the patients who could benefit most from these trials are taking hormones that make them feel better psychologically but ultimately may not control their cancer. Remember the silent progression of cancer, discussed above? This happens with step-up therapy, too. You may not feel it, but the cancer is still there, growing stealthily, and when it breaks out from below the medical radar screen, it can burst back into your life with a vengeance. Thus, you should ask yourself whether the good feeling you have now, that sense of doing something positive to fight the cancer, is enough to outweigh any second-guessing you may have later for not enrolling in a trial of a drug that would have fought the androgen-insensitive cancer cells when they were more vulnerable.

## Hormonal Therapy:
## Conclusions and a Look into the Future

Hormonal therapy doesn't work forever. But this is not to say that hormonal therapy does not work. *It does work. It does prolong life, and it does ease many symptoms of advanced prostate cancer.* The message here is this: there's no evidence that giving a man early hormonal therapy—intermittent or continual—or giving more hormonal therapy than is necessary works any better than giving adequate hormonal therapy *if and when the patient needs it.* Many men are told that early hormonal therapy will delay the progression of the disease. Unfortunately, as we discussed above, this is not true. The only thing delayed is your *knowledge* of the progression.

Hormonal therapy does not cure prostate cancer. And if a man lives long enough, his cancer will progress. If it were simply a matter of controlling the hormone-responsive cells, we'd have it made. But it isn't; it's the tricky hormone-insensitive cells—those are the ones we must learn to kill or at least disable. So what we need, urgently, is a better way to target this group of cells. As you will see below, many exciting new approaches for doing exactly this are being developed and tested.

## If You're on Hormonal Therapy, How Often Should You See the Doctor?

If you're on hormonal therapy—no matter what kind, and even if you feel perfectly fine—you should be followed closely. For most men, this means seeing a doctor every three to six months. At every visit, you should have:

- A careful history taken, to help your doctor spot subtle symptoms—such as back pain or other bone pain, difficulty with urination, or blood in the urine—that may suggest progression of cancer;
- A physical exam—to feel for any lumps or changes in the prostate or the prostatic bed; and
- Certain laboratory tests. This is mainly blood work—a PSA test to monitor the response to hormonal therapy and what's called a serum creatinine, a test to monitor kidney function. (An elevated creatinine level in the blood may signal that the cancer has silently obstructed the kidneys.)

Your PSA should fall to close to the undetectable range and remain that way. Hormones play a major role in the production of PSA; thus, when the male hormones are suppressed, hardly any PSA is being made. Many men assume that having a very low PSA level means the cancer is gone. Unfortunately, although the cancer has suffered a severe setback, it's still there, and the remaining cancer cells—the dreaded hormone-insensitive kind—don't make much PSA.

If your PSA stays at a very low level, you don't need any imaging studies, such as a bone scan or a computed tomography (CT) scan, unless your doctor detects something during a physical examination or you develop new symptoms. In fact, if a man is having a great response to hormonal therapy, a bone scan may look worse, because the bone, freed of cancer, is actually healing—and this new bone growth can make the bone scan light up like a Christmas tree. If, after a long period of remaining stable, your PSA level starts to go up, this usually means that the tumor is growing more actively. It usually takes a few months after this first elevation in PSA level before there are any signs or symptoms of progression or before a CT scan or bone scan may pick up new signs of cancer. However, if you started hormonal therapy before your scans showed any evidence of cancer, it may take a long time until your scans become positive, sometimes a year or even longer.

## If Your PSA Level Begins to Rise Now, What Should You Do?

First, let's make sure that the laboratory test is correct. Just about every doctor who treats men with prostate cancer can tell you that labs sometimes make mistakes. Have the test repeated in another laboratory. If the PSA level still comes back elevated, the next step is for you and your doctor to make sure that you're receiving the maximum benefit from hormonal therapy—that it's doing the job it's supposed to do and that it's not making things worse.

If you've been castrated, make sure that all the tissue was taken out. This is easier than it sounds; all you need is a blood test to measure your testosterone level. Similarly, if you're taking estrogens or an LHRH agonist, make sure you're getting the recommended dosage and getting your shots regularly (if you're not, the level of hormones may be fluctuating). Again, a blood test can confirm whether your testosterone level is at the crucial castrate range. In either case, if there's too much testosterone in the blood, this is probably the problem, and it can be fixed.

If your testosterone is in the castrate range and you're not on an antiandrogen, you should try taking one to see whether this makes your PSA level fall. Some men are helped by this. If, however, you already are taking an antiandrogen in addition to castration, estrogens, or an LHRH agonist, try stopping it (see above). In some men, going back and forth—stopping an antiandrogen, starting another one, stopping that one, restarting another one—causes repeated declines in PSA and stretches out the time that hormonal therapy can control cancer. For example, if you are taking Casodex (bicalutamide) and your PSA level begins to go up, you can try stopping it and waiting for about six weeks to see if your PSA level goes down. If it doesn't, or if it does and then rises again, you can try another antiandrogen and repeat the same sequence. Some men—especially those who respond to this sequence—will respond to other hormonal approaches, such as estrogens or phytoestrogens. Another option is Nizoral (ketoconazole), given along with corticosteroids (to block adrenal androgen production). As we mentioned earlier, ketoconazole is an antifungal agent that also happens to block the production of steroids. It has been reported that ketoconazole can lower PSA by at least half in 20 to 60 percent of patients. The usual dose is 200 to 400 mg a day (total daily dose 600 to 1,200 mg per day). However, for most men, this is not a good long-term option because of cost and side effects, which can include nausea, vomiting, and itching.

If it becomes clear that your PSA is no longer being controlled, it is time to act (see below). In a few men, prostate cancer can come back without the PSA level ever going up. This happens when the cancer returns as a small-cell carcinoma (discussed later in this chapter). When prostate cancer transforms itself into this kind of tumor, it behaves differently—often recurring as a large mass in the pelvis or as metastases to unusual sites, such as the liver or lung. If this is the case, a biopsy should be performed. It's important to know whether you have a small-cell carcinoma, because these cancers have a makeup similar to that of other small-cell cancers (of the lung, for example), and they respond to the same kinds of chemotherapy drugs used to treat those other small-cell tumors (see below). However, only about one-third of tumors that present this way turn out to be small-cell cancers, and unfortunately, only the small-cell cancers respond well to chemotherapy.

## What Happens If Hormonal Therapy Doesn't Seem to Be Working?

For decades, hormonal therapy has been the mainstay of systemic (treatment that affects the whole body, as opposed to localized treatment, which targets a particular area) therapy for prostate cancer. Hormonal therapy gave doctors a way to reach the cancer cells we knew were out there but couldn't even see—the cells that had slipped out of the prostate and escaped to distant sites. And even though hormonal therapy doesn't work forever, it does work quite well, often for years. However, the development of a hormone-independent state—in which the cancer is no longer controlled by hormones alone—happens to most men with advanced cancer over time. The hormones do keep working on the cells they have always affected—the cells that respond to hormones. But the androgen-insensitive cells continue to grow and multiply and develop devious new techniques until they finally take command.

The problem is similar to what can happen with antibiotics—the development of antibiotic-resistant organisms. It happens in other diseases, too, such as AIDS; just when doctors get a handle on the slippery virus, it outwits them. On the life-and-death battlefield of serious disease, it truly is survival of the fittest.

But we're getting better at guessing prostate cancer's next moves. As scientists have learned more about the biology of cancer—the intricate mechanisms involved in progression and metastasis—the links in the chain of advancing cancer—they have been able to develop new agents specially designed to target these specific links. Fortunately, many new approaches are in the works, and even more are coming along.

If you have been taking hormonal therapy and it no longer seems to be working, you need to see a medical oncologist, someone who is an expert in all of the new drugs and approaches we're going to talk about next. If your urologist doesn't suggest it, bring this up and say you would like to see someone who might be more experienced in some of the latest breakthroughs in the medical management of advanced prostate cancer.

## What Else Is Available Besides Hormones?

The idea that hormonal therapy is the only way to treat prostate cancer systemically is rapidly changing. Think back to the vinyl record or the videocasette—and how quickly compact discs and DVDs managed to supplant them, because they were better. What we're going to talk about now are new approaches to prostate cancer. Many of them have few side effects. None causes the long-term quality of life changes of hormonal therapy. One of these drugs, someday, is going to stop prostate cancer from advancing—or maybe even cure it altogether. For the first time ever, something new has entered the picture of treatment for advanced prostate cancer. More than hope, it's optimism.

As we have discussed in this chapter, hormonal therapy has not changed fundamentally over the last fifty years, and one conclusion is obvious: what's needed are approaches that kill both the hormone-dependent and hormone-independent cells. Over the last fifteen years, we have learned a great deal about the biology of cancer, and this new knowledge has led us to develop new drugs—and even new *kinds* of drugs—that are already making a difference in treatment. We have moved from the general concept that cancer represents an uncontrolled growth of cells, an unstoppable phenomenon that will eventually kill the person who has it, to the realization that cancer develops and progresses through a series of very specific events. There are steps within steps that define how cancer cells grow, spread, and cause different symptoms, such as bone pain.

One great boon here has been what's known as translational research. This is the transfer of knowledge from the laboratory to the clinic—or, as doctors say, "from the bench to the bedside." The Johns Hopkins oncologist Mario Eisenberger is inspired by one example in particular. In the 1960s, a scientist named Judah Folkman suggested that tumor growth and metastasis depend on the formation of new blood vessels, a process known as neovascularization or angiogenesis. It makes perfect sense that the spread of cancer cells from one place to another through the bloodstream would require blood vessels. Decades later, as we became able to use molecular biology to understand the body on the genetic level, we learned that a very potent substance called VEGF (for vascular endothelial growth factor; this is pronounced veg—as in *vegetable*—F) was a major stimulus for the formation of these new blood vessels. Scientists discovered that VEGF production goes up in cancer, because the cancer cells make VEGF to pave their way to other sites. And *this* discovery has led scientists to develop monoclonal antibodies—specifically targeted missiles that are "locked and loaded" on VEGF. One of these antibodies, called bevacizumab (Avastin), has been shown to work in many clinical situations and has already been approved for the treatment of advanced colon cancer. "In prostate cancer, Avastin in combination with a drug called Taxotere (see below) has shown very promising results and is currently being tested in a large study," says Eisenberger. If it performs as the researchers expect, it will likely be approved for use in prostate cancer. Also, he adds, other new drugs can affect the production of VEGF by cancer cells. These are small molecules—again, specifically designed and targeted—that interfere with the production of VEGF and other growth factors. "This is a good example of the kind of research that is under way in prostate cancer. Even though we are only in the beginning, we have already begun to reap the benefits."

So these are molecular approaches that target cancer. What about targeted approaches even more finely tuned to prostate cancer specifically? A good example here is the use of a protein called PSMA (for prostate membrane–specific antigen) that sits on the membrane of prostate cells—especially the most aggressive cancer cells. New antibodies tagged with a cancer cell poison (for example, a chemotherapy drug) that kills only prostate cancer cells seek out PSMA. One such antibody, developed by a urologist at Cornell University named Neil Bander, has been used to deliver both chemotherapy and radiation therapy for the treatment and even the diagnosis of prostate cancer. These studies are still in their infancy, but their potential is very exciting.

### The Key to Metastasis

Another entirely new approach was pioneered by the scientists Philip Beachy, David Berman, and colleagues at Johns Hopkins. They began with a mission to understand metastasis—specifically, wondering what gives some cells the power to slip away from the main tumor and cause trouble elsewhere. Recognizing that in many ways, the growth of a cancer is like the growth of cells in an embryo—the need to grow rapidly, for example—they looked at a common protein pathway normally responsible for embryonic development of the lungs, pancreas, prostate, part of the brain, and many other organs. The protein in question is called the Hedgehog protein (years ago, scientists discovered that when this protein was mutated in fruit flies, the insects were born with hedgehog-like prickles).

What they found in their breakthrough research, which was published in the journal *Nature*, was amazing: The Hedgehog pathway is not present in normal prostate cells—they don't seem capable of activating it—nor in most low- to middle-grade prostate cancer cells. But it's very active in metastatic deposits. It's also active in the cancer cells of men who were thought to have localized prostate cancer, but who later developed metastases. The scientists believe that the Hedgehog pathway is responsible for the stem cells in the tumor. Stem cells are the lifeblood of any organ; they give rise to new progeny. Consequently, if a tumor, using this pathway, develops immortality—the ability to regenerate itself—it is easy to understand how, with such apparent ease, it could escape the prostate to distant sites such as bone and set up a new home. What these scientists have done is nothing less than find the key to metastasis—a pathway as essential for a cancer cell to live outside its home-base environment as oxygen is to a deep-sea diver. Even more exciting: They have proven that they can block the pathway and stop metastasis in its tracks.

I tell my patients that this relationship is like soil and seeds. The soil is the stroma of the prostate, and the cancer cells are the seeds. If these cells spread but lack the proper soil, they can't survive. But if they can manufacture the Hedgehog protein, they can make the soil they need. They can pack their lunch and take it with them.

The next part of the story involves one-eyed sheep. In the 1950s and 1960s, several generations of sheep in the western United States were born with only one eye; they were called, understandably, Cyclops sheep. Their birth defect turned out to be caused by something their mothers were grazing on—a plant that was shown to contain a substance that, when purified, was appropriately called cyclopamine. When Philip Beachy knocked out the gene that makes the Hedgehog protein in mice, they produced Cyclops offspring as well. From this observation, he deduced and then demonstrated that cyclopamine must block the Hedgehog pathway. In laboratory experiments on mice with aggressive prostate tumors derived from cell lines established by the Johns Hopkins scientist John Isaacs, daily injections of cyclopamine slowed or reversed the cancer's growth and prolonged the animals' lives. When the scientists used human tumors, not only was the growth of the cancer stopped—eventually, they were able to discontinue treatment, and the tumors did not come back! By blocking the activation of stem cells, they were able to eliminate the tumor completely.

As you are reading this, scientists at Hopkins and elsewhere are actively working to find compounds that mimic the activity of cyclopamine—drugs that can be used in men with prostate cancer. Although the pregnant ewes that were eating the plants did not appear to be affected in any way, it is unclear whether the same will be true of men with prostate cancer, because cyclopamine appears to be active in a smattering of adult tissues, including the brain, and the substance's function in adults is not yet understood, according to David Berman. The potential here is unbelievable. This work shows a whole new approach to treating advanced prostate cancer: take away the soil, and the seeds die.

## And Finally, Don't Underestimate Serendipity

There is another way that progress happens, and it's not through dogged scientific investigation but through serendipity. The world of advanced disease can change on a dime. Many doctors—including myself—have seen it happen just like that. As a young doctor, I served for two years at the San Diego Naval Medical Center, caring for young men dying of metastatic testicular cancer. The picture was grim; in those days, chemotherapy cured only 10 percent of these men. And then came a miracle; a drug called cisplatin (Platinol) was discovered. A scientist noticed that bacteria did not grow around the platinum electrode on a battery and wondered whether platinum might have an effect on cancer. He developed a derivative of platinum and tried it on a number of mice that had tumors. It didn't work. But somebody noticed something unusual about the mice in this study—they had shrunken testicles—and asked another question: Could this compound have any effect on testicular cancer? Bingo. The response was electric, as it were—all of a sudden, 70 percent of men with this terrible cancer were being cured. Young men weren't dying of testicular cancer as often anymore.

Men with prostate cancer should understand this story well. There is hope that through serendipity, a similar discovery will be made. It could happen tomorrow. It might—if one or more of the tac-

## WHY HASN'T STANDARD CHEMOTHERAPY WORKED WELL IN PROSTATE CANCER— AT LEAST SO FAR?

In some cancers—leukemia is the best example—the proliferation, or growth rate, is speedy. And from a treatment standpoint, this is good—these cancers are highly susceptible to drugs that attack rapidly dividing cells. Not so with prostate cancer. Here, proliferation is sluggish—in fact, these slowpoke cells have plenty of leisure time to repair any hits caused by chemotherapy before they divide again. It's as if the damage never occurred.

In prostate cancer, the rate of cell division, or the birth of new cells, is very low. For example, in testicular cancer, 60 percent of the cells are proliferating; in breast cancer, the birth rate is 20 percent—but in prostate cancer, it's only 5 percent. So why is the cancer growing, if not from a cellular baby boom? The problem, instead, is that something happens to throw off the normal process of cell death. Many prostate cancer cells—the androgen-independent ones—have discovered the secret to immortality. So if scientists can't stop new cells from being born, maybe they can help these cells figure out how to die—or better yet, to die at a faster than normal rate. This treatment idea is being explored aggressively. Even a very slight shift in the balance can alter cancer's growth dramatically. If we could just decrease the number of cells proliferating and increase the number dying by a measly 2 percent, we could slow down the doubling time by sixty to ninety days. And this could open major new doors to controlling and even curing the disease.

tics we're about to discuss prove as successful as scientists expect—be happening already.

We write this with the great hope and expectation that there will be new treatments that will work like a high-powered rifle with only one target in its sights—prostate cancer cells. They will be specifically designed to target the biological mechanisms involved in cancer progression and metastasis. Here, now, is a rundown of where we stand today and what the future may hold.

## Conventional Cytotoxic Chemotherapy

*Cytotoxic* means cell-killing, and conventional cytotoxic chemotherapy drugs are drugs that actually kill cancer cells. They work by affecting the vital mechanisms of growing cells and can affect normal cells along with cancer cells. Recently, there has been a breakthrough in the use of chemotherapy—a drug called Taxotere (docetaxel), which works by interrupting an important process in cell division. It hinders the way cells multiply. Recently, Eisenberger and colleagues from twenty-four countries conducted a large study of 1,006 men taking hormonal therapy for advanced prostate cancer whose disease was getting worse. This study compared two different schedules of Taxotere (one group of men receiving the drug every three weeks, and one group receiving it weekly) versus treatment with a drug called Novantrone (mitoxantrone)—which, when given with prednisone, had been shown in previous studies to improve quality of life, but not to prolong life. The study showed that the men in the first group (taking Taxotere every three weeks) had an improved survival rate and quality of life compared with the men taking Novantrone. Both schedules of Taxotere reduced the men's PSA levels by at least 50 percent (in almost twice as many patients) and improved the men's quality of life. Taking Taxotere on the three-week schedule reduced the risk of dying from prostate cancer by 24 percent; the men in this group lived an average of 18.9 months, compared to 16.5 months in the Novantrone group.

Another study, conducted in the United States, compared Taxotere in combination with another drug called Emcyt (estramustine) to Novantrone and prednisone and showed virtually the same results. However, Emcyt (an estrogen combined with nitrogen mustard—the same type of compound used in poisonous gas in World War I) has a number of disturbing side effects, including blood clots, nausea, vomiting, feminizing effects, fluid retention, and heart failure. Because Emcyt did not add to the value of Taxotere, it is not being used in the United States. (However, it is used extensively in Europe.)

The demonstration that Taxotere works prompted the FDA to approve it for the treatment of men with prostate cancer. This was received with a great deal of enthusiasm—not only because if offered men a new treatment alternative, but because it confirmed that prostate cancer is a chemosensitive disease. Inspired by this, scientists are working to find other drugs that can be added to Taxotere to make it more effective. There are other cytotoxic chemotherapy drugs that have activity against prostate cancer. Included in these are Taxol (paclitaxel), Novantrone (mitoxantrone), Velban (vinblastine),

Cytoxan (cyclophosphamide), and Efudex (5-fluorouracil). These drugs are often used in men who do not respond to Taxotere. With chemotherapy, there are often side effects, many of which can be overcome. We will discuss these later in the chapter.

### Bone-Targeted Treatment

In 90 percent of men who have metastatic prostate cancer, metastasis happens in the bone; often, it happens *only* in the bone. As cancer sets up shop in bone tissue, many changes happen. Two different, similar-sounding cell types play a major role here: the osteoblast and the osteoclasts. Osteoblasts cause bone to thicken and become more dense. In prostate cancer, these cells are in overdrive; bone metastases are very dense, and the bone becomes hard, like concrete. These are called osteoblastic metastases. Osteo*clasts* constantly reshape, or remodel, bone by dissolving thick areas. In breast cancer—much more so than in prostate cancer—this is the predominant mechanism in metastases to bone. In these osteolytic metastases, the bone characteristically becomes very thin, brittle, and easily breakable. The embattled bones in prostate cancer can also be affected by the treatment itself—particularly by hormonal therapy. When the male hormones are withdrawn, there is increased osteoclastic activity. This creates an unfortunate situation: although hormonal therapy can kill prostate cancer cells, it can also weaken bones and make them prone to fracture.

However, this creates an opportunity for treatment as well. Because of the predilection of prostate cancer to spread to bone, bone-targeted treatment is an exciting new avenue of research. If prostate cancer likes bone—and bone, in turn, certainly seems to roll out the welcome mat for prostate cancer—how can we fix it so that this environment is no longer so hospitable? Because there are so many mechanisms involved in bone metastases, there are many new approaches under study. Some of these are discussed below.

### *Bisphosphonates*

We talked about these drugs earlier, in a different context—as a means of strengthening bone to prevent osteoporosis in men on hormonal therapy who are at high risk. These drugs work on the osteoclasts. One of these, called Zometa (zoledronic acid), reduces the incidence of bone pain, lowers the need for bone radiation because of pain, and reduces fractures and spinal cord complications. It also reduces the incidence and severity of osteopenia (loss of minerals in the bone). Zometa in general is very safe. It may cause a brief spate of flulike symptoms (aches, muscle pains) that lasts about a day. It can also cause a slight decrease in the red blood count and may change kidney function slightly. If you take Zometa, your doctor needs to monitor your blood count, and you will need to have a blood test that evaluates kidney function. All men who get Zometa should also take calcium (1,000 mg daily) and vitamin D (400 IU daily).

### Radiopharmaceuticals

These are drugs that contain radioactive particles and—like prostate cancer—have a special affinity for bone. There are several choices here, including strontium, samarium, and palladium. Radiopharmaceuticals are often used to combat bone pain. But there is a great deal of interest now in using these drugs earlier—either alone or with chemotherapy—in an attempt to get rid of cancer cells that may be hiding in the bone or bone marrow long before bone metastases develop. One preliminary study, done at M.D. Anderson Hospital in Houston, suggested that using strontium in combination with chemotherapy increased survival in men with bone metastases. Interestingly, new studies indicate that about 40 percent of men with bone metastases treated with samarium alone had significant drops in their PSA levels, suggesting that getting rid of whatever cancer lies in the bones means that the lion's share of the cancer has taken a huge hit. At Johns Hopkins and other hospitals, we are studying samarium given in combination with Taxotere, with great optimism. Taxotere and radiation are synergistic; they enhance each other.

### Side Effects

Radiopharmaceuticals can cause a drop in blood cells as a result of decreased production in the bone marrow. As a result, anemia can result.

## Endothelin Blockers

The chemical endothelin is made by endothelial cells, which line blood vessels, and although it undoubtedly has its good points, for men with prostate cancer, it's an enemy. It's awful. Endothelin is a vasoconstrictor, the most powerful one ever discovered, and is found in the bloodstream. During a heart attack, endothelin is one of several chemicals that cause an artery to spasm, or slam shut, cutting off the supply of blood and oxygen to tissue, resulting in terrible, sometimes crushing pain. But endothelin's concentrations are highest— about five hundred times greater—in semen; part of this fluid is contributed by the prostate.

Chemically, endothelin bears a striking resemblance to snake venom and to apamin, the compound that makes a bee sting hurt so much. Several years ago, pioneering research by Johns Hopkins urologists, led by Joel Nelson, linked endothelin to the excruciating, debilitating pain that comes when prostate cancer invades the bone. The Hopkins scientists also tied endothelin to the unique bone damage (caused by osteoblasts, as discussed above) found in some men with prostate cancer, in which the bone becomes unnaturally thick and rock-hard. Their idea that thwarting endothelin might ease terrible pain—which for years was simply assumed to be an inevitable part of the grim package of bony metastases—led to the first clinical trials of a new endothelin-blocking agent called an endothelin receptor antagonist. In those trials, the drug was given to men and women with advanced cancer that had metastasized to the bone, and it did indeed seem to relieve pain—as measured by a significant decrease in the patients' need for morphine or similar painkillers.

But we all hope for much more from endothelin blockers. The healthy prostate makes endothelin; the cancerous prostate does, too, even during hormonal therapy. Because endothelin is impervious to hormones—just like the hormone-insensitive cells in advanced prostate cancer—is it possible that blocking endothelin can also somehow slow the growth of cancer and prevent its damage? In laboratory studies at Hopkins, cancerous mice with higher levels of endothelin developed significantly more new bone growth (similar to the bone changes found in men with advanced prostate cancer) than other mice, while mice given an endothelin-blocker seemed to be protected against this growth.

With encouraging results from early clinical trials of an endothelin blocker called atrasentan (Xinlay), larger studies have gotten under way. The first of these to finish showed that Xinlay affected the biology of cancer progression; it also seemed to delay symptoms and slow the cancer. Men with bone metastases appeared to be most helped by the drug. Further studies are necessary before Xinlay can be approved for routine use in men with prostate cancer. But there is also the possibility that Xinlay could be even more effective if it's combined with other chemotherapy agents, and other clinical investigations will be needed to determine this.

### Interleukin-6 (IL-6)

IL-6 is a protein made by various cells in the body. Prostate cancer cells make it, too. What does this have to do with the bones? It turns out that osteoclasts stimulate the body to make more IL-6. It's also elevated in the blood of people with other problems, such as heart disease, inflammatory bowel disease, and arthritis (especially rheumatoid arthritis). Some scientists believe that it may be involved in metastasis. "A few years ago," says Eisenberger, "we studied a group of patients with bone metastasis and pain. We found that about two-thirds of them had very high levels of IL-6 in their blood." But there is an antibody called Remicade (infliximab), that lowers IL-6 levels in the blood by reducing one of the raw materials the body uses to make it. You may have heard of Remicade, which is already approved for the treatment of conditions including inflammatory bowel disease and rheumatoid arthritis—both of which involve very high levels of IL-6. At Johns Hopkins, scientists are testing the effects of Remicade and another antibody that works directly against IL-6 (Remicade actually works indirectly against this protein). "The preliminary results have been quite promising," says Eisenberger. At this point, an IL-6–specific antibody is being tested in combination with Taxotere at Hopkins and other institutions.

Other antibodies that target IL-6 are being developed as well. One of these, called Denosumab, shuts down osteoclasts—apparently even more effectively than do bisphosphonates. Denosumab is in full development as a treatment for prostate and breast cancer.

One exciting aspect of bone-targeted treatment is that many of these strategies have already proven clinically helpful on their own. It is very possible that, in combination, they may do even more. As we learn more about the mechanisms involved in bone metastasis, it is likely that we will identify even more ways in which we can target prostate cancer.

## Immunotherapy

### *Active Immunity*
Let's switch gears here and talk about another strategy for treating prostate cancer—helping the body become strong enough to help itself. The idea here is to even the fight. Imagine any great lopsided battle in history—like the ill-fated charge of the Light Brigade during the Crimean War—and say that you could somehow change the odds. What if those valiant Englishmen, the 11th Hussars, had worn bulletproof vests—or better yet, riot gear and helmets? They would still be outnumbered, but at least they'd have a fighting chance.

In about 70 percent of men with prostate cancer, advancing disease is accompanied by a substantial drop in lymphocytes—blood cells that make antibodies, which help the body's immune system fight off disease. The result is an underpowered immune system. Think of the scrawny, 97-pound weakling getting sand kicked in his face by the big, mean bully in the old ads for Charles Atlas's bodybuilding isometrics. In this case, to beef up the immune system, scientists have turned to a substance called granulocyte macrophage colony–stimulating factor (GM-CSF), a growth factor that stimulates the body's normal defense system. Among other things, GM-CSF appears to work as a growth factor for dendritic cells—crucial cells in the body's immune system that, in turn, stimulate T cells, warriors in the class of disease-fighters called lymphocytes, which zero in on tumor cells and eliminate them in various ways. Lymphocytes are activated by still other proteins (basically, the human body is one big string of proteins). In ingenious work, doctors at Johns Hopkins actually put GM-CSF directly into tumor cells and have used these cells as a souped-up vaccine.

The early studies of GM-CSF focused on men who underwent a radical prostatectomy, but still were not cancer-free. These men had micrometastases, as signaled by rising PSA levels within the first year after the operation. Some scientists believe this may be the ideal time to strike—after the cancer has been dealt a devastating blow and before it has had time to recover.

## GVAX

The original studies used prostate cancer cells that were taken and nurtured from each individual patient. This proved impractical, and a current vaccine, called GVAX, consists of cell lines of prostate cancer that have been irradiated and modified to make more GM-CSF. The early clinical trials showed that the vaccine was not only safe and without serious side effects, but there was a dose-dependent decrease in PSA. This vaccine is now in Phase 3 trials, and if it's successful, it could routinely be used—possibly in combination with other drugs, such as Taxotere—in men who have advanced prostate cancer or who are at high risk of developing it.

## Provenge

Another vaccine approach to cranking up the body's cancer-fighting ability is a drug called Provenge (sipuleucel-T), which recently made the news for its reported ability to prolong the lives of men with advanced prostate cancer. Provenge is made up of a patient's own blood cells, enriched by immune system cells specially engineered to kill cells that make an enzyme called acid phosphatase. "This is an earlier vaccine," comments Mario Eisenberger, who recently reviewed this study. More recent vaccines have been created to attack more specific targets, such as PSA or PSMA. For example, PSMA (prostate-specific membrane antigen) is a protein that's made on the surface of prostate cells and is highly expressed in advanced cancers. Antigens such as PSMA are pieces of protein that must pass inspection by the body. The body says, basically, "Friend or foe?" If the body decides an antigen is an enemy, it attacks by making special assassin cells to eliminate it. Because only prostate and prostate cancer cells make this protein, only they would be affected.

Unfortunately, Eisenberger notes, acid phosphatase, the focus of Provenge, is expressed ubiquitously in tissues throughout the body—which means there's a lot of it out there for the vaccine to target, and this may dilute its effectiveness. "We would not expect a vaccine generated against a generalized protein to be so powerful."

As it turns out, Eisenberger adds, the key to these results has much to do with the study itself. "The study was originally designed to look at men who had metastatic prostate cancer and who had failed hormonal therapy to determine whether treatment delayed progression of the disease. Unfortunately," he says, "it didn't cause a delay. There was no significant difference in the time it took cancer to progress—which means that the primary endpoint of the study was negative."

However, surprisingly, the men who had randomly been assigned to the vaccine group survived four months longer than men who were treated with placebo. "How could that be? How could there be a survival advantage if the vaccine failed to prevent progression of the disease?" The answer to the question may be in understanding *what else* these men received. In all of the men—those who received the vaccine and those in the placebo group—cancer progressed. When this happened, the men in the placebo group were treated with the vaccine. The men who had already taken the vaccine were immediately given Taxotere. Thus, what helped these men the most—getting the vaccine or receiving effective chemotherapy as soon as the cancer progressed?

Finally, this study was limited by its small number of participants—only 127 men. With this type of study, the larger the number, the more helpful the results, notes Eisenberger. For example, in one study of Taxotere plus prednisone whose results were published in the *New England Journal of Medicine*, 1,006 patients were required to show the effect on survival. The company that makes Provenge has now embarked on a larger study in an attempt to confirm these results and clarify the value of this vaccine.

As technology improves, we will certainly find better ways to boost the immune system or learn how to use these and other vaccines in combination with other treatments.

*Passive Immunity*

A second way to use immunotherapy is through what's called passive immunity, which involves antibodies. Antibodies are Y-shaped proteins churned out by the white blood cells, or B cells. We make them at the proverbial drop of a hat. You name it—germs, viruses, parasites, any unsavory pathogen that invades the body—and these B cells get busy, creating antibodies tailor-made for each specific enemy. Here's where the antibodies' peculiar shape comes in. The antibodies use the arms of the "Y" as grappling hooks that stick into proteins at the surface of the offending cells and disable them.

Scientists can create antibodies to proteins such as PSMA—which is present on nearly every prostate cancer cell in amounts that increase as the cancer becomes more aggressive—in mice. In the past, using antibodies such as this could cause a problem—an allergic reaction. The body has its own version of the old saying "Fool me once, shame on you; fool me twice, shame on me." The first time the body is exposed to something new, it absorbs the information and commits it to a vast memory bank; the body never forgets a face or an enemy. (In fact, by the time most of us reach adulthood, we may well have antibodies that can recognize more than 100 million different foreign invaders.) The second time, if the body recognizes this intruder as an enemy, it can develop an allergic response, which may be severe. But today, scientists have overcome this roadblock and are able to make genetically engineered, "humanized" (a hybrid of mouse and human) antibodies in mice that don't cause an allergic reaction. In exciting studies, these antibodies, called monoclonal antibodies (because they were all made from a single clone in research that won the 1984 Nobel Prize in Medicine), are being used to attack prostate cancer cells directly or to attack some of the growth factor receptors on those cells.

In prostate cancer, a number of monoclonal antibodies, or MABs, are being tested. The most advanced MABs are those that target PSMA and are tagged with radioisotopes—tiny bursts of radiation that, directed to specific targets by the antibodies, act as guided missiles. This is called radioimmunotherapy and, as we mentioned earlier, these were developed by Neil Bander, a urologist at Cornell University. Bander, who has developed a new, highly specific MAB to PSMA, has achieved remarkable success at making large tumors "melt away" in the laboratory. Now he is testing MAB treatments in several groups of patients, including men with hormone-refractory cancer. In one early trial, the MABs proved able to target all the cancer—even at some tiny sites that did not show up on bone scans. Many more trials are currently under way or in the works.

---

### ADJUVANT THERAPY:
### "THE TIME HAS COME FOR PROSTATE CANCER"

Imagine that you are looking at two boxes. Both contain weapons. One box reads "To be used as a last resort only. Open if all else fails, and hope for the best." The other says "Open at the first sign of trouble. Strike early, strike hard, and set your sights on victory."

Such is the transformation of chemotherapy for prostate cancer in recent years. It used to be that chemotherapy was the "Hail Mary pass," given to men of poor performance status—men who were in pain, often debilitated, who had lost weight and were too weak to tolerate strong doses of anything. Chemotherapy really wasn't given a fair shot—and we do not know for sure that in other, less beaten-down patients, it might not have worked better. But today, energized by scientists such as Mario Eisenberger—unsinkable, creative, stubborn, and above all confident that they can find the winning formulas—the field has undergone nothing less than a revolution.

One key to the change is the philosophical evolution in chemotherapy's role. Today's drugs are more targeted, with far fewer side effects than the devastating "scorched earth" drugs of old. And this means that instead of being stuck on the sidelines—waiting to be needed in case the A team treatments (radical prostatectomy and radiation therapy) and B team treatments (hormonal therapy) were not successful—chemotherapy is getting into the game sooner than ever.

"Radical prostatectomy cures many men with prostate cancer," says Eisenberger. "However, the disease comes back in about one-third of men, and many, unfortunately, will suffer from the symptoms caused by metastasis and die of their disease." The good news is that instead of waiting for this to happen, "we now have many factors to help us predict which men are more likely to have cancer recur after surgery." These factors include:

- The presence of tumor in the lymph nodes adjacent to the prostate;
- The presence of cancer in the seminal vesicles;

- The presence of cancer in the surgical margins;
- Gleason scores higher than 7; and
- A very high PSA level before surgery or a PSA that increased more than 2 ng/ml in the year before surgery.

*Success in Other Cancers:* Doctors treating cancer of the breast and colon have found, in patients at high risk of having a recurrence, that adjuvant treatment—starting chemotherapy and, in breast cancer, starting hormonal therapy as well, immediately after surgery—can delay the onset of metastasis and even prolong survival. "In fact," notes Eisenberger, "in these two tumor types, if the surgical specimen shows that the adjacent lymph nodes are positive, the use of chemotherapy is standard." In breast cancer, too, researchers have identified certain molecular markers that not only predict the higher risk of recurrence but have led to more specific ways of controlling the cancer.

"The time has come for prostate cancer," says Eisenberger. He is heading a massive study to determine whether adjuvant treatment can delay the return of prostate cancer in men at high risk. This investigation, called the TAX 3501 study, will involve about 1,700 patients from twenty-five countries worldwide. It will test whether immediate hormonal therapy using leuprolide acetate (Lupron), which stops the production of testosterone, with or without Taxotere, started right after surgery, works better than treatment with the same drugs given months or years later, when the cancer shows the first sign of recurrence (when the PSA level starts climbing). "Taxotere is the best chemotherapy for prostate cancer that kills both cancer cells, which respond to testosterone, and those that do not respond to hormonal therapy," says Eisenberger. Researchers in the TAX 3501 study also will collect patients' tumor tissue and blood samples in an attempt to discover, as in breast cancer, whether there are molecular markers to help define the biology of the cancer and even the design of new treatments.

## Gene Therapy

Cracking the DNA code has been, to the world of cancer research, the equivalent of discovering the Rosetta stone—the key that unlocked the meaning of Egyptian hieroglyphs. With gene therapy, again, the approach is exquisitely precise. Scientists are able to program the body's DNA like a computer chip, sending it on a selective search-and-destroy mission targeted only at prostate cancer cells.

*Lethal Viruses*

One of the most effective weapons may turn out to be a genetically engineered virus doctored to act as a Trojan horse, slipping into the body, attaching itself to prostate cancer cells, and exterminating them before they even suspect anything's amiss. On the outside, it looks like a normal virus. But on the inside, it's a revved-up cancer-killing machine, designed to deliver its special surprise package to prostate cancer cells.

At Johns Hopkins, scientists are testing several viruses. One is the adenovirus, an upper respiratory virus—remodeled so that it's switched on by the PSA promoter, a small stretch of DNA near the PSA gene in the body. The PSA promoter acts as a chemical switch that governs how PSA is produced. Perhaps, if prostate cancer has a saving grace, it's PSA. This enzyme, indispensable in diagnosing the disease and choosing the appropriate treatment, a marker for every stage of prostate cancer, and even a predictor of its course, is an excellent target for this new biochemical warfare. Scientists studying cancers elsewhere in the body—in the breast, for example, the colon, or the brain—would give their eyeteeth for a potential weapon as selective as this: nearly every prostate cell makes PSA. The fact that PSA is prostate-specific means no other cells need be harmed by this virus, which enters the body "locked and loaded," in effect, and programmed to fire only at PSA's signal. It is not activated in other cells. The virus doesn't care whether a cancer cell responds to hormones or is hormone-resistant. As long as it makes PSA, the virus will find it.

The virus—any virus—invades an unsuspecting cell, overpowers its defenses, and co-opts its machinery to do the virus's bidding. When it has consumed all the cell's resources—stripping it clean, like a locust in a wheat field—and has no more use for the cell, it destroys it and moves on. Normally, when the body realizes that a virus is on the loose, it sends its own powerful home guard—immune system warrior cells, such as those activated in immunotherapy (described above)—to fend off the intruder.

In a series of adenoviral gene therapy trials, the Johns Hopkins scientists Ron Rodriguez and Ted DeWeese tested the virus in men who had a local recurrence of prostate cancer after radiation treatment, detected by a rise in PSA level. This was a Phase I trial, designed simply to make sure a drug is safe for patients to take—not to measure any other results, such as changes found in PSA levels or biopsies. Nonetheless, "we've certainly seen some exciting things," says DeWeese, a radiation oncologist. The virus was well tolerated, with minimal side effects. And, "Several men had significant declines in their PSA," says the urologist Rodriguez. "Even in the ones who didn't—most of them have not had the increase in PSA that you would have expected."

DeWeese administered the virus using a highly accurate computer program he helped design to administer brachytherapy seeds—in fact, the technique is similar, except that instead of radioactive seeds, it's droplets of virus being placed precisely within the prostate, guided by transrectal ultrasound and a three-dimensional CT scan of the prostate.

The scientists opted to inject the virus directly into the prostate (instead of into the bloodstream) because they believe it's the best means of buying extra time for the virus to work—before the body's immune system spots the invader and attempts to knock it out. "We've all been exposed thousands of times to the common cold virus," DeWeese says. "Most of us have antibodies primed and ready to strike, to mount an immune response. So while all of these patients will get an immune response at some point, at least it's delayed long enough to allow some replication of this virus, and therefore killing, to occur."

These early trials have shown that viral gene therapy can kill prostate cancer cells; however, the activity in these studies has not been high enough to warrant use as an individual treatment. Surprisingly, Rodriguez and DeWeese have noticed that when these viruses are combined with radiation therapy, the net effect is far more potent than they expected. The combination of radiation and virotherapy is nearly seven times better at reducing tumor burden than the predicted sum of the two therapies. These findings have inspired the two investigators to try combining seed therapy with virus gene therapy; they're working to determine the best way to do this. Says Rodriguez, "Eventually, we believe that this sort of combination therapy will replace conventional seed therapy and pave the road for the development of new molecular therapies for prostate cancer."

However, the ultimate goal of gene therapy will be to treat men with advanced disease. For this to happen, they will need to develop better homing devices for the virus, so it will be able to track and find prostate cancer cells wherever they may be in the body, and beat the clock—attack the cancer cells before the immune system can stop the virus. For years, this immune clearance problem appeared insurmountable. But once again, surprising results came from a recent study, run by Rodriguez and another Johns Hopkins colleague, the medical oncologist Michael Carducci. In this study, virus injected into the bloodstream was able to find and kill enough prostate cancer cells before the immune system cleared the infection to make PSA levels drop in some men. "We interpret this finding as a very positive predictor—that if we can enhance the homing of these viruses, we can markedly improve their success," says Rodriguez. He and Shawn Lupold have been developing a new homing device to help the virus find and kill the prostate cancer cells quickly by targeting PSMA. These new changes in the virus have been "extremely difficult and tedious," but according to Rodriguez, who is known for his tenacity despite difficult odds, "we have made clear and persistent progress in this area and expect that at the current rate of progress, we should have the new viruses refined within a few more years. Once these new viruses are completed, we believe the real potential of this approach can finally be realized."

Gene therapy, Rodriguez adds, has always had to fight a certain amount of hype and expectations that "have been perhaps unrealistically high, given the intense media attention given to this nascent technology." But now, this technology has finally started to come into its own. In China, there are two commercially available adenoviral gene therapy drugs available for use against head and neck cancer; so far, more than two thousand patients have been treated with these drugs, with extremely encouraging early results.

### Activating Apoptosis

Another PSA-targeted approach works like a molecular grenade that detonates only in prostate cancer cells, causing them to kill themselves. This suicide process is called programmed cell death, or apoptosis— a Greek word that refers to leaves dropping off a tree.

"We're taking advantage of two attributes of prostate cancer here," says the Johns Hopkins scientist John Isaacs. "One is that it makes PSA, and the other is that PSA is an enzyme that can clip proteins, like a pair of molecular scissors." (This aspect of PSA is discussed in chapter 5, under Bound and Free PSA.) As part of its normal routine, PSA recognizes certain strings of amino acids, the building blocks of proteins, and cuts them up. (The specific proteins are involved in making a sperm-trapping gel that is part of semen; PSA's main job is to break down this gel.) Isaacs and colleagues are designing a drug by genetically altering a potent toxic molecule and hooking it chemically to this protein carrier—so that it's only activated when PSA goes into its protein-clipping mode. Then the PSA, recognizing this sequence of proteins that it's supposed to cut, will, in effect, pull the pin on its own grenade. One clip and *boom!*—out comes the toxic molecule.

The secret weapon here is an unlikely terminator, modified from a highly potent bacterial toxin called aerolysin. In its altered form, aerolysin's killing powers are severely limited; it's toxic only in the presence of PSA. "The treatment is highly focused," Isaacs explains. "PSA is only made by normal prostate and prostate cancer cells, and it only functions as molecular scissors within cancerous tissue—not in the bloodstream. This means that it will only target and kill prostate cancer cells and will leave normal tissues alone."

PSA detonates aerolysin by snipping off its tail, which allows the toxin to drill large holes in the cell membrane. These holes cause the cell to swell and then explode. Isaacs and his colleague Samuel R. Denmeade have tested their PSA-detonated bomb in mice that have human prostate cancer, with exciting results. Just one injection of the toxin into the center of the tumor leads to a dramatic reduction in tumor size. In one recently completed study, 60 percent of mice receiving a single injection had *no detectable tumor* fifteen days after the treatment. This agent is now undergoing Phase 1 clinical trials.

Denmeade and Isaacs are developing this therapy for injection into the prostate gland in men with prostate cancer that has returned after radiation therapy. In toxicology studies required by the FDA before the drug can be tested in humans, a single injection of the PSA-detonated toxin into the prostate of monkeys (the only other species besides humans that makes PSA) produced widespread destruction of prostate tissue without any significant side effects. Once these toxicology studies are completed, the first clinical trials in men with recurrent localized prostate cancer will be performed at Johns Hopkins by Ted DeWeese.

### Drugs That Block Tumor Invasion and Metastasis

This is the "class of drugs that make biologic sense," says the Johns Hopkins oncologist Michael Carducci, who is working to develop and test several of these. They are antimetastatic—they put roadblocks in the way of cancer's progress, hindering it from invading other cells, from developing new blood vessels, or from growing at all.

### *Angiogenesis Inhibitors*

One way to stop cancer is to cut off its supply line. The idea here is to put cancer on a leash. It may not die, but it won't get any bigger, either. There is great excitement in the scientific community about drugs that can accomplish this. They are called angiogenesis inhibitors.

Like Roman soldiers, advancing cancers pave the way before them, laying down a track of new blood vessels. This guarantees a ready-made supply of nutrients—nourishing meals for the road—which, it seems, the cancers absolutely cannot do without. Destroy this infrastructure, cut off the supply line, block the formation of these new blood vessels—and the cancer cells starve.

Cancer cells make new blood vessels grow by subverting a normal process involved in wound healing. "Usually, once you become an adult, your blood supply is pretty stable, and—except when your body's trying to repair an injury—you don't really need new blood vessels," explains the Johns Hopkins oncologist John Isaacs. "But in order for a cancer to grow, it has to stimulate its host to do a lot of things for it. A cancer isn't an autonomous machine that can grow anywhere; it's not like an air fern that just needs sunlight and water. It's very dependent on its host, and one of the major reasons why is because it needs vigorous growth of new blood vessels."

This process is called angiogenesis—and drugs to block it, angiogenesis inhibitors, already exist. The good thing about these drugs,

Isaacs says, is that "your other blood vessels—supplying your heart, lungs, brain, and normal tissue—are already fully developed. Inhibitors of angiogenesis don't really cause any damage to them. They target the blood vessels only in cancerous areas. The huge advantage of this group of drugs is that "there's really no way the cancer cell can become resistant to its requirement for blood vessels." That would be like a lung cell becoming resistant to oxygen.

The disadvantage of these drugs is that they must be taken continuously in order to block the constant stimulation of blood vessel growth by the tumor, just as someone with high blood pressure must take medication every day. But many men might find this a tiny price to pay for the potential benefits—putting a cancer's growth into slow motion for years, perhaps even decades. "Say a man has very limited, micrometastatic disease," says Isaacs. "We know that, untreated, it might take five or six years (or longer) for this cancer to produce symptoms. But an antiangiogenic medication might be able to prevent that from happening for twenty years. If the man is sixty years old, that may allow him to not die from prostate cancer. He may still have prostate cancer cells in his body—this doesn't eliminate all of them— but it will allow him to survive his cancer." Another advantage of these drugs is that they only block the formation of new vessels, they don't affect established vessels. And new vessels are the lifeblood, literally, of tumors. Unfortunately, however, they are also forming in the heart all the time, as a natural way to bypass blocked vessels. There is concern that this may be a major problem in the widespread use of these drugs against cancer, and doctors are approaching studies of them in humans with great caution.

Angiogenesis inhibitors are being tested in many forms of cancer. Scientists believe they will work best on men with micrometastases and that starting these drugs once cancer has become entrenched— when it starts producing such symptoms as bone pain—would be like closing the proverbial barn door after the horse has already galloped away: too little, too late. "If a man has very extensive disease, these drugs won't cause the tumor to melt away," explains Isaacs. (Another approach, such as gene therapy, may prove more effective for these men.) It may be that angiogenesis inhibitors will prove most effective when combined with other forms of treatment.

Remember VEGF, which we discussed earlier in this chapter? It's a potent substance made by cancer cells to increase their own blood supply. Some studies have shown that men with higher levels of VEGF are more likely to develop metastases and die from prostate cancer. These observations led to the investigation of angiogenesis inhibitors that lower VEGF levels and stop cancer from growing. Some angiogenesis inhibitors currently being tested include thalidomide (Thalomid) and a related drug, lenalidomide (Revlimid), bevacizumab (Avastin), sunitinib (Sutent), and sorafenib (Nexavar). All of these are taken orally, except Avastin, which is injected into a vein. Although Thalomid can combat prostate cancer and may have even better results when combined with Taxotere, the neurological side effects (nerve damage) and the higher risk of blood clots make this less than an ideal drug. Revlimid, which was designed to have fewer severe side effects than Thalomid, is being tested at Hopkins in men with only a rising PSA level after treatment for localized prostate cancer.

The drug Avastin—already approved for use against breast and colon cancers—is a monoclonal antibody that targets VEGF. Currently, a large Phase 3 trial is under way, comparing the combination of Avastin and Taxotere with Taxotere alone in men with advanced, metastatic, hormone-refractory cancer. Nexavar and Sutent, which have been approved for the treatment of advanced kidney cancer, are now being studied in clinical trials as well.

## Differentiating Agents

Here again, the idea is to slow down the cancer, to tame it—ideally, to make it revert to its former, slow-growing self. "Every cancer has cells that are dividing and cells that are dying," says Eisenberger. "If the cells are proliferating very actively—much more than the rate of dying—then the cancer is growing." Differentiating agents keep cancer in check by slowing down the booming birth rate, giving the death rate a chance to catch up. "This is not conventional chemotherapy," adds Eisenberger. "It's not one of those drugs that you give and destroy everything, and then hope that the healthy things come back very quickly and the cancer cells will not recover. It has a different mechanism."

*Differentiating Agents That Show Promise*

Differentiating agents that have worked well in early experiments include retinoids (vitamin A derivatives), vitamin D derivatives, and butyrates. In chapter 3, we talked about vitamin D's role in inhibiting cancer; in laboratory studies, it causes cells in culture to revert to a more differentiated state. Potent analogs of vitamin D are being tested to see whether they may work in men with more advanced disease. Calcitriol (Rocaltrol) is an example. Recently, a study of 250 men with metastatic, hormone-refractory cancer showed that when Rocaltrol was combined with Taxotere, the results, in terms of PSA response, were very similar to those in men taking Taxotere alone. However, men in the Rocaltrol plus Taxotere group seemed to have fewer side effects and to live longer. Because this was a small study, a larger, Phase 3 trial is now under way.

Over the last several years, the Johns Hopkins investigators Michael Carducci and Roberto Pili have studied several differentiating agents, starting with a drug called phenylbutyrate. These drugs, they found, work by putting cancer's growth, or proliferation, into slow motion. They do this by turning on genes that have been silenced by the cancer. Although phenylbutyrate showed promise as a differentiating agent, it required too many pills to be taken, and its availability has become limited. Pili and colleagues have shown that differentiating drugs may work better when they are combined with another agent—vitamin A (retinoids), which also slows down cancer's growth. (Low levels of retinoids are believed to increase a man's susceptibility to prostate cancer.) Together, retinoids and differentiating agents can hamper the growth of new blood vessels, shrink tumors, and prevent them from progressing.

A newer class of differentiating agents can block an enzyme called histone deacetylase (HDAC). These drugs (called histone deacetylase inhibitors) seem able to reverse at least one process in cancer; they can turn genes that cancer cells have switched off back on. Having these regulating genes back in place seems to check cancer's growth. Pili and colleagues are developing and testing several of these new drugs.

## Drugs That Inhibit Signal Transduction and Cell-to-Cell Interaction Mechanisms

Cells talk to each other through a bunch of signaling mechanisms involving highly specific receptors. There are several ways to interfere with these signals—to block the transmissions, throw static into the mix, or change the message. Scientists have decoded some of these transmissions; in breast cancer, for example, we know that one of these receptors is HER-2. A humanized monoclonal antibody (like the MABs discussed above) has been approved by the FDA as a treatment for breast cancer. This same compound, called Herceptin (trastuzumab), in combination with several others, is also being tested in prostate cancer. Similar approaches for inhibiting substances called growth factors, chemical switches that help promote cell division (some of which are believed to spur prostate cancer's progression) such as epidermal growth factor, are also under way.

### Small-Cell Carcinoma

Small-cell carcinoma is different from "regular" prostate cancer in many ways, although at first it looks just the same. Typically, a man who has small-cell carcinoma of the prostate appears to have the usual prostate cancer and may undergo surgery or radiation to cure it. Sometimes, however, the disease returns with a vengeance. Instead of a few stray cells causing a detectable PSA level, small-cell carcinoma bursts back on the scene as a rapidly growing soft tissue mass, often in the prostate bed. Worse, this is often quickly followed by spots of cancer in the lungs, liver, bone, and brain—and throughout all of this, a man may have only a low PSA level. The diagnosis of small-cell carcinoma can be confirmed with a biopsy of one of these areas. It is crucial to know whether you have this form of prostate cancer, because the same drugs that work on small-cell carcinoma elsewhere in the body work here as well. Many doctors prescribe combinations of cisplatin (Platinol) or carboplatin (Paraplatin) and etoposide (Vepesid), paclitaxel (Taxol), docetaxel (Taxotere), and topotecan (Hycamtin). Radiation can be very effective in targeting isolated metastases as well.

## Help If You're in Pain

Another issue in advanced cancer is the day-to-day business of palliative treatment—easing symptoms and pain and keeping up nutrition in men who don't feel like eating. In this area of treatment, thankfully, there *is* much that can be done, and *you have a right to demand everything possible*—medication or a procedure to ease pain or symptoms of urinary obstruction—to make your life better. Many men are amazed at how much better they feel when the individual symptoms of advanced prostate cancer are addressed and eased. And the intangible benefits of simply feeling more like your old self again—being able to go back to work, play a round of golf, or attend a family gathering—are beyond price.

"Pain is very closely associated with quality of life," says the Johns Hopkins oncologist Mario Eisenberger. "People in pain have a reduced appetite; they lose weight. They're often depressed. Sometimes they're bedridden, the pain is so bad. If we control the pain aggressively, we often see patients getting stronger and eating better. Aggressive pain management is clearly to the patient's benefit."

It's not only beneficial, it's your *right* as a patient not to suffer. Far too many men with advanced prostate cancer endure excruciating pain in the course of their disease. Several studies have shown that an average of 72 percent of men with advanced prostate cancer are in pain. In one study of 201 men with prostate cancer, 47 percent reported feeling pain that ranged from "moderate to very bad," despite the use of painkillers. This tells us several things. One is that, as diseases go, prostate cancer is more painful than most. Its particular patterns of spreading—metastases to bone and particularly to the spine—make it second only to cervical cancer in terms of causing severe pain. But this study also shows us something else. These 201 men were on analgesics—painkillers—yet they still hurt. Some of them even felt miserable pain. Does this mean that painkillers don't work? No. It means the doctors treating these men weren't giving them enough medication to make them comfortable.

There is no excuse for that. And often, both sides—doctors as well as patients—are at fault. An article by University of Colorado scientists cited some reasons why prostate cancer patients often are undermedicated. One is that many doctors just don't learn enough about pain medication in medical school and in their subsequent professional training; they learn how to save or prolong lives, but not always how to make their patients comfortable. (This situation is getting better, as medical schools and continuing education courses are doing a better job of teaching doctors how to manage patients' pain.)

But perhaps a bigger problem—and this also has to do with the way health-care professionals are educated—is the very real fear that patients will get addicted. This is hogwash. The sole purpose of these drugs is to alleviate pain, and frankly, few patients need these medications more desperately than people with cancer—especially men with metastatic prostate cancer whose pain is extreme. And yet every day all over this country, this study showed, some doctors prescribe painkillers at inadequate dosages, some nurses withhold doses of painkillers, and some pharmacists refuse to provide drugs.

In addition, some doctors worry about controlling the side effects of analgesics (see below). They worry about inadvertently precipitating a patient's death—or worse, being an unwitting part in a patient's suicide attempt if he overdoses.

Other problems listed in this study come under the category of communication failure. Some guidelines for drug dosages (printed in medical reference books and other sources) are not appropriate for the particular intensity of cancer pain. And sometimes—this is increasingly common—if a patient is being looked after by a group of physicians, there may not be a clear understanding of who's responsible for pain management. The pain may "fall through the cracks."

### You're a Patient: What Can You Do?

If you're suffering terrible pain, talk to your physician. If you're being treated by a group practice, demand that one doctor oversee your pain and other symptoms. If you're still not satisfied with the care you're getting, look for another doctor—preferably, someone who treats many cancer patients and is attuned to their particular, intense pain.

Another option is to contact the National Hospice and Palliative Care Organization, a group whose goal is to "enable patients to carry on an alert, pain-free life and to manage other symptoms," so their days "may be spent with dignity and quality at home or in a home-like setting." (For more on this, see Where to Get Help, at the end of this book.)

Most hospice programs—there are hundreds throughout the country—are directed by physicians, and care is administered by a spectrum of health-care professionals, including nurses, psychologists, members of the clergy, and social workers. Care is available twenty-four hours a day, every day, and it is centered on patients and their families.

There are also some regulatory issues, the University of Colorado study showed. When potentially addictive narcotics (strong painkillers such as morphine) are involved, so is the government. That's why most of these drugs are called controlled substances. Some governmental red tape can include limits on refills; however, this is not an insurmountable difficulty—it just means patients need to get their doctors to write new prescriptions when their medication runs out.

But finally, the study showed a variety of reasons why the *patients themselves* didn't ask for adequate pain medication. Some men aren't very good at expressing their symptoms or conveying the depth of their pain, the researchers found. Some men feel it isn't "macho" to admit that their pain is intolerable. (If you have a problem with this, it may help to take along a family member who feels no such hesitation when you go to see the doctor.) Other men are afraid of becoming addicted—and some of these men aren't helped any when zealous family members urge them to "just say no" to drugs!

Some men believe that the pain is just an inevitable part of having the cancer and that nothing can be done to help them. Others worry about the pain yet to come and want to save the "big guns," the strongest medications, until the pain becomes intolerable. (Actually, with heavy-duty painkillers such as morphine, relief always comes when doctors boost the dosage, so there is nothing to be gained by seeing how much pain you can stand.) Some men don't want to be labeled as "bad" patients by complaining about their pain. And finally, the study said, some men—ever the providers—worry that costly pain medication will use up all their families' resources. For these men, methadone may be a good option. At around $30 a month, it's the cheapest narcotic.

*The bottom line is that you—or a loved one with prostate cancer—do not need to suffer terrible pain. There is help available. Take it.*

## Drugs for Pain

It makes sense to treat each level and kind of pain differently. At the lowest level is mild pain that responds to aspirin, acetaminophen (Tylenol), or ibuprofen (Advil, Motrin). Next come such opiate drugs as codeine. As far as opiates go, codeine is considered weak. In terms of pain relief, it can't hold a candle to high-powered opiates such as morphine—the highest rung on the pain-relief ladder. (However, this milder opiate generally is sufficient to ease moderate pain.) The biggest advantage to strong opiates is "their lack of ceiling effect," as one study puts it. "Increasing the dose always increases the pain relief," although it can also increase the side effects.

In addition, other drugs not generally classified as painkillers— particularly corticosteroids—have proved helpful in reducing inflammation and bringing relief from some spinal pain. Corticosteroids given in high doses also work by interfering with the effects of substances made by the body, or maybe the cancer cells, that mediate pain. Sometimes the body's response to this is fast and dramatic. The problem is that nobody can use high doses of steroids for a long time because of side effects such as swelling, bleeding, ulcers, and muscle weakness, in addition to mood changes. Ask your doctor if one of these drugs might be right for you.

If you are elderly, have other health problems, or are taking other medications, certain painkillers may have a greater effect on you than on other men. Be sure to discuss these factors, the side effects of various drugs, and the form in which you should take these drugs—pill, liquid, rectal suppository, skin patch, or shot—with your doctor. If you need additional information, your pharmacist also may be able to provide you with the package insert sheets for various drugs. These generally are impenetrable, written in tiny print, and confusing—they contain more information than most people want to know. They also tend to list every possible side effect, even the unlikely ones. However, some people find this information helpful. (For more sources of information, see Where to Get Help, at the end of this book.)

*Complementary Approaches to Pain Management*

Talk to your doctor before you try any treatment, even if it seems "natural." Having said that, many people benefit from other, non-traditional forms of pain management, including prayer and meditation (discussed below), acupuncture, deep breathing, aromatherapy, relaxation techniques, massage therapy, biofeedback, hypnosis, yoga, and even laughter (also called humor therapy). Advocates of these therapies cite many good effects. They can lower blood pressure; reduce stress hormones, which cause the arteries to tighten; slow the heart rate; block or interfere with pain signals; stimulate the immune system; cause the body to release endorphins, its own natural painkillers, and improve blood circulation. Most important, the above therapies are not harmful. And all of these benefits—particularly those to the cardiovascular system—can improve your quality of life.

*Drugs for Milder Pain*

Listed here are some nonsteroidal anti-inflammatory drugs (NSAIDS) and some of their brand names. (Just because we don't mention the brand name here doesn't mean it isn't a good drug.) Over-the-counter drugs include aspirin, acetaminophen (brand names include Tylenol and Datril), and ibuprofen (brand names include Motrin, Advil, and Nuprin). Prescription drugs include diflunisal (Dolobid); choline magnesium trisalicylate (Trisilate); salsalate (Disalcid); naproxen (Naprosyn); naproxen sodium (Anaprox); indomethacin (Indocin); sulindac (Clinoril); and ketorolac (Toradol).

*Drugs for Moderate to Severe Pain*

Listed here are prescription drugs and some of their brand names. (Again, not all brand names are mentioned here.) They include fentanyl (Duragesic), propoxyphene (Darvon, Darvocet), codeine (Tylenol with codeine), oxycodone (OxyContin, Roxicodone, Tylox, Percocet, Percodan), meperidine (Demerol), methadone (Dolophine), hydromorphone (Dilaudid), and morphine (Roxanol).

**Treating Specific Pain**

Not too long ago, a widespread treatment called hemi-body irradiation was used to ease pain in prostate cancer patients with metastases to bone in several places. Hemi-body irradiation involved what radiologists call wide fields of radiation—large expanses of the body and comparatively high doses of radiation. The problem was that this often wiped out key blood-forming cells in the bone marrow and compromised the body's immune system, resulting in such complications as infection and the need for transfusions.

Now, for pain that is concentrated in one area—a portion of the spine, for instance—more specific pain treatment is a far better approach. Some of these are discussed below.

### Spot Radiation

This is localized external-beam radiation treatment targeted at one or several painful bone metastases. It won't prevent new metastases from cropping up in bone, but it generally helps ease pain in the sites it does treat. Spot radiation often results in several months of dramatic relief from pain, and it helps prevent spinal cord compression (see below). In recent studies, 55 percent of patients received complete relief from pain, 33 percent had partial relief, and only 12 percent had little or no response.

### Radiopharmaceuticals

Strontium-89 and samarium-153 (both of which we've discussed elsewhere in this chapter) are radioactive isotopes injected into the body as an outpatient procedure. They are specially tailored to relieve bone pain. Like calcium, they are taken up immediately by bone, as water is absorbed by a sponge—except these compounds tend to zoom right past healthy bone and zero in on metastatic cancer. Relief from pain has been reported in 50 to 80 percent of patients.

In two randomized studies, strontium-89 was shown to give better and more durable pain relief than limited radiation therapy, although in a more recent Dutch study, strontium was not found to be superior to local radiation therapy. The major side effect of strontium, as one might suspect, is damage to bone marrow, characterized by a drop in blood platelets. Samarium may be less toxic than strontium, because it has a shorter half-life and a shorter range of emitted energy. Because these agents can suppress bone marrow production, it is reasonable to use them in men who are not candidates for chemotherapy; bone marrow toxicity can be a rate-limiting factor in how much chemotherapy can be given.

Strontium-89 has a long half-life—fifty-one days—in the body; a single shot of the compound has proved effective at relieving pain for an average of six months. One advantage of this, as compared with spot radiation, is that it acts on new sites of metastasis that crop up while it stays in the body as well as the older metastases it originally was intended to treat. A European study suggests that strontium-89 may be even more effective if it's given earlier, before bone pain develops; this may help prevent progression of bony metastases and the need for spot radiation.

Also, strontium-89 can be used in combination with spot radiation. In one study, doctors found that this combined approach—strontium-89 plus spot radiation—delayed progression of pain seven months longer than did radiation alone.

### Bisphosphonates

We've talked about these drugs elsewhere in this chapter, but they can be helpful for alleviating bone pain, too. Drugs in this group, particularly pamidronate (Aredia), have shown promise in easing the pain of bone metastases in other forms of cancer.

## When Additional Treatment May Be Needed

In addition to causing extreme pain, metastases of cancer to bone can cause two other catastrophic complications—spinal cord compression and pathologic fracture.

### Spinal Cord Compression

About a third of men with metastatic prostate cancer are at risk for spinal cord compression. When cancer eats away at the spine, causing part of the spinal column to collapse, it traps and sometimes crushes nearby nerves. If you have severe pain in your back that accompanies leg weakness, loss of sensation (often beginning with numbness or tingling in the toes), trouble walking, constipation, or urinary retention, you may be at risk, and you need to get a magnetic resonance imaging (MRI) scan right away. An MRI scan is essential—it gives details of the spinal cord and can show early signs of compression. If spinal cord compression is an immediate danger, the MRI will show the cancer invading the dura, the membrane surrounding the spinal cord; this is called extradural compression. If your hospital doesn't have an MRI machine, it's worth it to make arrangements to travel to another hospital. *This is a very serious problem—a true emergency—and it requires aggressive, immediate treatment!* It is far better to treat potential spinal cord compression early than to try to repair the damage after it happens.

Patients in imminent danger of spinal cord compression should be treated with large doses of corticosteroids, usually a drug called Decadron (dexamethasone), for forty-eight hours. Then, depending on how the patient responds to this, the doctor will make a decision on what to do next—this could mean spot radiation treatment to the spine or something called surgical decompression, an operation to ease the pressure on the spinal cord.

If you have not yet begun hormonal therapy, now is an excellent time to begin—and fast—with immediate castration or treatment with an antiandrogen (see above). Giving an LHRH agonist alone in this situation is not a good idea, because it can cause a surge in testosterone that could aggravate the cancer sitting so precariously on the spine. This may be a unique job for drugs called LHRH antagonists.

Spinal cord compression is yet another blow in a series of unpleasant complications of prostate cancer, and it has the greatest potential to ruin quality of life—it can lead to paralysis with an accompanying loss of bowel and bladder function. Most significantly, it can result in the loss of a patient's independence and sense of dignity.

*If you begin to feel any of the warning signs mentioned above, call your doctor immediately; don't wait until your next scheduled appointment!* This may mean the difference between remaining able to walk and becoming bedridden.

*Pathologic Fracture*

When cancer invades bones, they become brittle. Brittle bones break. Therefore, men with metastatic prostate cancer are prone to broken bones (called pathologic fractures). Most susceptible are the bones that bear much of the body's weight, those in the hip and thigh. Sometimes, doctors can take steps to protect bones at risk—putting pins into the hipbone to strengthen it, for example. Such steps are a good idea when a bone has a large area of cancer (greater than 3 centimeters in diameter) that takes up at least half of the bone's outer shell.

## Other Complications

It may be the cancer, or it may be the drugs you're taking to treat it. In any case, you may experience some of the following symptoms or side effects. Some of the advice here comes from nurse practitioners at Johns Hopkins, Janet Walczak and Vicki Sinibaldi, who specialize in helping people undergoing chemotherapy.

*Fatigue*

Develop a healthy respect for fatigue. For many people with cancer—any kind of cancer—it's a ubiquitous shadow. Hard to measure and sometimes hard to see (particularly in men who make the extra effort not to show discomfort or admit any perceived weakness), fatigue can have profound effects. Wendy S. Harpham, a physician who has experienced this "on both sides of the stethoscope," in caring for patients and in her own battle as a long-term survivor of non-Hodgkin's lymphoma, coined the term postcancer fatigue. As she observed in the journal *CA: A Cancer Journal for Clinicians*, this fatigue can manifest itself in unexpected ways—difficulty concentrating or learning new information, forgetfulness, irritability or emotional swings, clumsiness, malaise, loss of interest in the world in general, miscommunication, mistakes, or decreased sexual desire. "Unlike the tiredness that healthy people feel, this fatigue is more difficult for patients to ignore, often impairs patients' ability to function well, and is not relieved with one night's rest. . . . The underlying physical problem . . . is that extra effort is required for even normal activities and social interactions." Because your energy levels may fluctuate from one day to the next or even from hour to hour, this may affect your ability to "pull your weight" at home or work—and this, in turn, may heap guilt or feelings of inadequacy on top of your other burdens. It may inevitably affect family and colleagues as well. "The situation may be compounded," Harpham adds, "if well partners, caregivers, or coworkers run out of steam. No matter how tired healthy people may be, they feel they can't complain or take a rest because [cancer] survivors are always more tired."

If any of this description strikes a familiar chord, talk about it with the people in your life, Harpham advises, so they can understand what's going on. A "tense facial expression or body language may cause bosses, friends, coworkers, and family members to believe that [you're] angry, sad, or upset when, in fact, simple tiredness is the culprit. Children may worry, mistakenly, that their parents are angry with them." Fatigue can fuel anxiety as well and magnify everything. But learning to recognize fatigue for what it is—and taking a few necessary steps to accommodate it instead of becoming frustrated with what you can't do—can help you deal with this problem. For more help, talk to your doctor.

### Urinary Tract Obstruction

If you're having any of these symptoms—weak urine flow, hesitancy in starting urination, a need to push or strain to get urine to flow, intermittent urine stream (starts and stops several times), difficulty in stopping urination, dribbling after urination, a sense of not being able to empty the bladder completely, or not being able to urinate at all—it's probable that the cancer has become extensive enough to block your urinary tract. Several procedures are available to ease these symptoms, including a TUR or the placement of stents.

### Weight Loss

What's wrong with losing weight, particularly if you've spent the better part of your life trying to do just that? The problem here is that people who have cancer need to eat. Losing weight means losing strength and the body's energy reserve for fighting off illness.

No appetite? Able to eat just a little at a time? The thought of taking vitamins makes you gag? Then eat less, more often—have small, nutritious snacks throughout the day. Make every calorie count. Empty calories in sugared iced tea or soda won't do your body as much good as the calories in juice, for instance; the same goes for the empty calories in a doughnut versus the calories in a muffin or slice of banana bread. Finally, if you just can't force yourself to eat as much food as your body needs, you may want to try a calorie-packed liquid nutrition supplement, such as Ensure or Sustacal. Most hospitals have nutritionists available to help you solve dietary problems like these. That's what these people are there for, so let them help!

In severe cases of weight loss, doctors can insert a gastrostomy tube, which bypasses the upper digestive tract and allows patients to get much-needed nutrition in liquid form. This tube provides a painless route for food to get to your stomach. It's comfortable and discreet—hidden by clothes—and can be removed when your appetite comes back and you don't need it anymore. Don't think the tube will be there forever. It is very common today for a gastroenterologist to insert a feeding tube at the beginning of someone's treatment with chemotherapy, and then to take it out again when the treatment has stopped and the patient feels like eating again.

## Constipation

This is another big problem for many men taking strong painkillers such as morphine, which sedate the digestive tract as they relieve pain. Many doctors prescribe mild laxatives or stool softeners at the same time they prescribe opiate analgesics. Another option is adding fiber supplements to your diet; these are available in a variety of forms, including mixtures you can add to fruit juice. You don't have to have a bowel movement every day, but you should be having one every two to three days—and when it does happen, it should not be uncomfortable.

## Nausea and Vomiting

These are side effects of several chemotherapy drugs, and they're the symptoms many men fear the most. Nausea is horrible. Some people feel it's even worse than vomiting—that feeling of dread, the heaviness that drains the life out of you and makes you flat-out miserable. This also becomes part of a bad cycle—you feel terrible, so you can't eat, and then your body becomes weak, which makes you feel terrible. Managing nausea can be a challenge for doctors, nurses, and patients; it often requires trial and error, patience, and determination. This is because different drugs to treat nausea and vomiting (called antiemetic drugs) work better for different people, and some people require more than one antiemetic drug at the same time. Some good antiemetics include dexamethasone (Decadron), dolasetron (Anzemet), granisetron (Kytril), ondansetron (Zofran), palonosetron (Aloxi), and prochlorperazine (Compazine).

You may feel like giving up, but you have to try, and keep trying, to get liquids and food down. If you don't, you could become dehydrated, and you may wind up in an emergency room or doctor's office, getting intravenous fluids. Some people with nausea look at a whole plate of food or even a full glass of juice and gag. You don't have to eat a whole plateful of food; just take a few bites now, and a few bites later, and a few more bites in an hour. If the smell of cooking bothers you, eat your food cold or at room temperature. (Speaking of smells, other odors that never bothered you before, such as perfume, air freshener, or pipe tobacco, may suddenly seem unbearable. Don't worry; this will go away when your treatment is over.) Stay away from fried, fatty foods; most of these require a strong stomach on a good day! You may find it's better to eat dry foods, such as cereal, toast, or crackers. Drink cool, clear, unsweetened juices, such as apple juice, or light-colored sodas, such as ginger ale. Although it's important to get plenty of rest, try not to lie flat for at least two hours after you have finished eating. Eat a light meal before treatment.

*Hair Loss*

This is another side effect of some—but not all—chemotherapy drugs, and it can happen to hair all over your body, not just on your head. This is almost always just a temporary problem. When your treatment stops, your hair will come back—and, as a surprise, it may come back with a different color or texture. Some drugs just cause the hair to thin slightly. Use low heat if you blow-dry your hair, and use a sunscreen or wear a hat to protect your scalp.

### Loss of Blood Cells and Platelets

Chemotherapy can destroy the cells in your bone marrow—your white blood cells, red blood cells, and platelets. This isn't good, because your white blood cells help your body fight off infection. If your white blood cell count falls, you may need antibiotics or even need to be admitted to the hospital for a brief time. If it falls too much, your doctor may decide to pause your chemotherapy or even decrease the dosage. If you have a low white blood cell count, stay away from crowds and especially from people who are sick. This can be hard, but remember, it's just temporary. Do your best not to cut yourself; wear gloves when you're gardening or cleaning. Remember, an open wound is a gateway for infection. If you feel sick or feverish, take your temperature; if it's higher than 100.7 degrees Fahrenheit or if you have chills, a productive cough, redness, or swelling (which could mean an infection), call your doctor or nurse.

If you have a low red blood cell count, you may feel weak, short of breath, tired, or dizzy, or have a fluttery, rapid heart rate. Your doctor may want to treat you with a drug called erythropoeitin, which will help boost your red blood cells. If your red blood cell count gets too low, you may need a blood transfusion.

If you have a low platelet count, you may have trouble with bleeding. If you develop sudden pain in your head, joints, or lower back, or if you experience sudden dizziness, call your doctor; you may be bleeding internally. If your platelet count becomes too low, you may need a blood transfusion.

### Diarrhea

This can be a result of some chemotherapy drugs that affect the cells lining the intestine. Some medications, such as Imodium (loperamide) and Lomotil (atropine and diphenoxylate), can help stop or slow diarrhea, but talk to your doctor before you start taking one of these. You need to replace the fluids you have lost through diarrhea; drink plenty of liquids, and eat small but frequent meals. Gatorade or Pedialyte can help restore electrolytes and help you avoid becoming dehydrated. Dairy products may make diarrhea worse.

### Sores in the Mouth

This is another temporary problem caused by some chemotherapy drugs. Sores in the mouth and throat can cause pain and infection. They can also hinder your ability to eat or drink. You must baby your mouth and throat during this time. Use a soft toothbrush; eat soft, soothing foods, such as ice cream, scrambled eggs, pudding, and Jell-O. Sucking on ice chips or Popsicles may be comforting as well. If your lips are dry, use a lip balm. Try gargling with a mixture of water, baking soda, and salt; ask your doctor or nurse about medicated mouthwashes (such as Magic Mouthwash or Gelclair) that may be helpful.

## Complementary Medicine

In chapter 4, we discussed many dietary approaches to preventing prostate cancer. Although the situation is different, the caveat still applies—even though something is complementary or alternative and you can buy it in a health food store, it can still hurt you. Remember, you can overdose on anything, if you get too much of it. Anything can be toxic, if taken improperly. Complementary medicine can include lifestyle therapy (some approaches are mentioned above in the section on pain) and dietary changes. At a minimum, these lifestyle approaches (including spirituality and prayer, discussed below) can change the way you perceive your illness. They can help you cope better, and there is a cascade of good events that can come from this—eating better, for one thing, becoming more rested, feeling stronger, and having a greater sense of well-being.

Changing your diet may help slow the course of prostate cancer, but nobody knows for sure yet. There is evidence to support this, which we'll discuss below. On the other hand, as we discussed above, it is dangerous to lose too much weight; this could seriously impede your body's ability to fight cancer. Also, studies suggest that as many as two-thirds of patients who use alternative therapies don't tell their doctors. This is bad; alternative therapies (even natural remedies

## PROSTATE CANCER AND DEPRESSION

Here are some of the things you already have to cope with—stress, fear, anger, anxiety, sweating out one PSA test after another, pain, fatigue, uncertainty, and the cancer itself. But at some point, an estimated one in four cancer patients battles depression as well. Although it's common, this is not a normal part of cancer, and it can be treated. Not treating your depression in a stoic attempt to ride it out or snap out of it can even shorten your life. This is something beyond the normal sadness that accompanies having cancer.

If you have any of these symptoms, see your doctor: sadness that won't go away; sleeping much more or much less than normal; waking early in the morning, worried, and being unable to go back to sleep; inability to be happy; eating much more or much less than normal; feeling tired all the time; inability to concentrate or make decisions; restlessness; listlessness; not wanting to participate in normal activities; feelings of worthlessness, helplessness, and guilt; thinking often about death or suicide.

The vast majority of people suffering from depression can be treated successfully. Because the problem—believed to stem from a biochemical imbalance or faulty communication in brain cells—differs in everyone, it may take a bit of trial and error for you and your doctor to find the treatment that works best. Be patient, and don't give up. It may also help for you to talk with other men who are going through this. Ask your doctor about support groups in your area. (For more, see Where to Get Help at the end of this book.)

such as plant extracts or botanicals) can change the effectiveness of other medications and cause side effects. If you choose to augment your diet with any supplements, be sure to tell your doctor.

### The Mind-Body Connection

The mind has a tremendous—and largely untapped—ability to influence the body for bad as well as good. With this in mind, let's take a moment to dispel some guilt. There are a lot of books out there—and countless seminars, articles, and self-help pamphlets—selling the idea that with the right attitude, mental state, spiritual serenity, or even diet, you can heal yourself or control your illness. But the flip side of this mind-set is that if your illness progresses, somehow you've messed up, that you're to blame—you haven't eaten enough vegetables, taken the right multivitamins or supplements, or gotten enough rest or exercise, or you just generally allowed negativity to compromise your health. This definitely is not true.

"The average patient generally does not have a clear grasp of the molecular biology of carcinogenesis," writes the physician and cancer survivor Wendy Harpham in *CA: A Cancer Journal for Clinicians*. "Even to those patients who understand that recurrence is due to mutated cells that escaped the earlier round(s) of cancer therapy, the possibility of having accelerated the recurrence can be disturbing. Just as believers in mind-over-matter worry that negative thoughts can cause cancer cells to multiply, those who want to believe that proper actions can control outcome worry . . . that they've set themselves up for progression of disease." Too often with cancer, Harpham adds, a vicious cycle of fatigue and anxiety can set in, each feeding off the other.

The British evangelist David Watson, who wrote about his own battle with cancer in the book *Fear No Evil*, points out how unproductive such thinking is: "Many times I have talked with those who are seriously ill, and I have found them anxiously wondering what they had done to bring about their condition. They blame themselves; or if they cannot live with that, they project their guilt onto others or God. It's someone's fault! The trouble is that either feelings of guilt, which are often imaginary, or direct accusations, which are often unfair, only encourage the sickness. Both hinder healing."

Above, we mentioned some therapeutic options that generally come under the heading alternative or complementary medicine (although these practices, many of them traditionally eastern, are becoming increasingly respected by western physicians). All of these have been helpful to somebody, and the way they help one person may not be the way they prove beneficial to you. But we know that using your *mind* to lower your blood pressure, to facilitate deep breathing and relaxation, can help your *body* in its battle with cancer. We also know that the "lone wolf" does not do as well as the man who has many connections—who is married; who has good relationships with family and friends; who goes to a church, mosque, or synagogue. Many studies have confirmed the importance of emotional connection—loving support—to good health. As Tedd Mitchell, director of the Cooper Clinic's Wellness Program, recently observed in a national magazine, "We are made not to live alone, but to interact regularly with others. . . . In my medical practice, it seems that patients with strong family ties cope better with illness."

### Faith, Prayer, and Spirituality

If you are religious—whatever your religion—you probably feel great comfort in knowing that you're not alone, that God is always with you. You can draw strength from prayer and from the prayers of others, and from seeking peace. You can surrender the burdens of illness, anxiety, fear, fatigue, and uncertainty—trade them all in for a greater serenity about the future.

If you are not religious but thinking about it, now is the perfect time to explore your spirituality. There are excellent reasons to support this decision. Numerous studies have shown that, among other benefits, religious people—those who put their faith in something larger than themselves—live longer, have lower blood pressure, and need fewer pain medications. But if you are not interested, then you should not feel pressured; extra pressure is the last thing you need in your life right now. You should be allowed that freedom, and family members and friends should respect your wishes. (However, you still may want to explore one or more of the complementary forms of therapy mentioned above for stress reduction, relief of pain, and an improved sense of well-being.)

So if you pray for God to take away your cancer, will you be healed? Maybe. But many religious leaders say that the better, far more effective, prayer is the "Thy will be done" kind—because you don't know the big plan for your life (if you believe there is one, that is). Nobody does. It may help for you to talk about this with your doctor as well, if you feel comfortable doing so. Ask your doctor if he or she believes in God and in prayer. You can also direct your prayers toward the greater good—to help the doctors taking care of you, the scientists working to find the cure, and all the men with prostate cancer and their families.

## Can Changing Your Diet Affect Your Cancer?

In chapters 3 and 4, we discussed the strong circumstantial evidence linking the development of prostate cancer to dietary factors. It also appears that diet can influence the development of prostate cancer throughout an adult's lifetime and that something about the Asian diet seems to prevent this progression of cancer.

Based on these facts, many men believe that once they have prostate cancer, they can slow it down or cause it to reverse itself by changing their diet. One of the most intelligent and vocal advocates of this is Michael Milken, who at the age of forty-seven was diagnosed with advanced prostate cancer. His story is well known because he has devoted his life and considerable resources to fighting this disease and finding a cure. In addition to receiving the standard forms of medical therapy for his disease, he also changed his diet; he drastically reduced the amount of fat he ate (to 9 grams a day) and stopped eating desserts and most dairy products. Furthermore, because the Asian diet is rich in soy protein, he made this a staple of his diet, substituting tofu or tempeh for meat and mixing soy protein isolate powder with water or fruit juice. To make his spartan diet more palatable, he worked closely with the chef Beth Ginsberg to create tasty meals. (These recipes are in *The Taste for Living Cookbook*, by Ginsberg and Milken.) The idea of finding a cancer-fighting diet strongly appeals to many men.

Recent findings from the Health Professionals Follow-Up Study gave some scientific support for this concept. Investigators studied 1,200 men who underwent treatment for localized prostate cancer between 1986 and 1996 to determine whether their diet affected their risk of developing an elevated PSA level following treatment. Men who consumed two servings per week of fish and tomato sauce had a 20 percent reduction in their risk for progression. The authors concluded, "These data suggest that diet after diagnosis may influence the clinical course of prostate cancer, and fish and tomato sauce may offer some protection against disease progression."

In fact, many men with prostate cancer spend a lot of time at the health food store, loading up on dietary supplements such as saw palmetto and zinc. Although it's probably not a bad idea to take vitamin E and selenium (see chapter 4), there is no good evidence that other supplements or herbals will help slow down the progression of established cancer.

Thus, we don't know the verdict on diet and advanced prostate cancer yet. There has been no scientific, objective study to examine this approach. We do know that in breast cancer—a disease that seems to parallel prostate cancer, with its low rates in Asian women and the increase in risk when Asian women migrate to western countries—the consumption of fat, red meat, or fiber after diagnosis has not been found to lengthen or shorten life. As we discussed in chapter 3, prostate cancer is believed to develop because of oxidative damage to DNA. Hit after hit—mainly from eating too many "bad" things or not enough "good" things—causes a series of irreversible mutations in DNA, which in turn lead to cancer.

It is not reasonable to assume that diet can reverse cancer after the fact—that it can "unring the bell." The best example of this is smoking—we know it causes lung cancer, but it's impossible to make lung cancer go away by stopping smoking. There are a number of studies that suggest that soy and rye bran can inhibit the development of tumors. However, in most of these studies, treatment with soy began at the time the tumors were implanted into the animals. Soy and bran contain significant amounts of phytoestrogens, and these plant-derived estrogens can act like other estrogens and suppress testosterone. Also, some of these cancer cell lines can respond to estrogen itself. Thus, it's unclear whether these experimental studies accurately predict what will happen to a man who has an established cancer who switches to a soy-based diet.

Having said all that, there are some reasons to believe that changing your diet may help. In chapter 3, we talked about the way the fat in red meat and dairy products can encourage the growth of prostate cancer cells. An enzyme that is crucial here is AMACR (see chapter 3). This enzyme is responsible for breaking down the complex fatty acid (called phytanic acid) that is present in red meat and dairy products. When a man with prostate cancer consumes red meat and dairy products, the cancer cells have the potential to gain more out of these foods than normal cells can. And something else happens, too. When the body metabolizes phytanic acid, it makes a toxic by-product, hydrogen peroxide, that can produce further oxidative damage, attack DNA, and cause mutations that lead to cancer or cause it to progress.

For this reason, it makes sense that men with progressing prostate cancer should avoid red meat and dairy products as much as possible. This, along with eating a nutritious diet and making efforts to watch your weight, makes sense. Antioxidants may help as well.

So what's the bottom line? If you want to change your diet to reduce your intake of fat and increase your intake of soy, you should do it. But be careful not to lose too much weight too quickly. A rapid 10 percent drop in weight can compromise your immune system—which may be the major self-defense mechanism that is holding your cancer in check.

## Note for Wives, Partners, and Caregivers— Take Care of Your Own Health, Too

Alice B. Baldwin, whose husband had a successful radical prostatectomy (but who died a few years later of colon cancer), became a reluctant expert on coping with a husband's illness. She has some excellent advice to offer wives and partners on this subject. "You may be tempted to skip meals, to lose sleep, to forgo exercise, to drive in bad weather, and generally to ignore your own health," particularly if your husband or partner is hospitalized.

But neglecting your own health now may mean you won't have enough strength and stamina left over for the longer haul. "Recognizing your needs and fulfilling them as adequately as circumstances permit is your obligation not only to yourself but also to your spouse and to all who love you."

- Eat right, and take a multivitamin. Baldwin learned this the hard way during her husband's recovery from liver surgery. "Because of my concern for his welfare, I skipped meals off and on for a few days. Suddenly, the corridor blurred, and I found myself gripping a water cooler to keep from falling. For a few awful moments, I was afraid I would faint. In a few minutes I felt better, and after eating a light lunch, I was perfectly all right. I realized what a serious mistake I'd made by skipping those meals." If you can't take time for a regular lunch, be prepared with energy-boosting snacks such as boxes of juice, cheese and crackers, raisins, peanuts, and granola bars. Just don't let yourself become run-down.

- Keep track of your weight. "We all react differently to stress, but you should note and quickly correct gains or losses of more than a few pounds."
- Get some exercise. Take a walk once or twice a day. You'll need your own strength and resilience now more than ever.
- Get some sleep. Your odds of sleeping better will improve if you keep up an adequate diet and get some exercise. Recognize that stress interferes with your body's normal patterns, and snooze when you can—even if it's not when you're used to resting. Relaxation techniques—listening to peaceful music, visualizing pleasant scenes, breathing deeply—may help you unwind. If it helps, "remind yourself that you've done the best you could; your spouse and the medical staff have done the best they could; and now the day has ended," says Baldwin, although she admits that some nights she was simply too upset to sleep. "My husband's condition, his doctors' anxieties, my fears of the future all outweighed my physical and emotional exhaustion. Even as I write this sentence, my stomach muscles tighten, my throat constricts, my palms begin to sweat, and I remember exactly how scared I felt."
- Ask family and friends for help—particularly if you're commuting to the hospital or doctor's office on unfamiliar roads or in heavy traffic. "At the hospital, you will benefit from their handholding and emotional support; on the road, they can handle the tricky turns."
- Check your own vital signs daily. Baldwin recommends asking yourself some basic questions every day, including: How do I feel today? Why do I feel that way? Tomorrow, I will take care of my need for (fill in the blank). What concern interfered with my sleep?
- Finally, when the treatment is over and life is getting back to normal, realize that your relationship has altered in subtle but significant ways, Baldwin says. "If we did not actually love one another more than we did before the illness, we now cherished one another more fully. Our children and our relationships with them were similarly changed. Perhaps the experiences we shared accelerated our normal maturation and led us all to appreciate one another more deeply.

"I recognize that I was physically and emotionally drained, and that I lost much of my resilience. Evidently this was obvious to our children, because I detected them going to new lengths to protect and to help me. My gratitude to them was tempered by my concern for them. Discussing this with the youngest, a recent college graduate, I said, 'We do not want our lives to interfere with your life,' and she replied, 'Your lives are part of my life.'"

# About the Authors

**Patrick C. Walsh, M.D.,** is best known for his thirty years' service as the Professor and Director of the Brady Urological Institute at The Johns Hopkins Hospital and for his pioneering work in the development of the anatomic approach to radical prostatectomy—nerve-sparing techniques that have greatly reduced the risk of impotence and incontinence. He has also made major contributions to the basic understanding of benign and malignant disease of the prostate. Along with co-workers, he was the first to describe the 5-alpha reductase enzyme deficiency, to demonstrate the influence of reversible androgen deprivation on BPH, and to characterize hereditary prostatic cancer. He is on the editorial board of the *New England Journal of Medicine* and is a member of the Institute of Medicine of the National Academy of Sciences. For twenty-five years he was the editor-in-chief of *Campbell's Textbook of Urology*, which has been renamed *Campbell-Walsh* in his honor. In 1996 Dr. Walsh received the Charles F. Kettering Medal from the General Motors Cancer Research Foundation for "the most outstanding recent contributions to the diagnosis and treatment of cancer." Dr. Walsh was honored as the 2007 National Physician of the Year for Clinical Excellence by *America's Top Doctors*®, and was the co-recipient of the 2007 King Faisal International Prize in Medicine. Together with Janet Farrar Worthington, he authored the bestselling books for lay people *The Prostate: A Guide for Men and the Women Who Love Them*, published by Johns Hopkins University Press (1995) and Warner Books (1997); and, more recently, *Dr. Patrick Walsh's Guide to Surviving Prostate Cancer*, Warner Books (2001 and 2007). Dr. Walsh served as the president of both the American Association of Genitourinary Surgeons and the Clinical Society of Genitourinary Surgeons.

**Janet Farrar Worthington** is an award-winning science writer.

# Glossary: A Guide to Medical Language of the Prostate, from A to Z

*Note: Most of the words here are nouns; where we thought it necessary, we indicated otherwise.*

**ablation:** a method of getting rid of something. Cryoablation, for example, is using freezing temperatures to get rid of prostate cancer. Hormonal ablation is getting rid of the hormones that nourish a prostate tumor.

**acid phosphatase:** an enzyme that, like PSA, is secreted by the prostate. Elevated acid phosphatase levels can signal that something is wrong with the prostate.

**acute bacterial prostatitis:** a form of prostatitis associated with urinary tract infections, positive cultures that identify bacteria in the prostate, and an abundance of white blood cells in prostatic secretions. Acute bacterial prostatitis comes on suddenly, accompanied by fever and symptoms that demand prompt treatment.

**adrenal androgens:** weak male hormones made by the adrenal glands. These include androstenedione, dehydroepiandrosterone (DHEA), and dehydroepiandrosterone sulfate (DHEAS), plus small amounts of testosterone. They are minor players, believed to make up only 5 percent or less of the total androgen stimulation to the prostate. Their total effect on the prostate is a controversial issue.

**adjuvant therapy:** an additional therapy. This is more than an extra precaution; ideally, it is designed to treat a problem before it starts. In prostate cancer, this means giving additional therapy, such as immediate radiation or chemotherapy, to high-risk patients *before* there is evidence that cancer has returned, with the hope that it won't return.

**age-specific PSA levels:** a new way to evaluate PSA tests using a man's age to determine the significance of his PSA reading.

**alpha blockers:** a class of drugs, originally designed to treat hypertension, that act on the prostate by relaxing smooth muscle tissue.

**alpha-linolenic acid:** a "bad" fat. It's found among the omega-3 class of polyunsaturated fats, in red meats, margarine, cooking oils, and mayonnaise.

**analgesics:** painkillers.

**analog:** a synthetic look-alike of a drug or chemical.

**anal stricture:** tight scar tissue that can interfere with bowel movements.

**anastomosis:** the site at which two structures are surgically reconnected after an organ has been removed. After radical prostatectomy, this refers to the connection between the reconstructed bladder neck and the urethra.

**androgen-dependent, or androgen-sensitive, cells:** cells in prostate cancer that are nourished by hormones, which can shrink dramatically when the hormones that nourish the prostate are shut off.

**androgen-independent, or androgen-insensitive cells:** cells in prostate cancer that are not nourished by hormones and therefore don't respond to hormonal therapy.

**androgens:** male hormones, such as testosterone.

**angiogenesis:** the process of forming new blood vessels. Advancing cancer paves the way by making new blood vessels.

**angiogenesis inhibitors:** drugs that block angiogenesis. The idea is to starve cancer by cutting off its supply line. Cancer may not die, but it won't get any bigger, either.

**antiandrogens:** drugs such as bicalutamide (Casodex), flutamide (Evlexin), and nilutamide (Nilandron), used in hormonal therapy to treat prostate cancer. These drugs block the effects of testosterone and DHT on prostate cancer cells by neutralizing their effect (they prevent testosterone and DHT from binding to the androgen receptor).

**antibiotics:** drugs that kill bacteria.

**anticholinergic drugs:** a group of drugs whose side effects include hindering urination. These may help some men with incontinence.

**anticoagulants:** medications that help prevent the blood from clotting.

**antimetastatic drugs:** drugs that put roadblocks in the way of cancer's progress, discouraging it from invading other cells or from developing new blood vessels (this process is called angiogenesis).

**antimicrobial drugs:** bacteria-killing drugs, such as antibiotics.

**apoptosis:** also called programmed cell death; the process by which cells kill themselves.

**arachidonic acid:** an unsaturated fatty acid found in red meats, whole milk and cheese, and egg yolks.

**arterial (adj.):** relating to the arteries.

**artificial sphincter:** an implanted device used to treat incontinence that has persisted for a year or longer and shows no signs of improving on its own.

**ASTRO definition:** a definition for relapse, or biochemical failure, after radiation therapy (determined by a panel from the American Society for Therapeutic Radiology and Oncology). According to this definition, failure after radiation means three consecutive rises in PSA levels (taken at least three months apart) after it reaches its nadir—the lowest point PSA reaches after treatment. The date of failure is backdated to the midpoint between the nadir and the first rise in PSA. (Many doctors now are using the nadir + 2 definition.)

**asymptomatic (adj.):** experiencing no symptoms. A man with asymptomatic prostate cancer doesn't notice anything out of the ordinary; he feels fine.

**atypical (adj.):** a finding on biopsy; this means the cells do not look normal but are not necessarily cancerous.

**benign:** harmless; not cancerous; not fatal.

**benign prostatic hyperplasia:** see *BPH*.

**biopsy of the prostate:** a means of sampling prostate tissue so it can be checked for the presence of cancer.

**bisphosphonates:** bone-targeting drugs used for several purposes. They strengthen bone to prevent osteoporosis in men on hormonal therapy; they also reduce the likelihood of bone pain, reduce the need for radiation to the bone because of pain, and reduce fractures and spinal cord complications.

**bladder:** a hollow, muscular reservoir that functions as a holding tank for urine.

**bladder neck contracture:** a constriction of the bladder neck caused by scar tissue. This can impede urine flow.

**bladder spasms:** painful, uncontrollable contractions of the bladder.

**bladder stones:** tiny formations made when crystals of uric acid or calcium precipitate out of urine.

**bloodless field:** a surgical term that means controlling bleeding within a patient to give surgeons a better view as they perform an operation.

**blood-prostate barrier:** a membrane that prevents many substances, including antibiotics, from entering the prostate. This barrier breaks down when a man has bacterial prostatitis, permitting most antibiotics to enter the prostate.

**bone scan:** also called *radionuclide scintigraphy*. Imaging test in which doctors inject into the bloodstream a radioactive tracer, a chemical that's attracted specifically to bone. The bone scan is an excellent means of finding out whether prostate cancer has spread to bone.

**bound PSA:** PSA molecules in the bloodstream that are chemically tied to proteins. Other PSA molecules are without these chemical ties; these are called free. If a man has a PSA test and most of the PSA is bound, the PSA elevation is probably coming from cancer.

**BPH:** benign prostatic hyperplasia, or enlargement of the prostate. A benign condition that occurs in most older men when prostate tissue begins to grow around the urethra, gradually compressing it and hindering urine flow.

**BPSA:** a particular form of free PSA produced by the prostate's transition zone, a thin ring of tissue that surrounds the urethra, in BPH. BPSA is more of a marker for BPH than for cancer.

**BUN test:** the blood-urea-nitrogen test, a blood test used to check kidney function.

**calculi:** see *prostatic calculi*.

**capsule of the prostate:** the outer wall of the prostate gland.

**castrate range:** the level to which testosterone drops after orchiectomy. This is an important point of comparison in monitoring hormonal therapy, as certain drugs are judged by their ability to reduce testosterone to this range.

**castration:** see *orchiectomy*.

**catheter:** a tube used for drainage or irrigation; most commonly used to drain urine out of the bladder.

**cell division:** the method through which the body's cells multiply. A single cell divides into two. Then those two cells each divide into two, and so on.

**chemical castration:** the use of drugs to accomplish the same effect as orchiectomy—that is, to lower the testosterone level to the castrate range.

**chemotherapeutic drugs:** a class of cell-killing drugs used to treat many forms of cancer.

**chronic bacterial prostatitis:** a form of prostatitis associated with urinary tract infections, positive cultures that identify bacteria in the prostate, and an abundance of white blood cells in prostatic secretions. This can be a recurring illness, coming back periodically for years after an initial episode of acute bacterial prostatitis.

**chronic prostatitis/chronic pelvic pain syndrome:** the most mysterious category of prostatitis. Nobody knows what causes the symptoms in this group (which used to be named by what it was not, nonbacterial prostatitis), and antibiotics don't help at all. In some men, the prostate may not even be the problem—the pain and other symptoms may be a result of spasms elsewhere in the pelvis, rectum, or lower back. This category has two subgroups—inflammatory and noninflammatory, based on whether any white blood cells (also called inflammatory cells) are found in the prostatic fluid.

**clinical stage of prostate cancer:** an estimation of the extent of a man's cancer, based on factors such as the digital rectal exam, PSA test, and bone scan. Pathologic stage is much more certain, but this can be determined only when a pathologist examines actual prostate tissue after surgery.

**clonal selection:** the process whereby the most poorly differentiated, rapidly growing, aggressive cells overtake the slower, well-differentiated cells as a tumor progresses.

**complexed PSA:** the PSA bound to a protein called alpha-1-antichymotrypsin (ACT). The complexed PSA assay is a way of looking at the separation of bound from free PSA.

**complementary medicine:** nontraditional medicine. In pain management, for example, this includes herbal remedies, prayer and meditation, acupuncture, deep breathing, aromatherapy, relaxation techniques, massage therapy, biofeedback, hypnosis, yoga, and even laughter (also called humor therapy).

**conformal radiation therapy:** a technique for delivering external-beam radiation that maximizes the dose of radiation to the prostate tumor while keeping the risk of damaging nearby tissue to a minimum.

**corpora cavernosa and corpus spongiosum:** spongy chambers in the penis that become engorged with blood during an erection.

**corticosteroids:** powerful drugs that reduce inflammation and, in men with advanced prostate cancer, bring relief from some spinal pain. However, because of their side effects, they are not good for long-term use.

**creatinine test:** a blood test (also called a serum creatinine test) that checks for impairment of kidney function.

**cruciferous vegetables:** vegetables in the cabbage and turnip family, including broccoli, cauliflower, cabbage, Brussels sprouts, bok choy, and kale. They can help lower the risk of developing cancer.

**cryoablation** *or* **cryotherapy:** using extremely cold liquid nitrogen to freeze the entire prostate, causing cancer cells within the gland to rupture as they begin to thaw.

**CT (computed tomography) scan:** a circular series of X-ray pictures taken by a machine that goes around the body. A computer puts the pictures together, generating images that, as in an MRI, are like slices of anatomy.

**cystometry:** a test that measures bladder pressure and function, done by passing a small catheter through the urethra into the bladder. Changes in pressure are monitored as the bladder fills with water.

**cystoscope:** a tiny, lighted tube that works like a periscope on a submarine. In cystoscopy, it is inserted into the tip of the anesthetized penis and threaded through the urethra into the bladder; this allows the doctor to inspect the bladder, prostate, and urethra for abnormalities.

**deep venous thrombosis:** condition in which blood clots form in the deep veins of the legs; it is a potential complication of major surgery, such as radical prostatectomy. At best, these clots can be painful. At worst, they can be fatal, if a chunk of a blood clot in the leg breaks free and shoots up to the lungs. These should be treated immediately.

**DES:** see *estrogens.*

**DHT:** (dihydrotestosterone), the active form of male hormone in the prostate. It is made when testosterone is transformed by an enzyme called 5-alpha reductase.

**DIC:** disseminated intravascular coagulation, a blood-clotting disorder that develops in some men with advanced prostate cancer.

**differentiating agents:** drugs that work by slowing down cancer's rate of growth.

**differentiation of prostate cancer cells:** how cancer cells look under the microscope. Well-differentiated cells have distinct, clearly defined borders and clear centers, and their growth is relatively slow and orderly. Everything about poorly differentiated cells is murkier and not as well defined. As cancer progresses, these poorly differentiated cells seem to melt together and form solid, nasty blobs of malignancy. These are the most aggressive cells in a tumor, and they are given a high grade (8, 9, 10) in the Gleason scoring system. Well-differentiated cells are called low grade (2, 3, 4). Moderately well differentiated cells fall in between (5, 6, 7), and it's hard to predict what these cells will do.

**digital rectal exam:** a very important part of the physical examination in which a doctor's gloved, lubricated finger is inserted into the rectum to feel for lumps, enlargement, or areas of hardness that might indicate the presence of cancer. It is uncomfortable but not painful, and it's generally brief, lasting less than a minute.

**diuretics:** drugs that work by altering the way the body metabolizes sodium; this causes the kidneys to absorb less water, so more of it leaves the body in the form of urine. For most people, taking diuretics means urinating more frequently and having a more forceful stream. Taking them can be disastrous for a man with BPH.

**diverticula:** pockets of the bladder lining that poke out like balloons through the bladder wall. (A single one of these is called a diverticulum.)

**DNA:** the genetic blueprint; vital information contained in the nucleus of every cell.

**dorsiflexion exercises:** pumping the feet up and down to exercise the calf muscles, a good exercise to do immediately after surgery to prevent deep venous thrombosis.

**double-blind study:** a study in which neither the doctor nor the patient knows who's receiving the placebo or the standard medication, or who's receiving the new medication being tested.

**dry ejaculation:** also known as retrograde ejaculation. This is a complication of some prostate procedures, including TUR. For most men, this has no effect on the pleasant sensation of orgasm. Dry ejaculation is pretty much what it sounds like: semen is not expelled out the urethra when a man reaches sexual climax. Instead, it goes the other way—back into the bladder. This happens because part of the bladder neck—a muscular valve whose job is to slam shut at the time of ejaculation, forcing semen out the urethra—is often resected along with the prostate tissue. When this area is damaged or missing, there's nothing to prevent semen from heading the wrong way. This also occurs after a radical prostatectomy or radiation therapy, because the prostate and seminal vesicles, which make the fluid, are either removed or dried up.

**ED drugs:** drugs used to treat erectile dysfunction. These are phosphodiesterase inhibitors (including Viagra, Cialis, and Levitra).

**edema:** swelling caused by fluid retention.

**ejaculate (noun):** semen, the fluid that exits the body during orgasm, or sexual climax. *Ejaculate* also is a verb.

**ejaculation:** emission of semen at the climax of sexual intercourse.

**endothelin:** a chemical that's believed to be the culprit in the excruciating, debilitating pain that comes when prostate cancer invades the bone. Endothelin-blocking drugs are now being tested.

**epididymis:** the "greenhouse" where sperm mature and are stored until orgasm.

**epididymitis:** an infection of the epididymis. This may occur after a surgical procedure that damages the ejaculatory ducts, allowing infected urine to back up into the vas deferens.

**epidural anesthesia:** a local anesthetic administered through a tiny plastic tube, inserted between the vertebrae of the spine, near the small of the back. The epidural anesthetic bathes the area outside the membrane lining the spinal cord, temporarily numbing the nerves in the lower body. Unlike spinal anesthesia, which is delivered in one dose, epidural anesthesia can be given continuously. The area of numbness can be adjusted; so can the degree of pain relief.

**epithelial cells:** cells in the glandular tissue of the prostate that secrete fluid that becomes part of semen.

**erectile dysfunction (ED):** the inability to have an erection sufficient for sexual intercourse.

**estrogens:** female hormones. Estrogens block the release of a signal transmitted by the pituitary gland called luteinizing hormone (LH), which stimulates testosterone. Oral estrogens, taken as hormonal therapy by men with prostate cancer, reduce testosterone to the crucial castrate range. The main oral estrogen used for this is DES (diethylstilbestrol).

**excise (verb):** to cut out; to remove surgically.

**expectant management:** in prostate cancer, this means to delay definitive treatment until it becomes clear that the tumor is growing—to wait for evidence that cancer is on the move, and then take action. This is different from the watchful waiting approach used in Europe.

**external-beam radiation therapy:** a curative treatment for prostate cancer. It involves beaming X-ray energy into a prostate tumor from the outside, a few minutes at a time, over the course of several weeks.

**fascia:** a thin blanket of connective tissue.

**5-alpha reductase:** enzymes in the prostate that convert testosterone to DHT.

**5-alpha reductase inhibitors:** drugs that block the formation of DHT. This causes the prostate to shrink and improves the obstructive symptoms of BPH. These drugs do not affect levels of testosterone, the hormone responsible for a man's libido and sexual function.

**fluoroscopy:** an imaging technique in which an X-ray image appears live on a screen instead of as a still photograph.

**Foley catheter:** a catheter inserted into the penis and threaded through the urethra into the bladder, where it's anchored in place with a tiny, inflated balloon. It removes urine from the body; it also can be used for irrigation to prevent blood clots.

**following expectantly:** see *watchful waiting*.

**free PSA:** PSA (this is also called percent-free PSA) that is not chemically bound to proteins in the bloodstream. If a man has an elevated PSA level and most of the PSA is free, then the elevation is probably due to BPH.

**frozen section analysis:** freezing, then slicing tissue into very thin sections to be examined under a microscope. In a staging pelvic lymphadenectomy, lymph nodes are removed, then rushed to a pathologist for frozen-section analysis to check for cancer.

**FSH:** follicle-stimulating hormone, made along with LH by the pituitary gland. FSH has its major effect on sperm production.

**gene therapy:** one of the most exciting nonhormonal areas of treatment for advanced prostate cancer. Scientists are now able to program the body's DNA like a computer chip, sending it on a selective search-and-destroy mission targeted only at prostate cancer cells.

**genetic drift:** as a cancer progresses and its cells double over and over again, the DNA becomes less stable. The cancer develops new mutations; it becomes more aggressive. As the tumor progresses, well-differentiated cells deteriorate into poorly differentiated cells. This downslide is called genetic drift.

**genetic susceptibility:** a complex of genetic factors that create a more hospitable atmosphere for cancer.

**Gleason score:** a way to classify the severity of cancer based on the way it looks under a microscope. Cells that are well-differentiated are given a low grade (2, 3, 4); poorly differentiated cells are given a high grade (8, 9, 10). Moderately well differentiated cells fall in the middle. See also *differentiation of prostate cancer cells*.

**glutathione-S-transferase-$\pi$ (GST-$\pi$):** an important enzyme that helps prevent oxidative damage, which can lead to prostate cancer.

**grade of prostate cancer:** see *Gleason score*.

**growth factors:** substances that activate processes that promote cell division.

**gynecomastia:** tenderness, pain, or swelling of the breasts in men. This is a common, easily treatable side effect of some forms of hormonal therapy for prostate cancer.

**Hedgehog pathway:** the path taken by a cancer in metastasis. Blocking this pathway may mean that we can prevent cancer from spreading.

**hemi-body irradiation:** a once-common form of radiation treatment delivered to ease pain in prostate cancer patients with metastases to bone in several places. It involves irradiating great expanses of the body.

**hereditary prostate cancer (HPC):** HPC is present in families if there are three first-degree relatives (a father or brothers) who develop prostate cancer, or two first-degree relatives, if both developed it before age fifty-five; or if prostate cancer has occurred in three generations in the family (grandfather, father, son). HPC can be inherited from either side of the family.

**heterogeneity:** the state of being diverse or varied; not uniform. In prostate cancer and BPH, heterogeneity refers to a "melting pot" of cells, all jockeying for position in one area.

**high-dose-rate (HDR) brachytherapy:** also called temporary brachytherapy, this is usually given along with external-beam radiation. As its name suggests, the seeds don't stay in; they're removed at the end of each treatment session.

**hK2:** human kallikrein-2, an enzyme made by the prostate that's a "cousin" of PSA.

**hormonal therapy:** the use of hormones to treat advanced prostate cancer. Hormonal therapy is aimed at shutting down the hormones that nourish the prostate. Some cells in a prostate tumor are responsive to this, but some aren't.

**hormone-dependent, hormone-sensitive:** see *androgen-dependent, androgen-sensitive.*

**hormone-independent, hormone-insensitive:** see *androgen-independent, androgen-insensitive.*

**hormone-refractory prostate cancer:** metastatic prostate cancer that has returned after months or years of being controlled by hormonal therapy.

**hot flash:** a sudden rush of warmth in the face, neck, upper chest, and back lasting from a few seconds to an hour; a side effect of some hormonal treatments for prostate cancer. Although hot flashes aren't harmful to a man's health, they can be bothersome.

**hydrogenation:** a means of preserving food. Hydrogenation helps keep shortening solid at room temperature. Hydrogenated foods raise cholesterol level and may contribute to oxidative damage.

**hyperplasia:** an increase in the number of cells in the prostate.

**hyper-reflexive (adj):** overly reactive; spastic.

**hypofractionated radiation therapy:** Higher doses of radiation delivered over a shorter time period—four to five weeks, for instance, instead of eight weeks.

**image-guided radiation therapy (IGRT):** radiation therapy in which the location of a man's prostate (which is never constant) is checked every day before treatment so that small adjustments in his position can be made, making the radiation as precisely targeted as possible.

**imaging (verb):** seeing and taking pictures inside the body using various forms of energy, including ultrasound, magnetic resonance (MRI), and X-rays.

**immunotherapy:** treatments designed to maximize the immune system's ability to fight cancer.

**impotence:** also called erectile dyfunction. This is the inabiity to have an erection, which, in most cases, is very treatable.

**incidental prostate cancer:** apparently dormant, small cancer cell clusters that reside in millions of men. In some men, this cancer never poses a danger. In others, however, it eventually does.

**incontinence:** also called urinary incontinence. It is the unintentional leakage of urine. (Another kind of incontinence, bowel or fecal incontinence, means having an unintentional bowel movement.)

**infectious prostatitis:** a term some doctors use to describe bacterial prostatitis. Bacterial prostatitis is not infectious; men can have a normal sex life without worrying about giving the disease to someone else.

**insulin-like growth factors:** a class of hormones that may influence the development of prostate cancer.

**intensity-modulated radiation therapy (IMRT):** an approach to external-beam radiation using multiple beamlets to "sculpt" the radiation dose to fit the individual contours of each man's prostate and pelvic region.

**intermittent hormonal therapy:** also called intermittent androgen suppression. In this plan, men start taking hormones early, before signs or symptoms of advanced cancer begin. Then, when their PSA levels drop, they stop taking them and get a little "vacation" from treatment. The men are monitored closely, and at the first sign that the tumor is growing, they start taking the hormones again.

**interstitial brachytherapy:** implanting radioactive "seeds," or minute radioactive chunks of material, into the prostate to kill cancer.

**intra-abdominal (adj.):** in the abdomen.

**intraurethral (adj.):** in the urethra.

**intraurethral therapy:** a pharmacological treatment for men with ED using agents that can be placed directly into the urethra.

**invasive (adj.):** involving an incision, the body is physically entered. In minimally invasive surgery, this incision may be a hole as small as a dime, or there may be no incision at all if the body's own passageways—such as the urethra in the TUR procedure—are used. A noninvasive procedure does not invade the body at all; many forms of imaging are noninvasive.

**irritative symptoms in BPH:** these include frequent urination, especially at night; a strong sense of urgency in urination; inability to postpone urination; and sleep disrupted by the need to urinate.

**isoflavones:** phytochemicals found in plants such as soy; one of these is genistein, which may help fight cancer.

**IV:** the abbreviation for *intravenous,* which means, literally, "through the veins." Medication, fluids, or nutrition supplements can be administered this way.

**IVP:** intravenous pyelogram, an X-ray of the urinary tract that works like a glow-in-the-dark picture. A special dye is injected, making urine visible, and its path from the kidneys and out of the body easily traceable. Any blockage becomes easy to see. Some men have severe allergic reactions to this dye.

**kidneys:** the body's main filters. They cleanse the body of impurities and, at the same time, salvage and recycle useful materials.

**laparoscopic pelvic lymphadenectomy:** dissection of the lymph nodes as a means of staging prostate cancer. Laparoscopic surgery is minimally invasive; there's a tiny incision, and much of the surgery is conducted through "telescopes."

**latent (adj.):** dormant; passive.

**lateral lobe enlargement:** a form of BPH that results when prostate tissue compresses the urethra from the sides.

**LH:** luteinizing hormone, a chemical signal transmitted by the pituitary. LH motivates the testes to make testosterone.

**LHRH:** luteinizing hormone–releasing hormone (also called GnRH, for gonadotropin-releasing hormone); a chemical signal made in the brain by the hypothalamus. LHRH tells the pituitary gland to make LH and FSH.

**LHRH agonists:** synthetic look-alikes of the body's chemical LHRH. These drugs shut down the pituitary's production of the hormone LH.

**LHRH antagonists:** these drugs work faster than LHRH agonists to lower testosterone without producing the brief testosterone "flare."

**libido:** sex drive.

**linoleic acid:** a fatty acid found in corn oil, baked goods, and many snack foods.

**localized prostate cancer:** cancer that is confined within the prostate and therefore considered curable.

**local recurrence of cancer:** when cancer returns to the prostate or nearby tissue after treatment.

**lycopoene:** an antioxidant found in tomatoes, red grapefruits, watermelons, and berries that fights oxidative damage, which may lead to prostate cancer.

**metastasis, metastases, metastatic:** a metastasis is a chunk of cancer that has broken off from the main tumor and established itself elsewhere. A distant metastasis means this new site of cancer is far from its point of origin. The word *metastases* is plural, and *metastatic* is an adjective that refers to a metastasis.

**micrometastases:** tiny, invisible (and undetectable) offshoots of prostate cancer.

**middle lobe enlargement:** a type of BPH in which a lobe of prostate tissue grows inside the bladder. When it reaches a critical size, it can block the opening of the bladder neck like a cork in a bottle. This explains how some men with a small prostate on rectal exam can develop major symptoms of urinary obstruction.

**minilap:** mini-laparotomy staging pelvic lymphadenectomy. The minilap begins with an incision slightly larger than the one made in the laparoscopic pelvic lymphadenectomy. If there's cancer in the lymph nodes, the incision is closed. But if the lymph nodes are cancer-free, this incision is lengthened, and the radical retropubic prostatectomy is performed under the same anesthetic.

**monounsaturated fats:** "good" fats not linked to the development of prostate cancer. Olive oil is a monounsaturated fat.

**MRI:** magnetic resonance imaging; a means of imaging that's painless, noninvasive, and does not use X-rays. It is time-consuming, however, often taking about forty-five minutes. MRI gives a three-dimensional scan of the body, producing images that are like slices of anatomy.

**nadir + 2 definition:** this defines treatment failure after radiation therapy as a PSA level that has risen 2 ng/ml higher than a man's PSA nadir (the lowest level it reached following treatment).

**nerve-sparing radical prostatectomy:** what some doctors call the anatomical approach to radical retropubic prostatectomy; they're referring to important modifications that reduce blood loss and allow men to remain potent and continent after radical prostatectomy.

**neurogenic bladder:** trouble in the bladder caused by a neurological problem, such as Parkinson's disease.

**neurotransmitters:** chemical messengers; signals sent from a transmitter in one nerve cell to a receptor in another.

**neurovascular bundles:** cordlike structures that run down the sides of the prostate near the rectum. The bundles contain microscopic nerves that are essential for erection; they also contain arteries and veins that help surgeons identify the location of these nerves.

**nitric oxide:** a substance released by nerve endings during erection, causing the smooth muscle tissue in the penis to relax.

**nocturia:** frequent urination during the night. A man has nocturia if he has to get up several times a night to go to the bathroom. This is often a symptom of BPH.

**nocturnal penile tumescence test:** an evaluation to determine whether a man has erections at night while he sleeps.

**nonhormonal therapy:** exciting new treatments for advanced prostate cancer specifically designed to target the biological mechanisms involved in cancer progression and metastasis.

**noninvasive (adj.):** not invasive; in other words, there's no incision.

**NSAIDs:** nonsteroidal anti-inflammatory drugs, which are used to treat mild pain. Available over-the-counter and in prescription form.

**nutraceuticals:** drugs extracted from specific nutrients.

**obstructive symptoms in BPH:** these include weak urine flow, hesitancy in starting urination, a need to push or strain to get urine to flow, intermittent urine stream (starts and stops several times), difficulty in stopping urination, dribbling after urination, a sense of not being able to empty the bladder completely, and not being able to urinate at all.

**omega-3 fatty acids:** fatty acids found in fish oils that may be helpful in preventing coronary artery disease and are not linked to the development of prostate cancer.

**orchiectomy:** surgical castration. A form of hormonal therapy involving removal of all or part of the testicles. This causes testosterone levels to fall to the castrate range.

**orgasm:** the climax of sexual intercourse.

**overflow incontinence:** when urine leaks out because the bladder is too full to hold any more.

**oxidative damage:** incremental damage caused over many years as free radicals (toxic by-products of everyday metabolism) attack the DNA in cells, causing mutations that lead to cancer.

**palliate (verb):** to ease or relieve. Palliative treatment makes symptoms, and therefore quality of life, better, even though it may do nothing to cure the underlying cause of these symptoms.

**palpable (adj.):** tangible. Palpable cancer in the prostate means there's a lump, lesion, or nodule that a doctor's gloved finger can feel during a digital rectal exam.

**pathologic fracture:** when cancer invades bones, they become brittle. Brittle bones break. Therefore, men with metastatic prostate cancer are prone to getting broken bones, called pathologic fractures. Most susceptible are the bones that bear much of the body's weight, those in the hip and thigh.

**pathologic stage of cancer:** the definitive extent of a man's prostate cancer. (The possibilities include organ-confined cancer, capsular penetration, positive surgical margins, invasion of the seminal vesicles, and/or involvement of the pelvic lymph nodes.) This is determined after prostate surgery, when a pathologist examines the actual prostate specimen and dissected tissue from the nearby lymph nodes instead of merely making guesses about how far the cancer has spread based on test results and a few cells from biopsies.

**pathologist:** a doctor who studies cells, tissue, and organs and makes determinations about them, answering such questions as "Is there cancer here?" and "Was all the cancer removed?"

**PC-SPES:** a "natural" preparation of eight herbs, most of them used in Chinese medicine. Some of these herbs are potent phytoestrogens (the word *phyto* means that they come from plants)

**penile (adj.):** relating to the penis.

**penile implants:** bendable, inflatable, or mechanical prostheses that enable an impotent man to have erections sufficient for penetration.

**perforation:** puncture.

**perineum:** the area between the scrotum and rectum.

**perineural invasion:** a biopsy term meaning that prostate cancer has been found in the spaces around the nerves near the edge of the prostate. Because cancer that has penetrated the capsule can still be cured, perineural invasion has no long-term impact on a man's prognosis.

**peripheral zone:** the largest part of the prostate and the area where most prostate cancer occurs.

**periprostatic tissue:** tissue just outside the prostate.

**Peyronie's disease:** a disorder of the connective tissue within the penis that can cause curvature during erection.

**phosphodiesterase inhibitors:** drugs such as Viagra that can help facilitate an erection.

**phytochemicals:** chemicals derived from plants.

**phytoestrogens:** estrogens derived from plants. The prefix *phyto* means "coming from plants."

**PIN:** prostatic intraepithelial neoplasia. Abnormal cells, found in a needle biopsy, that are strongly linked to prostate cancer.

**placebo:** a "sugar pill" often taken by participants in a medical study. Patients taking a placebo are compared with patients taking actual medications.

**placebo effect:** a phenomenon that happens often in medical studies, in which patients taking a placebo have an inexplicable improvement in symptoms.

**polyphenols:** chemicals found in black and green teas that are known to have cancer-fighting properties.

**polyunsaturated fats:** fats found in vegetable oils (corn oil, safflower oil, and other cooking oils), nuts and seeds, fish oils, and margarine. There are a lot of these polyunsaturated fats, and some are worse than others.

**pressure-flow studies:** tests to monitor bladder pressure changes as a man urinates.

**proliferation:** spread or growth.

**prostate:** a muscular, walnut-shaped gland about an inch and a half long that sits directly under the bladder. Its main function is to make part of the fluid for semen.

**prostatectomy:** an operation to remove all or part of the prostate.

**prostate massage:** an important test for prostatitis done during a digital rectal exam. A doctor vigorously massages or presses on the prostate to express, or force, fluid out of the prostate and into the urethra. It then is collected on a glass slide and examined under a microscope.

**prostate-specific antigen:** see *PSA*.

**prostatic (adj.):** relating to the prostate.

**prostatic abscess:** localized accumulation of pus, like a pimple, under pressure in the prostate.

**prostatic calculi:** the prostate's version of gallstones or kidney stones. They're usually tiny and harmless. But when they get infected, as they often do in men with chronic bacterial prostatitis, they can cause an infection to persist and symptoms of urinary tract infections and prostatitis to return again and again.

**prostatic urethra:** the part of the urethra that runs through the prostate.

**prostatitis:** inflammation of the prostate.

**prostatosis:** a vague, unhelpful term that means simply "a condition of the prostate."

**prosthesis:** an artificial replacement for part of the body that is either missing or not functioning properly.

**proton-beam radiation:** an approach to external-beam radiation therapy that uses charged particles instead of electromagnetic waves. The proton beam shoots in a straight line, but it can be stopped abruptly—for example, at the delicate rectal wall, just on the other side of the prostate, so the fragile tissue in the rectum can be spared.

**PSA:** prostate-specific antigen, an enzyme made by the prostate. Levels of PSA can be checked through a simple blood test; elevated amounts of PSA in the blood can signal prostate cancer.

**PSA density:** the blood PSA score divided by the volume of the prostate, as determined by transrectal ultrasound.

**PSA velocity:** PSA's rate of change from year to year.

**PSMA:** prostate-specific membrane antigen, a protein that is made on the surface of prostate cells.

**psychogenic erectile dysfunction:** erection problems that are psychological, not physiological, in nature. Doctors making this ruling if a man can't produce an erection during sexual activity but has several a night while he sleeps.

**pulmonary embolus:** a blood clot in the lungs, a potential complication of radical prostatectomy. This is extremely serious and can be fatal.

**pulsed Doppler evaluation:** a test that uses high-resolution ultrasound to evaluate the arteries' blood supply to the penis.

**quality of life:** Basically, this means how good a patient thinks life is. When quality of life is excellent, a patient is relatively untroubled by symptoms or pain. When it is poor, pain or symptoms have interfered with a man's ability to function, to pursue his daily activities, and to enjoy his life.

**radiation "seeds":** see *interstitial brachytherapy*.

**radiation therapy:** see *external-beam radiation therapy* and *interstitial brachytherapy*.

**radical prostatectomy:** the operation to remove the prostate, and the gold standard for curing localized prostate cancer.

**radionuclide scintigraphy:** see *bone scan.*

**randomize:** doctors use this verb when discussing medical studies in which some men are assigned one treatment or another at random.

**receptors:** highly specific "locks" in cells that are opened, or activated, only by certain hormones or chemical signals, which act as "keys."

**regeneration:** regrowth.

**resect (verb):** to cut out; to remove surgically.

**resectoscope:** an instrument used in the TUR procedure. Threaded through the penis, it shines a light that allows surgeons to view the prostate as they chip away at excess tissue.

**retreatment:** having to undergo a repeat procedure to treat the same initial problem.

**retrograde ejaculation:** see *dry ejaculation.*

**retropubic (adj.):** behind the pubic bone; a surgical approach. In retropubic prostatectomy, the surgeon makes an incision in the lower abdomen, separates the abdominal muscles, and moves the bladder aside, unopened, to reach the prostate directly (as opposed to the suprapubic approach, in which the prostate is reached by cutting through the bladder).

**robotic radical prostatectomy:** this technique (also called robotically assisted radical prostatectomy) is performed laparoscopically, using instruments designed to mimic the movement of human hands, wrists, and fingers. This allows the surgeon a greater range of motion and more precision.

**RT-PCR:** reverse transcriptase polymerase chain reaction, a technique by which scientists examine cells from the blood to determine whether those cells can make PSA.

**salvage therapy:** a medical term for "Plan B." It means a patient is undergoing another form of treatment because the first form of treatment the patient underwent, was not successful in curing the problem. In prostate cancer, this is mainly the use of radiation therapy, cryoablation, or hormonal therapy in men who develop a rising PSA level after surgery or radiation therapy for localized disease.

**saturated fats:** fats found in red meats and dairy. (The Asian diet has hardly any saturated fat in it.)

**selenium:** a mineral found in fruits and vegetables, meats, and fish that may help prevent prostate cancer.

**semen:** the fluid that transports sperm.

**seminal vesicles:** glands that, like the prostate, are sex accessory glands. Fluid secreted by these glands is critical for ensuring the proper consistency of semen.

**sex accessory tissues:** glands such as the prostate, seminal vesicles, and Cowper's glands, which produce secretions that become part of the fluid in semen.

**sextant biopsy:** an attempt to get a comprehensive picture of the prostate by taking six tiny samples of cells from throughout the gland—one each from the top, middle, and bottom of the gland on the right and left sides.

**sinusoids:** spongy chambers within the penis that become engorged with blood during an erection.

**small-cell carcinoma:** a variety of prostate cancer. Cells in these tumors have a makeup similar to that of other small-cell cancers (of the lung, for example), and they respond to the same kinds of chemotherapy drugs used to treat those tumors.

**spinal anesthesia:** a shot of local anesthetic delivered into the small of the back through the dura, the membrane lining the spinal cord, and into the spinal fluid. Within minutes, the patient feels numb, relaxed, and heavy from the waist down.

**spinal cord compression:** a very serious problem in men with metastatic prostate cancer. This happens when cancer eats away at the spine, causing part of the spinal column to collapse, trapping and sometimes crushing nearby nerves.

**spot radiation:** localized external-beam radiation treatment targeted at one or several painful bone metastases. It won't prevent new metastases from cropping up in bone, but it can ease pain dramatically in the sites it does treat.

**stage of prostate cancer:** the extent of the disease—how big it is and how far it has spread. The stage of prostate cancer has a major role in determining what treatment a man should receive. See also *clinical stage* and *pathologic stage*.

**staging pelvic lymphadenectomy:** dissection of the pelvic lymph nodes to see whether they contain prostate cancer. This procedure is generally performed just before a radical prostatectomy.

**statins:** drugs that lower cholesterol and reduce the risk of a heart attack or stroke.

**stents:** tubes implanted and left in place to hold open a space that would otherwise collapse or be compressed.

**step-up hormonal therapy:** a gradual approach to hormonal therapy. The idea here is to start modulating the male hormones with agents that have the fewest side effects, and then to escalate as needed if the disease progresses.

**stress incontinence:** condition in which when urine leaks during certain activities, such as running or playing golf.

**stricture:** a blockage caused by scar tissue.

**stromal cells:** cells found in the prostate's smooth muscle tissue, which contract automatically to launch secretions into the urethra.

**strontium-89:** a highly effective radioactive substance, injected into the body, that is specially tailored to treat bone pain in cancer patients.

**subcapsular orchiectomy:** a cosmetic approach to orchiectomy. In this operation, a surgeon opens the lining of the testicles and empties the contents of each testicle. The lining is closed again, and this empty shell is placed back inside the scrotum—so nothing looks different;

in other words, no one can tell from outward appearance that there's nothing inside the testicles.

**suprapubic (adj.):** above the pubic bone; a surgical approach to the prostate.

**surgical margins:** the edges of removed tissues. These are assessed when pathologists look at the edges of tissue that has been cut out during surgery. If no cancer appears on these edges, the margins are said to be clear or negative. If this is the case, it is likely that all the cancerous tissue was removed. If the margin is positive, the surgeon might not have been able to cut out all the cancer.

**sutures:** stitches used to close an incision.

**Taxotere (docetaxel):** a new chemotherapy drug that hinders cells multiplication.

**template:** a highly sophisticated map of the prostate that helps doctors know exactly where to insert radioactive seeds.

**testes or testicles:** housed in the scrotum, these are a man's reproductive organs and the main source of the male hormone testosterone and of sperm.

**testosterone:** the male hormone, or androgen, which is important to the prostate and is essential for sex drive and fertility. It is also responsible for such "manly" characteristics as postpuberty body hair and the deepening of the voice. Lowering testosterone levels is a major goal of hormonal therapy to treat prostate cancer.

**thermal ablation:** using heat to destroy tissue.

**three-dimensional conformal radiation:** approach to external-beam radiation in which many X-ray beams, shaped to fit the target area, are focused on the prostate, delivering a homogenous, high dose of radiation.

**three-glass urine collection:** an important test for prostatitis. When a man urinates, the first urine to come out contains fluid from the urethra. Urine collected in midstream comes from the bladder. The last collection of urine is taken after a brief prostate massage, and this contains fluid from the prostate.

**total androgen blockade, or ablation:** a form of hormonal therapy to treat prostate cancer. The theory here is that even low levels of testosterone and DHT, engendered by the adrenal androgens, can stimulate cancer in the prostate and must be stopped. This can be accomplished by combining whatever achieves a castrate level of testosterone—surgical castration, estrogens, or an LHRH agonist—with an antiandrogen.

**transabdominal (adj.):** through the abdomen.

**transition zone:** the innermost ring of the prostate; it is tissue that surrounds the urethra. This is the sole site affected by BPH.

**transperineal (adj.):** through the perineum.

**transrectal (adj.):** through the rectum.

**treatment-planning CT scan:** CT images that show the physical terrain of the target area, the prostate and surrounding organs, before radiation treatment.

**trilobar enlargement:** a type of BPH involving three (two lateral and one middle) lobes, in which obstruction can occur in the bladder neck as well as the urethra.

**TUR:** abbreviation for transurethral resection of the prostate, the gold standard operation to treat symptoms of BPH. It does not require an incision; instead, prostate tissue is reached, chipped away, and removed in tiny fragments through the urethra.

**Ultrasound:** a painless, noninvasive way of imaging that creates a picture with high-frequency sound waves, like sonar on a submarine. It may be done either from outside, through the abdomen, or transrectally, via a wand inserted in the rectum. Transrectal ultrasound can determine the size of the prostate and direct the needle used for biopsies.

**ureters:** muscular, one-way channels that work like toothpaste tubes, squeezing urine out of the kidneys and onward toward the bladder.

**urethra:** a tube that, like the prostate, is involved in both the urinary tract and reproductive systems. It serves as a conduit not only for urine but also for secretions from the ejaculatory ducts and the prostate.

**urethral sphincter:** the muscle responsible for urinary control.

**urethral stricture:** scar tissue that blocks the urethra.

**urethritis:** inflammation of the urethra, often caused by an infection. If left untreated, this can result in a urethral stricture or a nasty infection that progresses into the vas deferens and involves the epididymis.

**urge, or urgency, incontinence:** a condition in which a man knows he has to go to the bathroom, but some urine leaks as he's trying to get there.

**urinalysis:** microscopic and chemical analysis of urine.

**urinary retention:** condition in which the bladder stays completely or partially full. Acute urinary retention means someone can no longer urinate. This is a very serious condition that requires immediate treatment.

**urodynamic studies:** tests that measure urinary flow, pressure, and volume to find out whether urinary trouble is caused by BPH or a problem with the bladder.

**uroflowmetry:** a test to measure the amount of urine a man passes and the speed of his urinary stream.

**urologist:** a physician who specializes in the diagnosis and medical and surgical treatment of problems in the urinary tract and male reproductive systems.

**UTI:** urinary tract infection. The presence of bacteria in the urine, sometimes associated with fever.

**vacuum erection device:** an apparatus that creates suction using an airtight tube, which is placed temporarily around the penis. An attached pump withdraws air, creating reduced atmospheric pressure—a vacuum—around the penis, causing it to become engorged with blood. The penis becomes erect. Then a constricting ring similar to a rubber band keeps the blood trapped in the penis so the erection can be sustained.

**vascular (adj.):** involving blood vessels.

**vas deferens:** one of the two hard, muscular cords that wind their way from the epididymis to the base of the prostate, where they meet with the duct of the seminal vesicle to form the ejaculatory duct.

**vasectomy:** a surgical procedure that is a form of male contraception. When the vas deferens is cut, sperm cannot exit the penis through ejaculation and instead are reabsorbed into the body.

**vasodilators:** drugs that open up blood vessels, making a wider channel for blood to go through. In the penis, they also cause the smooth muscle tissue to relax and the veins to close; some vasodilators, injected in tiny amounts in the penis, are used to produce erections.

**venous (adj.):** relating to the veins.

**venous leak:** a common cause of erectile dysfunction. Even though the arteries fill the penis with blood, producing a partial erection, the veins don't clamp down to keep this blood trapped inside the penis, so a full erection can't be achieved.

**vitamin E:** an antioxidant that may help prevent prostate cancer.

**watchful waiting:** the most conservative treatment there is. It means following someone's symptoms closely, but delaying treatment until these symptoms become severe enough to warrant it.

**wide excision:** during a radical prostatectomy, this means that a surgeon cuts out as much tissue as possible surrounding the prostate in an aggressive attempt to get every bit of cancer.

**X-ray therapy:** see *external-beam radiation therapy.*

**zones of the prostate:** there are five distinct regions of the prostate. The two most commonly referred to are the transition zone and the peripheral zone.

# Where to Get Help

You're not alone: There are many sources of good information available to help you. Here are a few of them.

**American Cancer Society**
1599 Clifton Rd, NE
Atlanta, GA 30329
(404) 320-3333
(808) ACS-2345
www.cancer.org
This national, community-based organization provides comprehensive information and resources, referrals to treatment centers, free publications, and sponsors a support group called Man to Man.

**American Foundation for Urologic Diseases**
1000 Corporate Blvd
Linthicum, MD 21090
(866) RING AUA
(410) 689-3700
www.afud.org, www.urologyhealth.org
This foundation supports research and provides educational materials on prostate cancer, erectile dysfunction, and other urologic conditions. It also sponsors Us TOO, a support group for prostate cancer survivors and their families (see below).

**The Brady Urological Institute**
The Johns Hopkins Hospital
600 North Wolfe St
Baltimore, MD 21287-2101
(410) 955-6707
http://urology.jhu.edu/
This Web site has many news articles about the latest research in prostate cancer being done at Johns Hopkins, which we will update regularly.

**The Prostate Cancer Foundation**
1250 Fourth St
Santa Monica, CA 90401
(800) 757-2873
www.prostatecancerfoundation.org

The Prostate Cancer Foundation's (formerly CaPCure) mission is to identify and support prostate cancer research that will rapidly translate into treatments and cures. Its Web site has information about clinical trials.

**National Association for Continence**
(formerly Help for Incontinent People)
PO Box 1019
Charleston, SC 29402-1019
(800) BLADDER (800-252-3337)
www.nafc.org

**National Cancer Institute Cancer Information Service**
Public Inquiries:
Building 31, Room 10A31
31 Center Dr, MSC 2580
Bethesda, MD 20892-2580
(301) 435-3848
(800) 4-CANCER
www.cancer.gov
This is a national clearinghouse with an extensive health information database and educational materials, including information about clinical trials.

**National Hospice and Palliative Care Organization (NHPCO)**
1700 Diagonal Rd, Ste 625
Alexandria, VA 22314
(703) 837-1500
www.nho.org

**National Library of Medicine**
www.nlm.nih.gov
This Web site allows you to gain access to millions of scientific publications and abstracts.

**Prostate Cancer Support Network (PCSN)**
5003 Fairview Ave
Downers Grove, IL 60515
(630) 795-1002

**PCa Support Hotline**
(800) 80-Us TOO (800-808-7866)
www.ustoo.com
**E-mail:** ustoo@ustoo.org
PCSN, affiliated with the American Foundation for Urologic Disease, provides services for several support groups, self-help organizations, and their members, including Us TOO.

# Index